MW01054540

2025 Harvard Health Annual

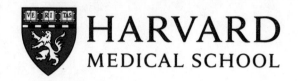

Harvard Health Annual 2025

Consulting Editor: Howard LeWine, M.D., Chief Medical Editor, Harvard Health Publishing,
and Editor in Chief, *Harvard Men's Health Watch*
Executive Editor: Kristie Reilly
Art Director: Mary Francis McGavic

Faculty Editors:
Christopher Cannon, M.D., Editor in Chief, *Harvard Heart Letter*
Toni Golen, M.D., Editor in Chief, *Harvard Women's Health Watch*
Anthony L. Komaroff, M.D., Editor in Chief, *Harvard Health Letter*

Contributing Editors:
Julie Corliss, Executive Editor, *Harvard Heart Letter*
Heidi Godman, Executive Editor, *Harvard Health Letter*
Maureen Salamon, Executive Editor, *Harvard Women's Health Watch*
Matthew Solan, Executive Editor, *Harvard Men's Health Watch*

Contributing Writers:
Francesca Coltrera, Charlie Schmidt, Robert Shmerling, Lindsay Warner

Publisher: Theresa Jankowski
Creative Director: Judi Crouse

Print ISBN 978-1-61401-385-3
Digital ISBN 978-1-61401-386-0
10 9 8 7 6 5 4 3 2 1

This publication is intended to provide readers with accurate and timely medical news and information. It is not intended to give personal medical advice, which should be obtained directly from a licensed health care provider. We regret that we cannot respond to individual inquiries about personal health matters. Websites listed in this book are accurate at the time of publication.

COPYRIGHT NOTICE
THIS BOOK IS COPYRIGHTED BY HARVARD UNIVERSITY AND PRESIDENT AND FELLOWS OF HARVARD COLLEGE AND IS PROTECTED BY U.S. AND INTERNATIONAL COPYRIGHT. ALL RIGHTS RESERVED. ©2025 Harvard Health Publishing.

Table of Contents

Foreword

Welcome to the 2025 edition of the *Harvard Health Annual!* Congratulations on taking this important step in learning about—and improving—your health. We hope this year's collection of informative, evidence-based articles and tips from Harvard Medical School supports your well-being and empowers you to live your best life.

As the world has emerged from the COVID-19 pandemic, medical research continues to advance at a rapid pace. As a result, many of us are living longer. Globally, the number of centenarians has doubled over each decade since 1950, and this population of "superagers" is projected to increase another five times in the next 30 years. Meanwhile, in the United

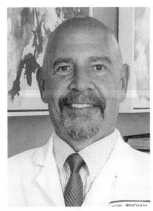

HOWARD LEWINE, M.D.
Chief Medical Editor,
Harvard Health Publishing

States, one in five people will be older than 65 by 2040, and the number of those older than 85 is expected to more than double in the same time frame.

That's why, for this year's annual, we're focusing on the theme "Living Longer, Living Well." As lifespans lengthen, quality of life—referred to as your "health span"—becomes increasingly important too. The chapters in this book will help you maximize your chance of maintaining good health and mobility throughout your years. Indeed, we believe your best years are still ahead of you.

A few highlights from recent research explored in these pages:

▶ Studies continue to show the major health benefits of not only your lifestyle choices, but your beliefs as well. In chapter 1, discover ways to boost your daily quality of life, such as picking up a hobby (page 8), gardening (page 11), and having a sense of purpose (page 13).

▶ Evidence is also building that managing stress wards off aging, which means all of us need to find healthy ways to cope with the challenges of life. In chapter 2, we stress the importance of exercise, breathing, meditation, and other proven techniques to help you do so.

▶ While the pandemic brought tragic loss, it also changed some of our patterns for the better. In chapter 3, read about how home-based blood pressure monitoring combined with telemedicine may actually be more effective—and is clearly a better use of your time—than periodic in-person doctor visits (page 64).

▸ Use of medical technology is increasing, but does it help? In chapter 11, read about the latest advances, including the pros and cons of trackers that measure sleep and activity and whether the newest weight-loss drugs are right for you.

Another powerful theme emerging from medical research: being part of a supportive community benefits mental and physical health—and is increasingly tied to longevity. For example, human and even pet companionship can reduce stress (page 17) and rates of cognitive decline (page 56). In chapter 2, learn about volunteering's significant effects on mood and overall well-being (page 46) and, in chapter 4, how being kind to others helps heart health (page 100).

As always, lifestyle choices also have a tremendous impact on overall health—and we're here to cheer you on as you make them. Making healthy changes could be easier than you think. In chapters 4 and 8, you'll learn, for example, that staying active throughout the day matters most (pages 95 and 191). Even simple household activities count!

Healthy habits can be harder to maintain when you're not feeling your best. It's especially challenging when symptoms don't point to a specific diagnosis, or a condition—such as long COVID—has features that change day by day. For many, managing chronic diseases like diabetes, arthritis, heart failure, or COPD can feel overwhelming. In chapter 6, learn techniques to ease stress and care for yourself that will help you cope with these health challenges and focus on thriving, not just surviving.

In other chapters, this year's annual explores the best diets for your heart, mind, and overall health and helps you figure out which foods to avoid—or embrace (page 101). We propose tips for navigating post-pandemic health care, including finding a primary care provider (page 292) and how to safely fill prescriptions online (page 315). And you'll learn the latest research on cancer prevention, including what to look for in a home skin exam (page 164), updated guidelines on breast cancer screening (page 176), and what kind of diet is linked to improved prostate cancer outcomes (page 179).

The *Harvard Health Annual* will convince you that healthy living is possible at any age—and you can start now. As one Harvard doctor we spoke with this year said: "Maintaining a healthy and positive mindset as you age is one of the best things you can do for a longer life" (page 9). Armed with the information in this book, you'll be well prepared to live your best life for years to come.

To your health,

Howard E. LeWine MD

Howard LeWine, M.D.
Chief Medical Editor, Harvard Health Publishing

Chapter 1

Living Longer, Living Well

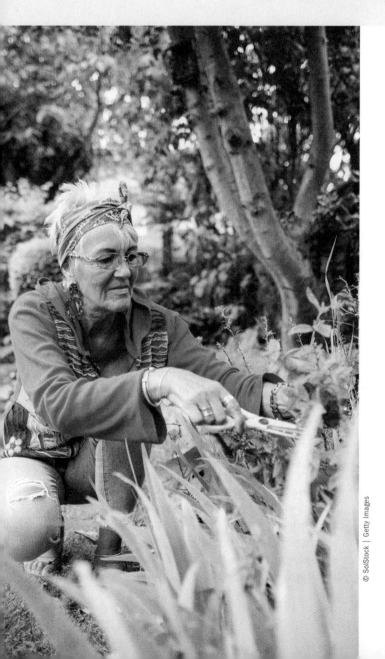

© SolStock | Getty Images

Healthy Habits! 5 Things You Can Do Now

1 **Wash your hands.** It's one of the best ways to prevent illness. (page 5)

2 **Pick up a hobby.** They're tied to health, happiness, and more. (page 8)

3 **Cultivate a positive attitude about aging.** Research suggests it could lead to a longer life. (page 9)

4 **Tend a garden.** Gardeners reap mood- and immune-boosting benefits, along with reduced anxiety. (page 11)

5 **Walk with a friend.** Pairing socializing with activity offers multiple rewards. (page 14)

Lessons learned from COVID

Living through the pandemic has changed many people's health habits, sometimes for the better.

More than four years after COVID emerged, people are resuming their pre-pandemic lifestyle. But don't let yourself return to all of your old habits. "Even though COVID brought stress and anxiety, it also changed how we live and approach our health, and in many ways, for the better," says Dr. Edward Phillips, founder and director of the Institute of Lifestyle Medicine at Harvard-affiliated Spaulding Rehabilitation Hospital. "The experience of living through COVID can be a teachable moment about how to continue the healthy habits we adopted during the pandemic."

Here's a look at four areas of health maintenance affected by COVID and the positive changes they created.

Exercise

With gyms and fitness centers closed, people had to find ways to stay active. Home workouts, online classes, and outdoor solo outings became the norm.

Keep it going. "The plus side of being forced out of your exercise routine is that it may have shown you new activities that you enjoy," says Dr. Phillips. For instance, some people have discovered that they prefer working out at home on their own schedule. Others have tried a new endeavor, like Peloton membership, and found it offers excitement and motivation they previously lacked. Even if you decide to return to your pre-COVID exercise style, consider expanding your repertoire.

"Be mindful that you are a different person now and may have new fitness goals and interests," says Dr. Phillips. For example, if you like gyms, try a new one that offers different classes, perhaps yoga or Pilates. Or explore boot camps that center around structured group workouts, or invest in short-term personal training sessions. If you've been power walking or cycling alone, consider joining a group or signing up for an event.

Diet

At the start of the pandemic, takeout delivery was popular. But over time, and to cut down on expenses,

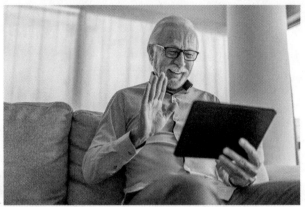
© Milos Zivojinovic | Getty Images

The pandemic showed people how to stay socially engaged using video calling.

more people turned to home-cooked meals. "And anything you make at home is almost always healthier," says Dr. Phillips.

Keep it going. Online grocery shopping was helpful during COVID, as it was safe and convenient. It also encouraged healthier shopping habits, according to Dr. Phillips. "You are less likely to make unhealthy impulse purchases when ordering online compared with shopping in person," he says. Try to continue online shopping, or at least mix it in with your regular grocery shopping. "Buying groceries online also can inspire you to try new healthy meals, expand your palate, and build your cooking skills," says Dr. Phillips.

Medical check-ups

A CDC study found about 40% of adults avoided routine medical care and check-ups during COVID. Make a list of your recent physicals, blood work, dental cleanings, eye and ear exams, and dermatology visits. Then go through the list and make appointments, starting with the most overdue.

Keep it going. A bright spot from COVID was the emergence of telemedicine, or virtual health care, in which you can consult with a doctor or nurse via video using your computer, tablet, or smartphone. Many people enjoyed the simplicity and time savings of telemedicine compared with office visits, and studies showed a surge in virtual appointments during the pandemic.

Telemedicine works well for follow-ups and consultations for minor issues, as well as routine check-ins for conditions requiring constant monitoring, like high blood pressure and cholesterol. "But you'll still have to do in-person visits for some routine check-ups and specialized care," says Dr. Phillips.

Social connections

Regular social interactions dropped off during the pandemic. The upside? COVID may have revealed your most valuable relationships by showing which people you really missed—and which ones you didn't, says Dr. Phillips. "You may have found you value some friendships more than you thought, and now you can invest more in them."

Group interactions also may have changed. For instance, you may find you don't miss larger gatherings but now cherish smaller, more intimate settings. "In this case, devote time to those gatherings that you find comfortable and enjoyable," says Dr. Phillips.

Keep it going. Zoom, Google Hangouts, Microsoft Teams, and other videoconferencing platforms are here to stay. "They helped people stay connected during the lockdowns, and now they can serve to continue social relationships regularly," says Dr. Phillips. "You don't need to wait until the next face-to-face opportunity."

A trend during COVID was "virtual happy hour," where co-workers got together after working hours to mingle on video calls. "Continue this by scheduling a weekly virtual visit with friends or family members to strengthen your social life," says Dr. Phillips. 🛡

Warding off germs: What's helpful, what's not

Have you adopted additional anti-germ habits since the pandemic? It's time to rethink some of them.

If we've learned anything about harmful microbes in the past few years, it's that we need to be proactive about avoiding them. That's especially true during the winter months, when we see an increase in cases of common colds, COVID-19, influenza, respiratory syncytial virus (RSV), and "stomach" bugs (such as norovirus).

How vigilant do you need to be to escape infection from those bugs? It's time to learn what does and doesn't keep you safe, so you can decide which habits to keep and which to let go.

Primary transmission

Harmful microbes spread in several ways.

Respiratory viruses—those that infect the upper respiratory tract (the nose, mouth, throat) or the lower respiratory tract (your windpipe and lungs)— are spread primarily when sick people cough, sneeze, or talk, sending infectious agents into the air. If you inhale them, you can get sick.

It's also possible to contract a respiratory virus by touching recently contaminated surfaces and then touching your eyes, nose, or mouth, although the risk is considered low.

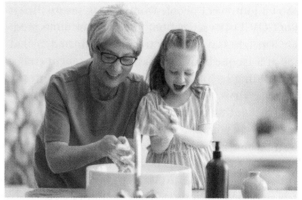

© konstantin yuganov I Getty Images

Getting your hands soapy and scrubbing for 20 seconds is still one of the best ways to avoid infection.

"Stomach" bugs infect the stomach or intestines. These microbes are spread when microscopic particles of feces or vomit from an infected person get into your nose or mouth. This can happen when you have direct contact with infected people, share eating utensils with them, eat food that's prepared or handled by them, eat food or drinks contaminated with infected particles, or touch contaminated surfaces and then touch your mouth or nose.

▶▶

Strategies that can protect you

Here are the best ways to protect yourself.

Wash your hands regularly. Wash them after shaking someone's hand; as soon as you get home from being out; and throughout the day before touching your face (especially your nose or mouth), preparing or eating food, taking medication, or blowing your nose. Get your hands soapy and scrub for 20 seconds. "Soap causes virus particles to burst open. Gastrointestinal viruses are hardier than other germs, which is why you need to wash your hands a little longer to protect against them," says Dr. Daniel Kuritzkes, chief of the Division of Infectious Diseases at Harvard-affiliated Brigham and Women's Hospital.

Wear a face mask. Face masks, especially those labeled N95 or KN95, help keep viruses from entering your nose or mouth. "Consider wearing a mask in crowded indoor settings, such as a theater, where germs move easily from person to person," Dr. Kuritzkes says. This is particularly true if you have lung or heart disease, which make you more vulnerable than most people if you get a respiratory infection.

Get vaccinated. Vaccinations for COVID-19, RSV (for people ages 60 or older), and the flu have been shown to prevent people from getting severe illness. For COVID-19 vaccination, "the data look quite good," Dr. Kuritzkes says. "If you are fully vaccinated, including at least one booster, you have an excellent chance of avoiding serious symptoms if you do get infected with the virus."

Use caution around sick loved ones. If family members in your home have a respiratory or gastrointestinal bug, Dr. Kuritzkes advises that you avoid close contact, wear a mask when you're near them, and wear rubber or latex gloves to clean up after them. To disinfect surfaces contaminated by respiratory viruses, use commercial disinfectants or a 70% isopropyl alcohol solution. To disinfect surfaces contaminated by gastrointestinal bugs, use products that contain bleach or quaternary ammonium. Don't use both at once (they produce toxic fumes), and be aware that bleach can damage certain surfaces, such as wood.

What you don't need to do

It's natural to want to do as much as possible to stay healthy. But some practices, such as removing your shoes before entering your home, probably won't keep you safe from winter bugs, although it will help keep your rugs and carpets clean. "Removing your shoes is a custom in many cultures, but there's no infectious disease basis for it. You won't catch anything from walking around your house with shoes on," Dr. Kuritzkes says.

Here are other anti-germ approaches that probably won't make a difference.

Washing your groceries or packages. "It's true that, in lab studies, a virus can be recovered from surfaces for a few days, but that's done under special circumstances," Dr. Kuritzkes says. "In reality, there's no concern about getting a respiratory virus by touching items at a supermarket or packages delivered to your home. Is it possible that you could contract a gastrointestinal bug if you pick up groceries or packages that were handled by someone who has norovirus? It's possible, but unlikely. Just wash your hands."

Cleaning your smartphone. Dr. Kuritzkes says it would be extraordinarily rare for you to get sick because you touched a contaminated surface and then touched your smartphone, which you put up to your face.

Changing your clothes when you get home. Some people don't want to sit on a bed or sofa in the same clothes they wore outside the house, such as at work or on the bus or subway. But there's no evidence that you'll contract respiratory or gastrointestinal bugs if you do.

Wearing a rubber or latex glove to touch a bank ATM machine or gas pump. Yes, lots of people have touched that ATM or gas pump before you, but all you need to do after touching it is use hand sanitizer, avoid touching your face, and wash your hands with soap and water when you can.

The takeaway

We all have to work hard to stay healthy. That includes maintaining good anti-germ strategies and taking care of ourselves—getting seven to nine hours of sleep each night, eating a healthy diet, limiting alcohol consumption, not smoking, and staying active. The combination of those habits keeps the immune system robust and ready to fight invading microbes.

Should you give up some anti-germ habits if they're probably unnecessary? It's your decision. It won't hurt to follow them, as long as they don't cause you distress.

"Just try to be aware of your actions," Dr. Kuritzkes says, "and don't let your guard down."

10 habits for good health

These strategies can support your wellness journey.

The foundation of a healthy lifestyle consists of lasting habits like eating right, watching your weight, exercising regularly, managing your mental health, and getting routine medical exams. But even daily, small steps toward these goals also can have a significant impact.

Here are some practices that can help support your ongoing health journey. While you might find it unrealistic to follow them all the time, try to include them in your daily life as much as possible.

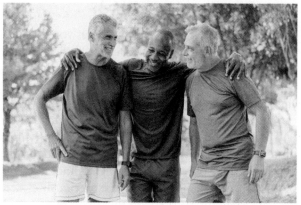

© andreswd | Getty Images

Daily social connections can stave off loneliness and help protect against cognitive decline.

1 Do a morning stretch

Stretching before getting out of bed wakes up the body, improves circulation, and promotes relaxation, helping to set the day's tone. While you're still lying in bed, move the covers aside, then flex and release your lower limbs several times. Bend your knees and lift your legs into the air. With your legs still elevated, flex your feet up and down and rotate them side to side. Next, sit up and slowly look left and then right. Roll your shoulders several times. Flex your wrists up and down, and open and close your hands repeatedly.

2 Stay hydrated

Proper hydration supports digestion, improves brain performance, and increases energy, among other health benefits. Drink a big glass of water after you wake up and a glass with every meal.

3 Floss

Maintaining good oral health includes daily flossing, but make sure you do it right. First, wrap the floss around your middle fingers, which helps you reach the back teeth. Then loop the floss around one side of a tooth, so it makes a C shape. Beginning at the gum line, slide it up and down the tooth several times. (Don't move the floss back and forth in a sawing motion. You miss cleaning the entire tooth, and the friction can irritate the gum.) Repeat on the other side of the tooth, and then the other teeth.

4 Apply sunscreen

Sunscreen is the best defense against skin-damaging rays. After washing your face in the morning, apply a facial moisturizer that contains sunscreen with an SPF (sun protection factor) of at least 30. Or blend equal parts sunscreen and a regular moisturizer. Use one or two nickel-sized dollops to cover your entire face, neck, ears, and any bald or thinning spots on your head.

5 Go nuts

When you crave a snack, reach for unsalted nuts and seeds like almonds, walnuts, peanuts, and cashews. They contain many beneficial nutrients and help prevent cravings for highly processed foods. Nuts are high in calories, so keep to a palm-sized portion.

6 Nap

Afternoon naps can recharge a weary body and may boost cognitive function. A 2021 study published by *General Psychiatry* found that nappers scored higher on cognitive tests than non-nappers. The researchers found that shorter and less frequent naps—lasting less than 30 minutes, no more than four times a week— were associated with the most benefit. Schedule naps for the early afternoon, then use a timer so you don't oversleep.

7 Bust some moves

Break up bouts of sitting with small bursts of movement. For example, dance across a room instead of walking. When you brush your teeth, suck in your lower gut for 30 seconds, which activates your abdominal muscles. Do 10 air squats or push-ups (on the ground or against the kitchen counter). Make it a habit to stand up "twice" each time you stand up—that is, get up, sit back down, and then get back up.

▶▶

▶▶ 8 Take a breather

Alternate-nostril breathing, in which you breathe through one nostril at a time, is believed to help reduce stress by slowing your breathing rhythm and forcing you to take deep, full breaths. Using a finger or thumb, close one nostril and slowly breathe in and out through the open nostril. After about five to 10 breaths, switch and close the other nostril and repeat the breathing pattern. For a variation, try inhaling through one nostril with the other closed, changing finger/thumb positions, and exhaling through the previously closed nostril. Then, inhale through that one, close it, and exhale through the other nostril. Go back and forth like this for a few minutes.

9 Enjoy a hobby

A study published in 2023 by *Nature Medicine* suggests that having a hobby is good for people's overall health and mood. Hobbies involve creativity, sensory engagement, self-expression, relaxation, and cognitive stimulation. One way to pick up a new hobby is with a project kit designed to teach you a skill like gardening, building a model, carving wood, or making beer, soap, hot sauce, or jewelry. The kits come with instructions and all the materials you need to start. You can find kits at local bookstores or hobby stores, or go online: just type "how-to kits" or "project kits" into a search engine.

10 Be social

Social interactions can stave off loneliness and protect against depression and cognitive decline. Strive to have some kind of social engagement every day: make a phone call, send an email, or chat with a neighbor. Another option is to create your own "social club"—a small group that you interact with regularly, like meeting for coffee or conversing over a Zoom call. Even casual conversations are beneficial; for example, chat with a grocery store employee or interact with a stranger on the street. ▮

IN THE JOURNALS

Having a hobby tied to happiness and well-being

Check those holiday gifts: if you received one that can get you started on a new hobby, it might be the gift that keeps on giving. A study published in 2023 by *Nature Medicine* suggests that having a hobby is good for your health, mood, and more. Researchers combed through five large studies involving more than 93,000 people across 16 countries (including the United States, Japan, China, and a dozen European countries). Participants were all ages 65 or older, and more than 60% had longstanding mental or physical health conditions. They periodically answered questionnaires about their health and well-being and were followed for four to eight years. Compared with people who didn't have hobbies, those who did reported better health, more happiness, fewer symptoms of depression, and higher life satisfaction. The findings were similar across all countries. The study is observational and doesn't prove that hobbies caused people to be healthy and happy. But the researchers say hobbies—such as arts and crafts, games, gardening, volunteering, or participating in clubs—involve creativity, sensory engagement, self-expression, relaxation, and cognitive stimulation, which are linked to good mental health and well-being. Plus, taking part in hobby groups keeps you socially connected, which helps reduce loneliness and isolation.

Can you feel younger than your age?

A positive attitude about aging can help your mind and body feel younger and healthier.

You've probably met some older people who boast "I feel like I'm 30!" or "I don't feel my age!" They tend to be positive, optimistic, and energetic.

But do they actually feel young and healthy, or is it wishful thinking?

"People with more positive attitudes about growing old tend to live longer and healthier lives than those with negative thoughts about aging," says Dr. David Sinclair, professor of genetics at Harvard Medical School.

Thoughts on aging

Research backs this up. A study published in 2022 in *JAMA Network Open* looked at the differences in aging satisfaction over four years among 14,000 adults over 50. The researchers found that the people with the highest satisfaction with aging had a 43% lower risk of dying from any cause over the four years than those who were the least satisfied.

The study also found that people more satisfied with the aging process had a lower risk for diabetes, stroke, cancer, and heart disease. They also had better cognitive functioning and were less lonely and depressed. People who embraced this positive mindset were also more physically active and slept better. "If you feel younger, you are more likely to act younger," says Dr. Sinclair. "Maintaining a healthy and positive mindset as you age is one of the best things you can do for a longer life."

Ways to feel younger

What can you do to feel younger in your mind, body, and spirit? Here are some suggestions from Dr. Sinclair:

Reduce anxiety. Anxiety becomes more common with age, so adopt practices to help manage it. "Daily meditation, reading stoicism [a philosophy that teaches how to maximize positive emotions and reduce negative ones], and simply spending some quiet time each day expressing gratitude are good places to begin," says Dr. Sinclair.

Have a sense of purpose. A strong sense of purpose means continuing to pursue goals and to feel life is worthwhile. Explore interests centered on self-development, growth, and connecting with others.

For example, learn an instrument or a language, volunteer for a cause you support, mentor a young person, or take college classes in subjects that stimulate your mind. Or learn new skills, such as public speaking, cooking, or auto repair. If you need further inspiration, revisit your youth. What did you enjoy doing when you were younger? Did you build model trains or enjoy certain sports?

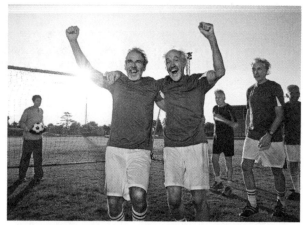

© Uwe Krejci | Getty Images

Joining a sports club is one way to build confidence and increase social connections.

Stay connected. Socializing keeps our minds active and engaged. Studies also show that personal connections help curb feelings of low self-esteem that dampen a positive mindset. Men often find it most natural to bond over a shared activity or interest, so consider joining a walking group, golf or bowling league, card or chess club, service club, or men's club at a community center.

Another option is to create your own "pod"—a small, intimate group you interact with regularly. Schedule weekly, bimonthly, or monthly meet-ups with friends in person or via Zoom or a conference call.

Challenge yourself. Find a physical challenge that you can realistically complete, create a plan of execution, and then work to meet that goal. For example, train for a 5K race, hike a trail, complete a series of boot camp classes, or walk a mile daily for a month. Regular exercise builds confidence in your ability to be active, and setting a challenge helps you experience ▸▸

a feeling of accomplishment. Both can make you feel more youthful.

Get a job. The workplace offers the chance to actively use your mental skills, such as problem-solving and breaking down complex tasks. It also shows that you still have value to others and the world and that what you contribute is needed.

Reject stereotypes. Ageism—the socially pervasive idea that you are too old to do certain activities—can put a damper on your mindset. "It can be tough to overcome, but constantly remind yourself that your age does not dictate whether or not you have the necessary ability, skills, or desire to succeed at something," says Dr. Sinclair. ♥

by **HOWARD LeWINE, M.D.**, Editor in Chief, *Harvard Men's Health Watch*

Do past lifestyle habits affect future health?

Q *I worry how much permanent damage my prior smoking and heavy drinking did to my body. I quit both five years ago. Will my past behavior affect how I age?*

A It's never too late to make healthier lifestyle choices. Some of the health risks of using tobacco and overusing alcohol begin to drop within days after you stop using them. To what degree the amount and number of years of tobacco and alcohol use affect how long you live or the quality of your life is difficult to predict. It also depends on genetics, which we continue to explore.

Regarding your alcohol use, blood tests and perhaps a liver ultrasound to evaluate your liver status and function might reassure you. If you currently have no damage to your liver or other organs from alcohol, then it is unlikely you will have alcohol-related problems in the future.

Smoking is not so straightforward. Quitting can reduce your risk of heart disease back to baseline after five years. The risks of chronic lung disease and smoking-related cancers, especially lung cancer, have already gone down since you quit. And your risk will continue to drop with each passing year. However, the increased cancer risk and the chance of developing chronic lung disease never completely go away if a person has smoked regularly for many years.

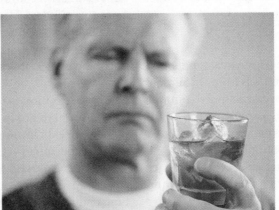

© Image Source | Getty Images

Many health risks from drinking can decline soon after you stop.

Sowing the seeds of better health

Growing evidence fortifies gardening's bumper crop of physical and mental benefits.

Katherine Rosa copes with winter's gloom by meticulously planning her summer flower garden, giddily anticipating pops of color and fragrance to shift her focus toward radiant days ahead.

"It lifts the spirit and keeps my sense of vitality alive in the dark of winter," says Rosa, a family nurse practitioner and researcher at the Benson-Henry Institute for Mind Body Medicine at Harvard-affiliated Massachusetts General Hospital, who's been gardening most of her life. "It's a little bit of joy."

Therapeutic horticulture—the practice of gardening as a means to promote better health and well-being—has existed since the 19th century. But the mind-boosting benefits Rosa reaps from digging holes, planting seeds, and pulling weeds join a veritable harvest of freshly documented health advantages.

Gardening yields much the same effects on body, mind, and soul as traditional exercise, Harvard experts say. And its appeal seems to be pollinating: as of 2015, an estimated 117 million Americans—one in three—kept gardens. Another 18 million took up the activity during the COVID pandemic, according to the National Gardening Association.

"Gardening is rarely something someone is forced to do. Most people garden because they love it," says Dr. Beth Frates, director of lifestyle medicine and wellness in the Department of Surgery at Massachusetts General Hospital. "It's an activity where you literally reap what you sow."

Bodywide bonuses

A growing body of new and established evidence offers a bouquet of reasons our bodies gravitate to gardening.

It gets you moving. A study published in 2023 in *The Lancet Planetary Health* suggests that gardening simply makes us move more. Researchers split 291 adults (82% women) who hadn't gardened previously into two groups; half were assigned to a community gardening group, and the others were asked to wait a year to start gardening. Both groups took periodic surveys gauging their nutrition habits and mental health. They also wore activity monitors.

The people in the gardening group increased their physical activity levels by about 42 minutes each week,

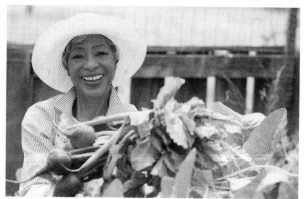
© Pauline St.Denis | Getty Images
Gardening can tone our minds and bodies.

more than a quarter of the standard recommendations of at least 150 minutes per week of physical activity. The CDC lists gardening as a moderate-intensity exercise that burns about 330 calories per hour, a rate similar to hiking or dancing.

"The joy of gardening allows for physical activity that feels fun and rewarding for many, especially those who don't consider themselves athletes," Dr. Frates says. "Some people think running, biking, or swimming are the only forms of aerobic activity, but this is a narrow view. Take advantage of the gym outside your window."

It improves your diet. The same study also found that participants in the gardening group ate about 7% more fiber each day—possibly because they're eating what they're growing—compared with people who didn't garden. Average daily fiber intake among American adults is about half of the recommended 25 to 30 grams per day, so the additional 1.4 grams eaten each day by the gardening group proved substantial, researchers said. Fiber can improve digestion, inflammation, and immune response.

It may fight off illness. A 2021 study published in *The Journals of Gerontology: Series A* suggests that people who garden may experience less age-related decline in immune system effectiveness. They also have lower levels of low-grade inflammation common among older adults that can heighten risks for cardiovascular disease, cancer, and inflammatory diseases. "Since gardening may cut stress, that also helps our immune systems to function optimally," Dr. Frates says. ▶▶

▶▶ Mental tonic

Along with potentially reducing your stress, gardening produces other key mental health benefits.

It smooths mood. Connecting with nature's calm can interrupt rumination, or repetitive thoughts that can contribute to depression. A 2022 study published by the journal *PLOS One* suggested that gardening lowered stress, anxiety, and depression in otherwise healthy women who attended twice-weekly gardening classes for four weeks. None of the 32 women in the study had gardened previously; half were assigned to the gardening sessions, while the other half went to art classes. They reported their levels of anxiety, depression, and stress. While both groups reaped mental health benefits, the gardeners reported less anxiety.

"Instead of focusing on the to-do list, the disagreement with a colleague, an argument with a loved one, or a difficult interaction at the grocery store, the gardener can set these worries aside to become fully immersed in the task at hand," Dr. Frates says.

It sharpens your brain. A 2019 study in the *International Journal of Environmental Research and Public Health* suggests even a single burst of gardening significantly improves levels of brain nerve growth factors important to staying sharp. The analysis involved 41 older adults (68% women) who spent 20 minutes tending to a garden plot. Blood samples were taken before and after the gardening activity to measure brain chemicals.

"When you're gardening, you need to be focused, and you're also relying on your memory," Rosa says. "You're continually stimulating your brain cells."

It fertilizes relationships. When your tomato plants produce far more of the fat, juicy orbs than you can eat, what do you do? Pass along the extras to friends and family members—strengthening bonds in the process, Harvard experts say. Gardening also turns into a social activity when done in community plots and with garden clubs, helping relationships bloom. "If gardening is one of your social networks, you're keeping relationships that are critically important to your happiness," Rosa says. 🛡

More evidence that aging might be reversible

It seems that every living thing ages—that aging is inevitable. Yet studies in animals have suggested that aging may, at least, be slowed. Scientists have been able to track this using genetic biomarker tests known as DNA methylation clocks, which indicate how rapidly body cells are aging. In a 2023 study published in *Cell Metabolism*, researchers found that when the blood supply of an old mouse was connected to the blood supply of a young mouse for three months, the organs of the young mouse aged dramatically. When the joined blood supplies were disconnected, the organs of the young mouse became biologically younger: in other words, the aging process could be accelerated and then reversed. The scientists then found that in people going through severe COVID-19, surgery for a hip fracture, or pregnancy, the clocks showed a sudden acceleration of aging followed by a reversal. This study did not identify the factors that cause or reverse aging, and we are still a long way from being able to slow human aging more powerfully than we can through living a healthy lifestyle. But this kind of research offers hope that, someday, we will understand the aging process well enough to slow it.

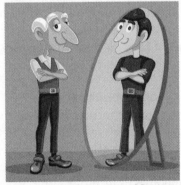

© nicoletaionescu | Getty Images

10 ways to find purpose in life

Try these exercises to reflect on your experiences, abilities, and interests, and discover a new way to make life meaningful.

Job burnout, an empty nest, retirement, the loss of a partner—any one of those can lead you to feel like you've lost your sense of purpose or reason to get up every morning. It's a common experience, especially as we get older. "When you lose something that's shaped you, it's a threat to your identity, and you wonder who you are without it," says Matthew Lee, a sociologist and research associate at Harvard University's Human Flourishing Program. The question is—will you do anything about it, or will you languish? Your response could affect your health.

The importance of purpose

Having a sense of purpose is associated with many health benefits, such as sharp memory and thinking skills, mood control, reduced risks of chronic disease and disability, and longevity.

Why is purpose so potent? "Several studies suggest that, compared with people who don't have a sense of purpose, those who do tend to perceive stressors as being less difficult and cope better with stress. That might help them avoid some of the physiological effects of chronic stress that contribute to heart attack, stroke, and early death," Lee says.

And some studies have found that people with purpose are likely to engage in healthy behaviors, such as keeping up with health screenings.

Finding purpose

Purpose can spring from something simple, like a hobby, or more complex, such as contributing your service to your community in some way. While there's no one formula to find that inspiration, there are ways to cultivate it. Here are 10 suggestions to get you started, adapted from the Harvard Special Health Report *Self-Care* (www.health.harvard.edu/scshr), with additional insight from Lee.

1. Zero in on your strengths. Ask friends, family, and your partner what comes to mind when they think of you. Do they find you entertaining, compassionate, or artistic? Use their feedback to think about how you can apply these attributes in a way that would give meaning to your life and the lives of others.

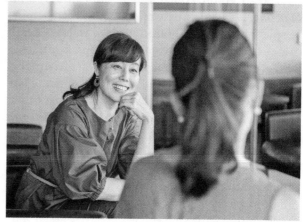

© Taiyou Nomachi | Getty Images

Becoming a mentor and sharing your skills can enrich your days and give you renewed purpose.

2. Think about the obstacles you have overcome in your life. Can you find ways to help others who are going through the same thing? "This can be profound," Lee says. "Your life experience can help others, which is inherently purposeful."

3. Draw up a purpose timeline. Your purpose changes as you age. Think about what it was at different points in your life, with particular focus on periods of evolution or transition. Did you learn any lessons that you can apply to your current situation?

4. Look for role models. Are there people whose work you admire? Can you learn how to do something similar?

5. Become a mentor and share your knowledge and skills. People often cite the encouragement and wisdom they've obtained from others who took the time to care about their careers. "A mentoring relationship is a caring one that enables us to give and receive love," Lee says. "Reciprocal, caring relationships are often what's missing as we get older."

6. Think about what the world needs. There are a great many needs on this planet, and different people will prioritize different ones. Are you concerned about world hunger? Climate change? Injustice? Identify a cause that's meaningful to you, and think about how you could help. "There are probably a million needs in your community that aren't being met. Maybe some of those needs require your skill set," Lee says. ▶▶

▶▶ Why not call a local group that interests you and ask about volunteering opportunities? Or visit Volunteer Match (www.volunteermatch.org) for ideas.

7. Read Viktor Frankl's book _Man's Search for Meaning._ It's a quick, easy read, and it's been helping people for decades. "Frankl noticed in Nazi death camps that people who were generous, connected with others, and found meaningful ways to support others were more vital and survived longer. They found a way to relate in a loving way to each other, and there was purpose in doing that. It may inspire you," Lee says.

8. Write your own story. Your own lived experience is also worthwhile. Recall the best stories from your childhood and write them down with all the detail you can think of. Include answers to important questions about yourself—the kind you wish you had asked your own parents and grandparents. Give the stories to your kids and grandkids.

9. Write your own obituary. You can do this at any age, maybe not for publication-just for yourself or your family. What do you want to be remembered for? Can any of that inform your purpose now? If you haven't yet achieved something you're especially proud of, remember that it's not too late.

10. Picture yourself winning the lottery. What would you do without financial concerns standing in the way? Would you travel the world? Volunteer? Figure out ways to do elements of those same things without a financial windfall. For example, if you've always wanted to visit Asia, see if you can sign up with a volunteer organization like the Peace Corps (there's no age limit!).

How to start

Don't feel pressured. "Explore the possibilities," Lee says. "It gets you moving again, and momentum can take you further in ways that you may find rich, rewarding, and even surprising." ▮

Better together: The many benefits of walking with friends

Walking with others has a host of health perks and helps you stay motivated.

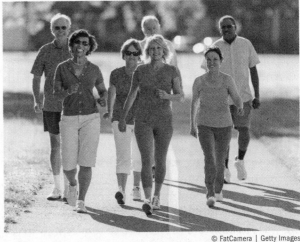

© FatCamera | Getty Images

Walking in a group is safer than walking alone. Plus, it adds socialization and accountability to your routine.

There's an old saying: if you want to go fast, go alone; if you want to go far, go together. One good example is exercising, especially brisk walking—the kind that gives your heart and lungs a workout and boosts overall health. The activity is easy to do with family and friends, and the team approach can pay off in many ways.

It's a great social activity

Going for a brisk walk with one or more friends is a form of socializing, which is essential for good health. Socializing helps stave off isolation and loneliness, which are associated with heart disease, diabetes, arthritis, depression, chronic stress, and premature death. Socializing also helps exercise the brain, which protects your thinking skills. When you socialize, your brain interprets people's facial expressions, speech, emotions, and body language, and then powers your reactions—turning your thoughts into words, facial expressions, and body movements.

That extra effort from socializing, even if you're unaware of it, promotes brain cell connections, which keeps thinking and memory sharp.

The physical work of a walk also stimulates the growth of new brain cells. So when you socialize while you walk, you get a double dose of brain-health benefits.

It gets you on a schedule

Have trouble sticking to an exercise regimen? You're not alone. "Humans aren't designed to exercise. We're designed to conserve energy. We love to sit around. That's our nature," explains Dr. Edward Phillips, associate professor of physical medicine and rehabilitation at Harvard Medical School and Whole Health Medical Director at VA Boston Healthcare System.

You'll have better luck staying on a walking routine if you go with friends, primarily for two reasons.

Accountability. "Friends have expectations, and we tend not to want to let them down. We jump through hoops to be there for others. So if you agree to walk with a friend, you're more likely to do it," Dr. Phillips says.

Motivation. "When you walk with someone else, you challenge and encourage each other. Imagine that you hit a wall while walking, but other people around you are still going. That makes you realize that it's doable, and you keep walking," Dr. Phillips says. "The other piece is that being with others is fun, and you might be more inclined to go for a brisk walk if you think about it as spending time with friends rather than a chore. You'll want to go."

It's practical

Walking with a buddy is safer than walking alone. "There are more eyes watching for hazards you may miss. And you'll be more visible to drivers when you walk in pairs or a group. Also, if you experience any kind of health problem while walking, or if you fall, a friend can take care of you and call for help," says Dr. Phillips says.

Having a person on hand who can help you is especially important if you have a chronic condition that

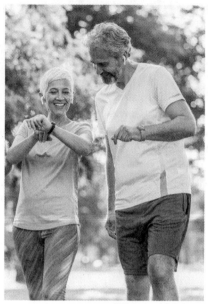
© filadendron | Getty Images
Note how long it takes to get from here to there, then challenge each other to go faster.

can lead to sudden symptoms, such as heart disease, asthma, or a balance disorder.

One caution: Don't leave your phone at home and assume you'll use someone else's in an emergency. If that person is unable to speak and share the phone's passcode, you'll be out of luck. It's better if each person on the walk brings a fully charged phone.

Techniques and drills

Make the most of your walk with friends by challenging and coaching each other. You can challenge yourselves by trying a different style of walking, such as Nordic walking, which uses poles. Doing new things is fun, good for your thinking skills, and easier with a buddy. Or try improving your walking times. "Note how long it usually takes you to get from here to there. If it's 32 minutes, try to do it in 31 minutes the next time, and 30 minutes the next," Dr. Phillips says.

To do a little coaching, Dr. Phillips suggests making a deal to keep each other in good walking form. Make sure all walkers are swinging their arms and keeping poles (if using them) at a 45° angle.

Maintaining the pace

You can easily adjust your pace to stay in step with just one friend. But what if you're walking in a group? "If you'd all like to walk at the same pace, use a metronome app, and play it loudly on your phone. Or clap your hands or beat a small drum. Take turns being the person who maintains the pace," Dr. Phillips suggests.

Or, if the group is comfortable with it, let the faster walkers get ahead. "After a little while, they can take a break and stretch while they wait for the others to catch up," Dr. Phillips says. "Or the faster walkers can slow down by making their routines more intense. They can raise their arms up and down while walking, wear a weighted vest, or carry other people's water bottles. Have fun with it and enjoy the journey. You're not just there for exercise. You're there for camaraderie. The fact that it comes with health benefits is icing on the cake." 🛡

To elevate your exercise routine, take a hike

Varied terrain, hiking poles, and natural landscapes can add physical and mental benefits to an outdoor workout.

Autumn is often an ideal time to go hiking, after the crowds, heat, and insects of summer have died down a bit. You can choose a location that suits your abilities, whether that's a tree-lined path near your home or a more challenging trail in a state or national park. And compared with brisk walking, hiking gives you a little more bang for your buck in terms of health-related benefits, says Dr. Luke Apisa, an emergency medicine physician who recently completed a fellowship in wilderness medicine at Harvard-affiliated Massachusetts General Hospital.

"Hiking on uneven terrain is an efficient way to build muscles in your lower body, which helps improve stability and balance," he says. Hiking uphill works the muscles in your hips and buttocks, while going downhill builds up the quadriceps, the muscles in the fronts of your thighs. Plus, a route that includes some gain in elevation will force your heart to work harder, which boosts cardiovascular fitness without requiring you to jog or run. If you have any joint-related issues in your knees or hips, walking on a trail is far less taxing than running on pavement.

Pick up some poles

Using trekking poles (also called hiking poles) when you hike can also reduce strain on your knees and ankles. "Poles allow you to offload some of the pressure on your legs, especially when you're going downhill, which can be jarring to the knees without extra support," says Dr. Apisa, who used trekking poles

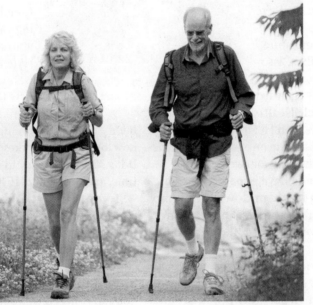
© FatCamera | Getty Images

Using poles while hiking provides added stability and strengthens your upper body.

himself while running the Everest Marathon in May 2023. Trekking poles, which have sharp metal tips that work well on rocky, uneven, and mountainous terrain, enhance your stability and reduce your risk of falling.

Trekking poles are similar to Nordic or walking poles, most of which come with attachable rubber tips for use on concrete or asphalt. While trekking poles have loose wrist straps, Nordic poles have special glove-like straps that allow you to use your palm to help propel yourself forward as you stride.

Using poles of any type, but especially Nordic poles, adds an upper-body workout to your hike, toning your arms, shoulders, and back. That translates to a higher heart rate and increased calorie burn, although you won't necessarily feel like you're working any harder than walking without poles, research suggests. Consider purchasing your poles at a store specializing in outdoor gear, where an employee can advise you on the best poles for your purposes, help you adjust the height, and give you a quick primer on their use.

Natural stress relief

The restorative and stress-relieving powers of being outside in nature are yet another potential benefit of hiking. Spending time in green space—nature preserves, woodlands, and even urban parks—may ease people's stress levels, according to several small studies. The traditional Japanese practice of *shinrin-yoku*, or "forest bathing," encourages people to experience the pleasures of being in nature. Research suggests the practice improves health and well-being and even appears to reduce levels of the stress hormone cortisol compared with being in urban environments. Chronic stress contributes to high blood pressure and heart disease risk, so anything you can do to counteract stress is likely helpful.

High-altitude hiking

What about ascending to high elevations while hiking? The higher you go in altitude, the less oxygen you take in with each breath. Your body responds by raising your heart rate and the amount of blood pumped with each beat. This temporarily boosts blood pressure. Fully adapting to the lower oxygen level can take several weeks.

If you are generally healthy and your blood pressure is under good control, a good rule of thumb is to go no higher than 8,000 feet in the first leg of the trip and stay there for at least one night. Take it easy for a day or two before any strenuous hiking, and pay attention to how you feel. If you're feeling fine, then you should be okay to go 1,000 to 2,000 feet higher each day. But if you have heart or lung disease, check with your physician for more specific advice before traveling to a high-altitude destination, Dr. Apisa advises. ▼

Healthy social connections help relieve stress

Researchers have found that social interactions help relieve harmful levels of stress, which can adversely affect coronary arteries, gut function, insulin regulation, and the immune system. One study, which examined data from more than 309,000 people, found that lack of strong relationships increased the risk of premature death from all causes by 50%—an effect on mortality risk roughly comparable to smoking up to 15 cigarettes a day, and greater than obesity and physical inactivity. Caring behaviors may also trigger the release of stress-reducing hormones. In addition, evidence suggests that the life-enhancing effects of social support extend to the giver as well as to the receiver.

All of this is encouraging news because caring involvement with others may be one of the easiest health strategies to enact. It's inexpensive, it requires no special equipment or regimen, and we can engage in it in many ways.

Making new friends and social connections can sometimes be a challenge. Try these three ways to meet new friends:

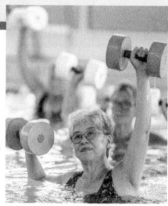
© FatCamera | Getty Images

Social connections have measurable effects on health—and benefit both giver and receiver.

Join a gym. Many YMCAs and fitness centers offer group classes. If you take the same class with any regularity, and you're open to starting conversations, you'll eventually get to know your fellow fitness enthusiasts.

Attend a local church, synagogue, or mosque. If you're spiritual, your religious institution is the perfect place to get to know people in your community. Take advantage of potluck suppers and other get-togethers where you can mingle.

Volunteer. Pick a cause that's important to you. Offer to assist with a local politician's re-election campaign. Work in a soup kitchen. Help children learn to read. Or volunteer at your local pet shelter. Getting out in the community is a great way to meet people.

Eating high-quality carbohydrates may stave off middle-age weight gain

Hoping to avoid middle-age weight gain? Steer clear of low-quality carbohydrates and starchy vegetables such as peas, corn, and potatoes, a Harvard-led study suggests.

The 2023 study, published by *The BMJ,* evaluated weight changes in 136,432 adults 65 or younger (average age 50, 83.5% women) who were tracked for up to 28 years. Although participants gained an average of more than three pounds every four years, the quality of carbohydrates they ate appeared to play a role in weight control. A daily increase of 3.5 ounces of low-quality carbohydrates—such as sugar-sweetened drinks, refined grains, and starchy vegetables—was associated with gaining up to three pounds over a four-year period. But an increase of just one-third of an ounce of fiber in participants' daily diets was linked with gaining 1.7 fewer pounds over four years. The associations were especially strong in women and in people with excess body weight.

While consuming too much sugar is unhealthy, refined carbohydrates such as white pasta, white bread, white rice, and chips appeared more problematic, contributing even more to middle-age weight gain, the study authors said.

Want to stay out of the hospital? Exercise a bit more

If an apple a day keeps the doctor away, what can an extra dose of daily exercise accomplish? It may keep you out of the hospital, according to a recent analysis.

Adding 20 minutes of moderate-to-vigorous physical activity—including walking, cycling, or swimming—to your daily routine can cut your risk of being hospitalized for a variety of common medical problems, the study suggests.

The 2023 study, published by *JAMA Network Open,* used data from nearly 82,000 U.K. adults (average age 62, 56% women) who wore an activity tracker for one week. Over the following seven years, those who'd shown greater levels of physical activity—particularly moderate-to-vigorous exercise—were less likely to be hospitalized for nine of the 25 most common reasons people are typically admitted: diabetes, gallbladder disease, urinary tract infections, stroke, pneumonia, blood clots, anemia, diverticular disease, and colon polyps.

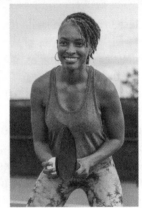

© Lpettet | Getty Images

An extra 20 minutes of exercise cuts the odds of being hospitalized.

How might exercise promote this effect? Some likely reasons are that it helps us control weight and blood pressure as well as improve inflammation levels and immune response. "With diabetes, for example, it's clear that blood sugar control is better if people are getting more physical activity," says Dr. David Bates, chief of the Division of Medicine at Brigham and Women's Hospital. "For conditions such as blood clots and pneumonia, if you're more active, the risk is also lower."

"The very safest thing to do is stay out of the hospital," he adds. "More and more, we know that physical activity is strongly associated with better outcomes across a range of factors."

Ways to maximize your energy

Lifestyle tweaks and a little planning will help reduce fatigue and give you more oomph for everyday activities.

The boundless energy we took for granted in youth usually fades as we age. While we once had the ability to tackle lots of strenuous or stressful tasks in a day, now even a few bursts of activity can leave us feeling flat-out fatigued. So what happens to our energy? Can we rev it back up? And how can we make the most of the energy we have?

Why energy changes

Your energy level can decline as a result of aging, illness, or other factors. Here are some of the main ones.

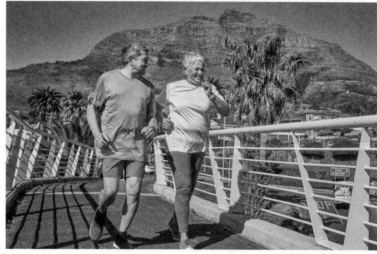

© Charday Penn | Getty Images

If you're too tired for a workout later in the day, schedule it earlier, when you have more energy.

Age-related changes. As we get older, we lose energy-producing engines in the cells (mitochondria), and as a result we make less adenosine triphosphate (ATP)—the molecule that delivers energy to cells throughout the body. We also lose muscle mass, resulting in fewer cells, fewer mitochondria, and lower ATP production. If you're too tired to be active, it compounds the problem by further weakening and shrinking muscles.

Chronic illness. Many illnesses, such as depression, rheumatoid arthritis, and heart disease, cause fatigue, making it hard to get through daily activities.

Medication side effects of medications. Many drugs can make you drowsy, such as antidepressants, antihistamines, anticonvulsants, and some blood pressure drugs (beta blockers, for example).

Poor diet. Are you eating too much processed food or simply not consuming enough calories? That's not helping your muscles, organs, or mitochondria. They all need nutrients and fuel to work properly.

Other lifestyle factors. Poor sleep, chronic stress, and social isolation also have physiological consequences that can sap energy at the cellular level.

Boosting energy

Fortunately, a healthier lifestyle can help give you more energy. That means eating a diet low in added sugars and processed foods, with enough calories and nutrients to meet your needs; getting seven to nine hours of sleep each night; managing stress; and (if necessary) talking to your doctor about medication side effects.

And perhaps the fastest, most important way to boost your energy is to move more. The recommended amounts of exercise are at least 150 minutes of aerobic activity (such as brisk walking) per week and at least two muscle-strengthening workouts per week. But studies have shown that any amount of exercise is beneficial.

For example, a 2023 review of almost 200 randomized controlled trials of resistance training, published by the *British Journal of Sports Medicine*, found that people who did any strength training at all increased muscle mass and physical function compared with people who didn't do strength training. The most effective regimens for strength included higher-weight loads and more repetitions.

Be frugal with energy

In addition to boosting your energy, it's essential to use what you have wisely. Think in terms of "energy dollars" and be more frugal about the way you spend them. Strategies known as the "four P's" can help.

Prioritizing. "Think about what you need to accomplish in a day versus what you want to accomplish, ▶▶

▶▶ and make the necessary activity your priority," says Erin Krey, a physical therapist at Harvard-affiliated Spaulding Rehabilitation Hospital. "For example, maybe you have a doctor's appointment in the afternoon, but you wanted to go shopping in the morning. Instead, go shopping on another day, and take it easy in the morning so you'll have the energy to get to the afternoon appointment."

Planning. Planning how to use your energy will help you accomplish more. "Planning could be scheduling just one major errand or appointment per day as opposed to three errands, which you know will leave you exhausted the next day, or cleaning just one room in your house per day as opposed to several," Krey says.

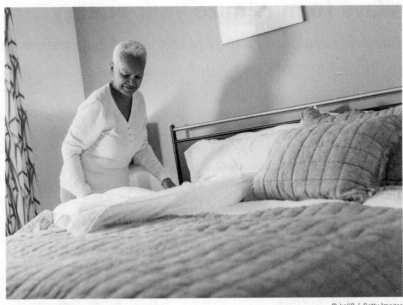

© kali9 | Getty Images

To pace yourself, break large jobs, such as tidying up the house, into smaller tasks, and rest in between each one.

Planning could also mean that you schedule rest breaks, or that you gather all the ingredients you need to prepare a meal and place them by the stove before you start, so you won't have to keep going back and forth across the kitchen. Or planning could involve asking for help from family members or friends in advance of a job that will be too taxing for you alone.

Pacing. Don't try to rush through activities, which can use up all of your energy quickly. "Rushing leads to fatigue and increases your risk of falling," says Kim Stuckart, an occupational therapist at Spaulding Rehabilitation Hospital. "Remember that slow and steady will win the daily race. Spread out your activity to give yourself time to recover in between tasks."

What might that look like? "Break up a large task, like cleaning a room, into smaller tasks such as dusting, vacuuming, or making a bed, with breaks in between," Krey says.

Positioning. Maintain good posture when you're sitting or standing. "You'll expand your lungs so they can take in more oxygen," Krey says. "And it might help to sit down during activities to reduce the amount of energy you're using. You can apply this to anything that makes you feel tired while standing. Try sitting at a table when you do meal prep, or sitting in a shower chair when you bathe. These little attempts to save energy will eventually add up so you feel better and you can stay active longer." ▮

by **HOWARD LeWINE, M.D.**, Editor in Chief, *Harvard Men's Health Watch*

Is it possible to prevent arthritis?

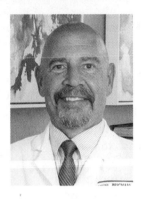

Q *So many of my relatives and friends have arthritis. I have been fortunate so far. Is there any proven way to prevent it?*

A You may be able to lower your risk for three of the most common types of arthritis: osteoarthritis, rheumatoid arthritis, and gout. Here's a brief description of each and how to possibly prevent them.

Osteoarthritis, the most common type, occurs when the cartilage of a joint erodes (breaks down). Bones begin to rub against each other, causing pain and difficulty moving the joint. It's also the most common reason for knee and hip replacements. Take these steps to lower your risk:

▸ Maintain a healthy weight. Osteoarthritis becomes more common with age and tends to run in families. But millions of cases might be prevented by avoiding excessive weight gain.

▸ Avoid trauma. Injury also increases the risk of osteoarthritis. Some ways to avoid injury include exercising regularly, doing resistance training, and not taking unnecessary risks at work or at play.

▸ Prevent and treat conditions that might contribute to joint damage like gout (see below) or an infection.

Rheumatoid arthritis is a chronic inflammatory disease that causes pain, stiffness, warmth, redness, and swelling in joints. Over time, the affected joints may become misshapen, misaligned, and damaged. Rheumatoid arthritis usually occurs in a symmetrical pattern, meaning that if one knee or hand has it, the other usually does, too. Ways to reduce your risk of rheumatoid arthritis include avoiding tobacco and improving your oral health. Gum inflammation (gingivitis) caused by certain bacteria has been linked to many health conditions, including rheumatoid arthritis. Good oral hygiene and regular dental care may lower the risk (see "Rinse, brush, floss, scrape, and repeat," page 28).

Gout occurs when crystals of uric acid get deposited in one or more joints and trigger inflammation that causes pain, swelling, and redness. You can reduce your risk by doing the following:

▸ Eat a healthy diet. Avoid any foods that seem to trigger gout attacks, such as liver and sweetbreads. A heart-healthy diet such as the Mediterranean diet may reduce the risk of gout in some people.

▸ Limit alcohol. Stick to no more than one drink per day, and avoid binge drinking.

▸ Stay well hydrated.

▸ Lose weight if you are overweight or obese.

▸ Avoid diuretics (water pills) if possible (but discuss all medication changes with your doctor).

If you notice joint pain, joint swelling, or difficulty doing activities, see your doctor. Early diagnosis and treatment can make a big difference in your future joint health.

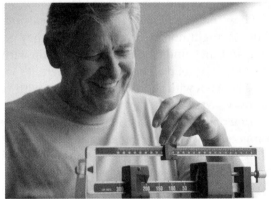

© Jose Luis Pelaez I Getty Images

Maintaining a healthy weight can help prevent osteoarthritis.

3 group housing trends for the 60 and older set

Living together offers benefits for both health and finances.

The kids are grown, the house is empty, and you (and your partner) are wondering if you'll be spending the next few decades living alone—risking loneliness, social isolation, and chronic health problems. If the prospect is unappealing, you have options—and they're not limited to retirement facilities. Here are three trends to consider.

1 Specialized communities

A specialized community is sort of a private mini-neighborhood with dwellings clustered around common spaces. The units might be individual houses or cottages built around recreational areas, gardens, parking, and a common house for gatherings and planned activities. Or they could be apartments in a tall building with a courtyard and a "common house" on the first floor. The communities are run by the people who live there or by nonprofit organizations. Residents might own their homes or rent them.

There are several different types of specialized communities, such as those that are intergenerational (with a mix of young families and older adults), those only for people ages 55 and older, and those that are mission-oriented—with everyone in the community committed to a shared goal, such as providing stable lives for foster children (children live with young families and interact with older residents regularly).

"These communities might be more affordable than traditional housing. They promote socialization and active involvement with neighbors. People look out for each other and share activities. They might drive a neighbor to a doctor appointment, or maybe help kids with homework. We've heard many reports of people benefiting from the model," says Jennifer Molinsky at Harvard's Joint Center for Housing Studies. She leads research exploring housing challenges for the aging population.

Hundreds of these communities are already established in the United States or are just being built. For more information, visit the Cohousing Association of the United States (www.cohousing.org).

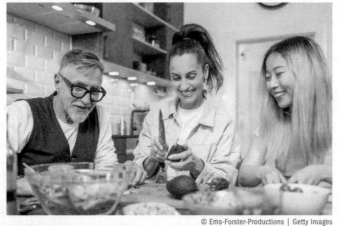
© Ems-Forster-Productions | Getty Images

A young adult boarder might share meals with you or help out around the house.

2 Home sharing

For many people, sharing a home with other adults makes good sense: they can take on a boarder, earn money to help pay the bills, and gain instant companionship.

You can find mature boarders through groups such as Silver Nest (www.silvernest.com) or the New York Foundation for Senior Citizens (www.nyfsc.org). The groups help you list your space, conduct background checks on potential boarders, set up leases, and more.

There are also companies that connect you to younger boarders. For example, Nesterly (www.nesterly.com) helps older homeowners rent space at below-market prices to young adults, such as graduate students, who agree to pay rent and help out around the house.

"These engagements can be very meaningful. Students might not know anyone when they get to town, and they find a home and friendship with an older person or couple. For the homeowners, it's someone to help out with chores or share meals with you," Molinsky says.

If you're uncomfortable sharing your home with strangers, consider sharing a home with friends or siblings. You might charge rent, or you could even buy a home together.

Another benefit to living with friends or siblings is sharing the costs of services you both may need, such as private-duty care for help with daily activities, such as dressing or cooking.

3 Residential care homes

If you need more than just part-time assistance and you'd like to live with others in a homey atmosphere, consider a residential care home (or group home). It's set up like a small assisted living facility in a private home that's licensed by your state.

A group home looks like any other house on the block, but inside it has four to 10 residents and qualified staffers available 24 hours a day. Some staffers might live there. Services include assistance with bathing, dressing, meal prep, cleaning, and transportation.

Each resident typically has a private or shared bedroom and bath. There are also common areas such as a kitchen and living room. The setting naturally invites socializing, friendship, and quality time with others.

Costs are similar to assisted living (starting at $3,000 per month, depending where you live), and are based on the amount of care you need.

Keep in mind

Don't wait to figure out your future housing. "Look ahead. Think about what you might need and want in the future, including opportunities for socializing, help around the house, or added income," Molinsky says. "Consider your finances and your circumstances, and start investigating while you have time to plan. It's best to be proactive."

Hearing aid use linked to longer life

Hearing loss is a known risk factor for premature death. So will using hearing aids improve your longevity? Previous studies on the subject have been mixed. But new evidence published in 2024 in *The Lancet Healthy Longevity* offers hope. Researchers evaluated the hearing test results and questionnaire answers of almost 9,900 people (average age about 49 when the study began) who were followed for more than 10 years. After adjustments for participants' age, race, gender, level of hearing loss, medical history, socioeconomic status, other medical conditions, and type of insurance, the risk of premature death was 24% lower among people who used hearing aids regularly, compared with people who never used hearing aids. The study was observational and doesn't prove definitively that hearing aids protect people from early death; we'll need more evidence for that. However, we know that hearing aids can help people hear conversations again, which may help ward off loneliness and social isolation—two risk factors for many chronic diseases (including dementia) and early death. If you haven't been hearing as well lately (or, at least, if that's what your family is telling you), it's best not to put off a hearing test.

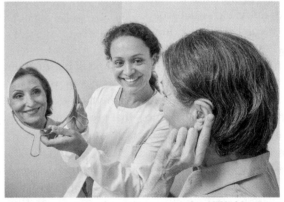

© peakSTOCK | Getty Images

By helping to maintain social connections, hearing aids may aid more than just your hearing.

Bonds that transcend age

Intergenerational friendships can yield surprising health benefits.

Most friendships fall into the "birds of a feather flock together" category, joining people who mirror each other's traits and interests.

But what happens when feathered friends are very different ages? An intergenerational friendship—which typically involves an older adult and one who's 15, 20, or more years younger—is a rare bird, but it can deliver a stimulating balance of experiences, attitudes, and approaches and produce intriguing health benefits.

Making friends isn't always easy, and the effort can seem harder still if age feels like a barrier. But confining ourselves to alliances within our peer group is a mistake, says Ronald Siegel, an assistant professor of psychology at Harvard Medical School.

"We're like a fish in water with our usual social group, but it's potentially very limiting," he says. "Intergenerational friendships require us to let go of biases about generations and approach the other person with curiosity. You realize there are all different types of intelligence, insight, and awareness that are fascinating and rich because the person came of age in another era."

Boosting mind and body

Like all friendships, those between people of diverse ages appear to help our bodies and minds. A study published in 2023 by the journal *Social Psychological and Personality Science* suggests good friends and good health go hand in hand, lowering stress and blood pressure levels and taming spikes in blood pressure during periods of stress. "When people have relationships in which they trust one another, they thrive," Siegel says.

Younger pals might also help us maintain a more youthful outlook. Older adults with friends more than 10 years younger feel younger themselves and are more satisfied with the aging process, according to a 2022 study published by the *European Journal of Aging*. And this self-perception can lead to health advantages that include living longer, earlier research suggests.

While acknowledging this potential benefit, Siegel urges a broader view. "I'm more inclined to want us to be able to embrace whatever age we are and live that to the fullest," he says. "Friendship is more about sharing our gifts and learning from one another."

Indeed, May-September friendships can open our eyes to social and cultural shifts and how they affect others at different life stages. "We can learn enormously from each other, because the same way that each culture has a wisdom and perspective others don't, each age group has that too," Siegel says. "There's tremendous value in that."

Siegel has noticed that people who don't have these types of bonds tend to cling to narrower opinions because "they're simply not exposed to views that shake them up." But a flexible mindset, he says, is a cornerstone of psychological health.

"Life is always changing, and if you're only using the same old coping strategy for every challenge, it will probably fail. But if you're able to adapt—including with aging—you're going to thrive," he says. "Anything that makes us more flexible psychologically contributes to our well-being."

Friend-making tactics

If you're interested in making friends of diverse ages, Siegel offers this advice.

Tap familiar settings. Younger and older adults often work and mingle in the same places, whether the office, community or religious groups, or exercise classes. Use your shared workplace or activities as a springboard for a deeper connection.

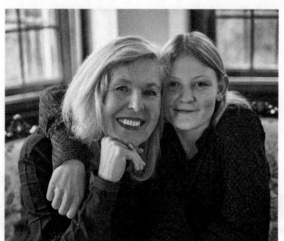

© Oliver Rossi | Getty Images

May-September friendships can benefit body, mind, and soul.

Take a chance. "If you're thinking about reaching out—talking to someone, inviting them to lunch, connecting in some way—but you're afraid of rejection because you're a different generation, risk it and see what happens," he says.

Aim for genuine connection. Worry less about making a good impression and more about showing true interest in the other person's life and experiences. "We should do this with same-age contacts, but it's perhaps even more important when there's a bit of a divide based on age," Siegel says. "This will form a feeling of trust and goodwill that leads to grabbing lunch, going on a walk, or hanging out together." 🛡

Why you should "Walk with a Doc"

These free, physician-led walks—available in 560 locations throughout the United States—offer benefits beyond boosting physical activity.

You know that walking helps your heart. So does spending time with other people, being outside in nature, and learning about ways to improve your health and well-being from a professional. Want to get all four at once? Show up at a Walk with a Doc event.

Launched in 2005, this nonprofit organization sponsors free, doctor-led walks in mostly outdoor venues (usually public parks) across America. Today, Walk with a Doc is in 34 countries worldwide, including 560 communities around the United States. In surveys and focus groups, participants give the program high marks. Nearly all of the responders—96%—say they strongly agree that Walk with a Doc has helped them lead a healthier lifestyle, according to a 2020 article in *Current Cardiology Reports* co-authored by Walk with a Doc founder Dr. David Sabgir.

The program's initial inspiration was to encourage people to be less sedentary. But the informal teaching that happens before and during the walks is a boon for patients and doctors alike, says cardiologist Dr. Simin Lee, associate physician at Harvard-affiliated Brigham and Women's Hospital. "In our current health care system, most of the care is compressed into a short office visit," she says. Walk with a Doc gives physicians time to discuss important health topics—such as exercise, diet, and stress management—in greater depth. Dr. Lee started the Walk with a Doc chapter in Jamaica Plain, the Boston neighborhood bordering the Longwood Medical Area, which is home to Harvard Medical School and many of its affiliated medical institutions.

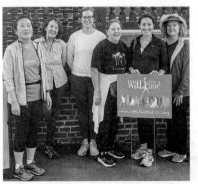

Photos courtesy of Walk with a Doc

(Above) Walk with a Doc events, like this one held in Columbus, Ohio, usually take place in public parks and last between 30 and 90 minutes.

(Left) Harvard cardiologist Dr. Simin Lee (holding sign) started a Walk with a Doc program near the Harvard Medical School campus.

Walking and talking

"Most of the chapters do monthly walks, but I wanted to encourage continuity and habit formation, so I did my walks every week," says Dr. Lee. The walks, which are currently led by her Brigham and Women's colleague Dr. Catherine Hwang, feature a 1.5-mile loop around Jamaica Pond every Wednesday evening at 5:30 pm. In general, weekday walks are usually about 30 minutes long; weekend walks may last 60 to 90 minutes.

About five minutes before starting the walk, the doctor speaks on various topics of interest, including those requested by the participants. For her initial talks, Dr. Lee focused on the recommended "dose" of exercise. During the walk, she demonstrated what moderate-intensity exercise looks like. "I'd tell people to notice how I ▸▸

▸▸ could still talk in full sentences but that my breathing was a little heavier than when we were just standing around," she says.

During later walks, she taught interval training by cueing the group to pick up their walking pace for a few minutes, and to then pull back and return to their normal walking speed. Interval training is a good way to add variety to your workout and is especially helpful for improving cardiovascular fitness, she notes.

"Sometimes, it can feel futile to just rattle off some basic counseling about exercise during an office visit. It's so much more powerful when you can demonstrate it in person," she says. As much as we appreciate all the medications we have at our fingertips to manage cardiovascular disease, people really are interested in doing things for their health that don't involve taking pills, Dr. Lee says. She also did a series of talks about how exercise benefits many chronic health conditions, including high blood pressure, diabetes, heart disease, dementia, and cancer.

Camaraderie and pleasant scenery

As Dr. Sabgir wrote in his article, most Americans are living lives that are sedentary, lonely, and not connected with nature. Many Walk with a Doc programs, including Dr. Lee's, have helped foster social connections and forged friendships among the participants. The walks she led often included 10 or more people, who would sometimes bring friends or family members along. "Creating a shared sense of community is a really important aspect of the program," she says.

So is the stress-relieving power of spending time in nature, which has become less and less common. Research suggests that over half of all Americans spend fewer than five hours outdoors each week. "In our increasingly digital world, where people spend a lot of time inside in front of screens, it's just lovely to be outside to get fresh air and witness a beautiful sunset and the changing seasons," says Dr. Lee. For more information about Walk with a Doc, including how to find a location near you, go online to www.walkwithadoc.org. ▼

Get out of your slump

Posture can worsen as you age. Here are some ways you can stand up to it.

Remember how your mom measured your changing height with pencil lines on a door frame? If you did that now, the line from your maximum height will likely have dropped an inch or more.

People typically lose almost one-half inch every 10 years after age 40, with height loss becoming more rapid after age 70. The main reason is Father Time.

"It's natural for people to lose some height with age, as over time the discs in the spine wear down, causing them to compress," says Dr. David Binder of the Orthopaedic Spine Center at Harvard-affiliated Massachusetts General Hospital. Other factors can contribute to a shrinking height, such as osteoporosis, which can begin in men around age 65 and decrease bone density, especially in the spine.

But perhaps the leading contributor is poor posture caused by weak and inflexible muscles. "Weak muscles, especially in the upper back, chest, and core, encourage

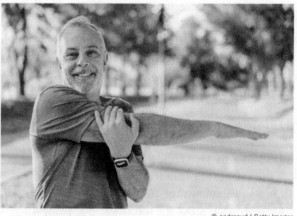

© andreswd | Getty Images

Exercises like the arm-across-chest stretch help strengthen posture-supporting muscles.

slumping, which tips your body forward," says Dr. Binder. "And inflexible muscles decrease range of motion."

The good news: you can take simple steps to improve your posture. The first is to adopt an all-around strength training program. "A personal trainer or physical therapist can design an exercise routine that fits your needs and addresses your specific areas of muscular weakness," says Dr. Binder.

Next, do regular stretching. Yoga and tai chi are ideal activities, as they help strengthen posture-supporting muscles and teach proper alignment and body awareness, so you can feel when your body is not in a healthy position. You also can add specific back, chest, and core stretches to your regular workouts, or do them periodically throughout the day—especially after long periods sitting at the computer, watching TV, or driving.

Here are four posture-supporting stretches to get you started.

Shoulder blade squeeze

Sit up straight in a chair with your hands resting on your thighs. Keep your shoulders down and your chin level. Slowly draw your shoulders back and squeeze your shoulder blades together. Hold for a count of five; relax. Repeat three or four times.

Abdominal pull-in

Stand or sit. Inhale, then exhale slowly to a count of five, pulling your lower abdominal muscles up and in as if moving your belly button toward your backbone. Relax and breathe normally. Repeat a few times.

Tips for a healthier posture

Many simple lifestyle choices can help improve your posture. For example:

▶ Be mindful of your posture throughout the day, and realign yourself regularly.

▶ To prevent muscle fatigue, avoid staying in one position for too long. Shift positions or get up and move around every 30 minutes to an hour.

▶ Have your vision checked. Poor eyesight can make you thrust your head forward to read.

▶ Move your TV closer to you. You may subconsciously lean in or hunch over if your television screen is too far away.

Check your posture

What does a healthy posture look like? Here's a test from the American Physical Therapy Association. It can help determine if you need to be evaluated by a physical therapist.

▶ Start by standing with your back against the wall and your heels about three inches from the wall.

▶ Place one hand flat against the back of your neck, with the back of the hand against the wall.

▶ Place your other hand against your lower back, palm facing the wall.

▶ If you can move your hands forward and backward more than an inch or two, you may need to adjust your posture.

Arm-across-chest stretch

Raise your right arm to shoulder level before you and bend the arm at the elbow, keeping the forearm parallel to the floor. Grasp the right elbow with your left hand and gently pull it across your chest so that you feel a stretch in the upper arm and shoulder on the right side. Hold for 20 seconds; relax both arms. Repeat to the other side. Do three times on each side.

Wall slide

Stand against a wall so your tailbone, shoulder blades, and head are pressed against the surface. Place the backs of your hands on the wall at shoulder level with your elbows bent at 45° and palms facing forward. Slowly extend your arms up the wall, raising your hands as high as comfortably possible while keeping your tailbone, shoulder blades, and head stationary and in contact with the wall. Slowly return to the starting position. You should take about five to 10 seconds to reach up and another five to 10 seconds to lower your arms. Repeat eight to 12 times (or just three to five times if you have shoulder issues). ▉

Rinse, brush, floss, scrape, and repeat

A thorough daily dental care routine can protect against gum disease and other serious health issues.

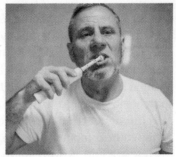

© Nes I Getty Images

Using an electric toothbrush can help remove more plaque than using regular brushes.

One of the best things you can do for your overall health as you age is a daily routine you've followed since childhood.

"Maintaining good dental health not only protects against gum disease, but also helps ward off many other age-related diseases," says Dr. Leonard Brennan, co-director of the Harvard School of Dental Medicine's Geriatric Fellowship Program. "Good oral health helps you enjoy life by allowing you to chew, taste, swallow, speak, and smile. The chances are in your favor that you can keep your teeth for a lifetime if you maintain your oral health." It can even help protect your health during a hospital stay (see "6 things to do when heading for the hospital," page 298.)

The most common form of gum disease is gingivitis (gum inflammation). It begins when bacteria buildup in the mouth causes plaque and tartar to form on teeth, which, if not removed, can lead to tooth decay. "The amount of bacteria in the mouth doubles every four to five hours," says Dr. Brennan.

Gingivitis also can lead to red, swollen, and bleeding gums. If left unchecked, gingivitis can advance to more serious periodontitis, which can cause bone deterioration and tooth loss and reduce the ability to speak and chew properly.

Gum disease can affect other aspects of one's health. Research suggests it can increase the risk of diabetes, cardiovascular disease, stroke, and dementia.

Because regular dental care can be expensive (particularly for older people, as Medicare doesn't routinely cover dentist visits), self-care is the best preventive medicine. "Daily dental care to remove bacteria from the teeth, gums, and tongue is relatively inexpensive compared with costly dental treatments," says Dr. Brennan.

A proper dental routine consists of five steps: rinsing, brushing, flossing, tongue scraping, and a final rinse.

Rinsing

Before you brush, dislodge food particles by thoroughly swishing and rinsing your mouth with plain warm water.

Brushing

Brush at least twice a day, suggests Dr. Brennan. With brushing, focus on quality rather than quantity. "Focusing on how well you brush the front and back of each tooth can help remove the most bacteria," says Dr. Brennan.

Dr. Brennan recommends using an electric toothbrush over a regular one. "Studies have found that they are better at removing plaque, as you can get more strokes from the brush's vibrations than from your hand motion," he says. Use a brush head with soft or extra-soft bristles and replace every three to four months, or more often if the strands are visibly matted or frayed.

To brush properly, tilt the toothbrush at a 45° angle. Beginning with the upper teeth, take several up-and-down short strokes from the gum line to the chewing surface of the tooth. Do one tooth at a time before moving on to the next. To clean the inside surfaces of the front teeth, hold the brush vertically and make several up-and-down strokes. Repeat the process for the lower teeth.

If you have arthritis that makes it hard to hold a toothbrush, or if it's challenging to reach the back teeth, invest in grip aids that slide over your brush's handle. (You can find them at drugstores or online.) "They make it easier to hold the brush and extend the length to help with the hard-to-reach back teeth," says Dr. Brennan.

For toothpaste, choose one with the American Dental Association (ADA) Seal of Acceptance, which verifies it contains decay- and plaque-fighting fluoride. While the ingredients can differ slightly, all toothpastes have the same general components: mild abrasives, humectants, flavoring agents, thickening agents, and detergents.

Natural toothpastes are also popular, but again, look for the ADA seal. The word "natural" indicates certain ingredients are omitted, such as artificial flavors, colors, preservatives, and sweeteners. It also means that certain active ingredients that help with cleaning are derived from plant sources. Toothpaste comes in gel, paste, or powder forms. They all work equally well, so choose the one you like best. Some brands also contain other ingredients that improve oral health. They might reduce tooth sensitivity, combat gingivitis or tartar buildup, prevent enamel erosion, or whiten teeth. Ask your dentist for a recommendation for these specific issues.

Flossing

Dr. Brennan says you can floss before or after brushing using either waxed or unwaxed floss. "But, if possible, try to floss routinely after a meal to remove food particles that can hasten bacteria buildup." To floss correctly, wrap the floss around your middle fingers, which helps you reach the back teeth. Loop the floss around each tooth so it makes a C shape. Beginning at the gum line, slide it up and down the tooth several times. Avoid just moving the floss back and forth in a sawing motion. You miss cleaning the entire tooth, and the friction can cut and irritate the gums.

"If gum bleeding occurs, don't stop flossing; just be more gentle around that area," says Dr. Brennan. (Bleeding will usually subside after a week or so, but if it doesn't, make an appointment to see your dentist.) If traditional flossing is difficult, try over-the-counter tools, such as floss picks, pre-threaded flossers, tiny brushes that reach between the teeth, or water flossers.

How often should you see your dentist?

Most people should see their dentist for a regular checkup at least once a year, but ideally twice for cleanings and x-rays as needed. Still, the frequency depends on your overall oral health. "If your teeth and gums are healthy and you don't have issues, you can often stretch out dental exams to once a year," says Dr. Leonard Brennan, co-director of the Harvard School of Dental Medicine's Geriatric Fellowship Program. "The ideal interval for routine dental exams is not clear cut and depends on the dental and medical health of each patient."

Tongue scraping

Next, do tongue scraping, which can further eliminate bacteria. Sold in drugstores and online, tongue scrapers are small tools made of stainless steel, silicone, or plastic. (You could also use a spoon.) Make a gentle raking motion several times from the back of the tongue to the front.

Rinse again

Finish up with another rinse using an over-the-counter alcohol-free mouthwash with fluoride, which can help protect against tooth decay. "Some products are available that help reduce tooth sensitivity and strengthen teeth," says Dr. Brennan. Ask your pharmacist or dentist for suggestions. 🛡

Health-savvy house hunting

After the nest empties, certain home features can promote your comfort and safety.

After decades of kid wrangling, life is all about you again—and so is your home. For many people in their 50s and 60s, an empty nest prompts visions of travel and time with grandchildren, along with thoughts of moving to a new space to optimize the next phase of life.

But house hunting later in life also brings a new set of considerations. Your needs are different now—you may want less space and upkeep, for example—and

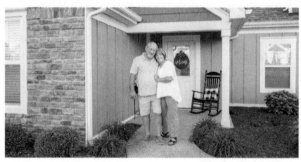
© Courtney Hale | Getty Images
Smart home-buying decisions now can help you live well in the next phase of life.

your capabilities may be different as well. It's time to consider what architectural features can make your ▸▸

▶▶ new home a "forever home" that enables you to age in place if you become less mobile or agile. (See "Want to age in place? Tap technology," page 272.)

Perhaps you think it's overly cautious to make home-buying decisions based on changes that may never come to pass, especially if you feel vigorous and plan on staying that way. But since change is the only thing we can count on, Harvard experts say it's smart to embrace this mindset now, before a mishap at home threatens your independence.

"People really dig their heels in and refuse, and we hope whatever breaks that cycle isn't a broken hip," says Katherine Lyman, a geriatric nurse practitioner at Harvard-affiliated Beth Israel Deaconess Medical Center. "It's wise to take the long view. We're all younger in our minds. I don't see this as giving in; I see it as really solid future planning."

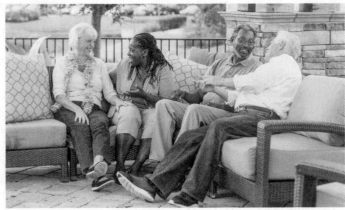
© kali9 | Getty Images

Living in a vibrant community can expand your social options.

Choosing an age-friendly home

Home sweet home will seem even sweeter if it's also age-friendly. Cast a critical eye on the following details when you're house hunting.

Exterior stairs. Even a couple of stairs leading into a home can impede your comings and goings if you should someday need a walker or wheelchair. "A no-step entry is ideal," Lyman says. "It sounds basic, but even two stairs can be problematic for someone who can't let go of support to walk."

Interior stairs. Avoid these, too, if possible. A single-story home eliminates the problem if climbing stairs becomes difficult. But even if you do choose a two-story dwelling, there are ways around this issue. Look for a first-floor primary bedroom and bathroom suite. "Visitors and grandkids can stay upstairs," says Dr. Suzanne Salamon, clinical chief of gerontology at Beth Israel Deaconess. Any stairs should be covered with carpet and not just wood, Dr. Salamon notes. "I see a lot of people who slip and fall on nice, shiny wood floors. And make sure there's a banister—preferably two."

Lighting. Spaces that are bright and sunny not only are mood lifters, but also keep you safer. Hallways, especially, should be well lit (whether naturally or artificially).

Layout. An open, flat floor plan with wide hallways and doorways allows people to move fluidly through the home, and can more easily accommodate a wheelchair or walker later.

Kitchen. Avoid cabinets that are too high. "The last thing I want to see is an 85-year-old on a step stool reaching up to get a chafing dish," Lyman says.

Another small but pivotal detail: the placement of the dishwasher. It's ideal if this appliance is situated in a corner, so you don't have to navigate around it repeatedly when it's being filled or emptied. "When the door is down, people bang their legs into it," Lyman says. "I can't tell you how many leg injuries I've seen."

Bathroom. With its slick surfaces, the bathroom is the site of a large proportion of home falls. But perhaps the biggest hazard is a bathtub-shower combo that requires you to climb in and out. "Have the lowest possible step up into the shower," Dr. Salamon advises, "and make sure there's room enough for a shower chair."

Location, location, location

What's outside and nearby can be just as important as what's inside a dwelling. With this in mind, Harvard experts suggest strategies to home in on a sound choice.

Aim for amenities. Aging in place is easier if you're near health care facilities, stores, pharmacies, and parks to walk and relax in. "You need to anticipate that you may not be able to drive later on, or may not want to drive at night," Dr. Salamon says.

Prioritize interaction. Look for a vibrant community that expands social options even if you're not venturing far, such as a 55-plus neighborhood with a fitness center and clubhouse. "For people who like getting together, that creates a built-in social life," Salamon says. ♥

Chapter 2

Mind, Mood, and Memory

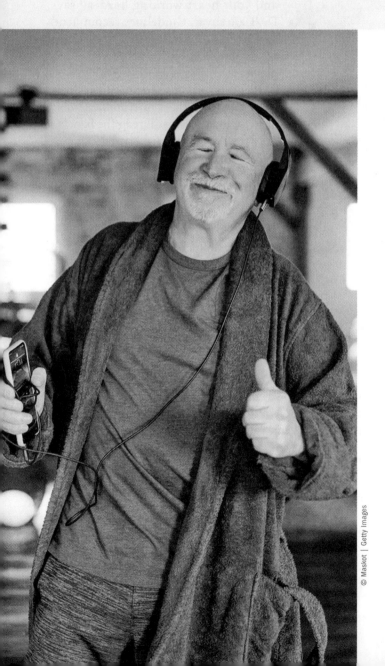

© Maskot | Getty Images

Healthy Habits!
5 Things You Can Do Now

1 **Consider a multivitamin.** Evidence increasingly suggests they may help protect the brain. (page 37)

2 **Limit TV—but feel free to browse online.** Internet use is linked to a reduced risk of dementia. (pages 41 and 43)

3 **Get moving, particularly in nature.** Both offer a significant mood boost. (page 45)

4 **Help others.** Doing good deeds is also good medicine, research shows. (page 46)

5 **Adopt a pet.** Animal companions reduce stress, isolation, and risk of cognitive decline. (page 55)

What's the Best Medicine for Your Brain?

The three basics of healthy living: exercise, diet, and sleep.

The diagnosis of dementia is based on a set of symptoms, including memory loss, confusion, changes in personality, a decline in cognitive skills, and inability to perform everyday activities. But can you do anything to lower your risk?

An estimated 3% of adults ages 65 and older currently have dementia, and that proportion rises substantially as people age. By age 85, about one-third will be diagnosed with some form of the condition.

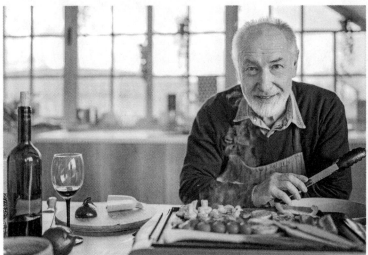

Eating a plant-based diet has been shown to support brain health.

© Pekic | Getty Images

"The most convincing evidence continues to be for the boring stuff—aerobic exercise, a brain-healthy diet, and quality sleep," says neuroscientist Dr. Daniel Daneshvar, chief of the division of brain injury rehabilitation with Harvard-affiliated Massachusetts General Hospital. "Even people with a family history of dementia could lower the risk by investing more in these basic healthy lifestyle habits." Here's how they help with dementia prevention.

Aerobic exercise. The buildup of beta-amyloid protein in the brain is a key hallmark of Alzheimer's disease, the leading cause of dementia. Another common form, vascular dementia, stems from damage to brain cells that occurs when narrowed or hardened blood vessels lead to insufficient brain blood flow.

Aerobic exercise increases blood flow to the brain, supporting blood vessels and decreasing the risk of blood vessel damage. It also helps reduce inflammation, thought to be one of the main factors linked to excess beta-amyloid buildup.

Although most aerobic exercise—defined as any activity that increases your heart rate—requires you to move your entire body, the main focus should be on your heart and lungs. "Activities like walking, running, swimming, cycling, even dancing, if done at sufficient intensity, get you breathing faster and your heart working harder," says Dr. Daneshvar. Guidelines recommend adults do at least 150 to 300 minutes of moderate-intensity aerobic exercise per week.

It's never too late to begin, either. "Even older people who have rarely done aerobic exercise before can still reap the benefits once they start," says Dr. Daneshvar.

Brain-healthy diet. There are several extensively studied diets that promote brain health, like the Mediterranean, DASH (Dietary Approaches to Stop Hypertension), and MIND (Mediterranean-DASH Intervention for Neurodegenerative Delay) diets. "These diets are linked to lower levels of brain-damaging chronic inflammation," says Dr. Daneshvar. (For more on these diets, see "Protecting yourself from Alzheimer's disease," page 33.)

Quality sleep. During sleep, the brain clears out harmful beta-amyloid proteins. But the cleaning process can't do a complete job if sleep is regularly disrupted—by insomnia, sleep apnea, or other issues that cause you to wake during the night. "Eventually, this can cause or exacerbate abnormal protein buildup," says Dr. Daneshvar.

If you regularly don't feel rested upon waking or have trouble falling and staying asleep, speak with your doctor. It's important to address any sleep disorder or other health issues that interfere with sleep, like acid reflux. Taking multiple medicines, depression, and changes in the bedroom environment (for instance, in temperature, noise level, smartphone usage, or light exposure) also can disrupt sleep. 🛡

Exercise your brain—and increase longevity— by socializing

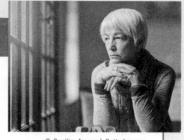

© Cecilie_Arcurs | Getty Images
Social connections can influence lifespan.

Social aspects of older adults' lives may influence their longevity, a recent study suggests. In the Harvard-led study, published in 2023 by *Proceedings of the National Academy of Sciences*, researchers interviewed 8,250 adults ages 65 and older. Within the next four years, 22% died. The researchers found that eight of 183 possible factors predicted participants' deaths within those four years: feeling isolated; meeting with their children less than once a year and not being active in their lives; living in an unclean neighborhood; feeling little control over their finances; not working for pay; not volunteering; and being treated with diminished courtesy or respect.

The results suggest that social lives are as important as medical conditions in helping predict how long someone will live, the study authors said.

Another 2023 study published by *JAMA Neurology* found that socially isolated older adults have a 27% higher chance of developing dementia than those who aren't isolated. "Regular interactions activate mental processes, including attention and memory, which can bolster cognition," says neuroscientist Dr. Daniel Daneshvar with Massachusetts General Hospital.

Have your social connections slipped? Here are some ways to increase engagement—and benefit your overall health at the same time:

Get into group dynamics. Join a group activity, such as a walking club, a golf or bowling league, a book or chess club, or a continuing education class at an adult education center.

Schedule friend time. If you have a circle of friends but don't see them regularly, take the initiative and schedule routine get-togethers or video chats. Designate a day, time, and place for coffee, lunch, or any type of gathering designed for easy conversation.

Engage in "weak ties." Casual interactions, known as "weak ties," are important too. For example, strike up a brief conversation with a stranger or employee at the grocery store or coffee shop. Even social media conversations and texting qualify.

Protecting yourself from Alzheimer's disease

There is no cure (yet), but there may be ways to reduce your risk.

Alzheimer's disease is the most common type of dementia: between 60% and 80% of patients with dementia have Alzheimer's disease. The disease is associated with excessive accumulation of tangles and clumps of protein in and around brain cells. These tangles and clumps, which make it difficult for brain cells to communicate with one another, may be the reason for the cells' eventual demise.

Scientists don't fully understand what causes some people to get Alzheimer's and others not. Some factors, like advancing age and family history, are clearly associated with a higher risk (see "Can we fix Alzheimer's genes?" on page 286). Though some drugs can reduce certain symptoms and others may slow disease progression, Alzheimer's disease as yet has no cure (see "Drugs for Alzheimer's disease," page 36). Still, ▸▸

recent research suggests that it's possible to lower your risk for developing the disease, no matter your age or family history.

"For people without changes in the brain, it's never too late to reduce one's risk, and even for those with early changes, it's possible to change the odds in your favor and slow cognitive decline," says neurologist Dr. Seth Gale, co-director of the Brain Health Program at Harvard-affiliated Brigham and Women's Hospital.

Imperfect science

It's important to note that most factors linked to Alzheimer's disease come from population-based studies. Researchers look at the behaviors and medical conditions of people in their 40s, 50s, and beyond and then see who develops Alzheimer's later in life. This allows them to determine if those who get the disease (or those who don't) share specific features or followed particular lifestyle practices.

"It's not perfect, and the findings only show association, rather than direct cause and effect. But they paint an important picture that certain factors are linked with a lower risk," says Dr. Gale. Here are the factors that stand out. Dr. Gale notes that following a combination of the strategies listed here over many years offers the best protection.

Exercise. Multiple studies find that people who engage in regular physical activity have a lower risk for Alzheimer's than those who don't. It's not clear why exercise helps, but the leading theory is that activity increases blood flow to the brain, which likely helps maintain the supply of vital nutrients and energy needed to protect the brain from deterioration over time. "In this way, exercise helps preserve the hippocampus, one of the brain regions responsible for memory," says Dr. Gale.

He adds that studies have not pinpointed whether certain aerobic activities, done for a specific duration, are better than other ones. "Still, a good guideline is to aim for 150 minutes of light- to moderate-intensity exercise per week, like brisk walking, cycling, or tennis," he says. "More is better, and doing something is always better than nothing."

Other research has suggested that doing short bouts of high-intensity exercise may offer the same or greater protection. In a study published in 2023 by *The Journal of Physiology*, researchers found that six minutes of high-intensity exercise (in this case,

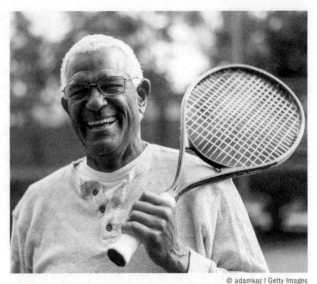

© adamkaz | Getty Images

Regular aerobic exercise is one of the best ways to keep an aging brain healthy.

cycling) increased the production of a specialized protein called brain-derived neurotrophic factor (BDNF). BDNF helps with learning and memory and might protect the brain from age-related decline and dementia. While lighter-intensity cycling also done for six minutes increased BDNF, the brief, vigorous exercise was more effective.

Diet. People who follow a plant-based diet like the Mediterranean or MIND diet appear less likely to develop Alzheimer's. While the two eating plans are similar, the Mediterranean diet recommends vegetables, fruit, and three or more servings of fish per week, while the MIND diet prioritizes green leafy vegetables like spinach, kale, and collard greens, along with other vegetables. The MIND diet also endorses berries over other fruit and recommends one or more servings of fish per week. A 2023 study published in *Neurology* found that people who followed either diet had fewer of the Alzheimer's-associated protein clumps and tangles in their brains compared with people who did not consume such diets—and other research suggests incorporating even some of its elements may be associated with a reduced risk of dementia.

Blood pressure. Over time, high blood pressure can damage blood vessels throughout the body, including the brain. Scientists have found that lowering high blood pressure can protect against dementia, though there is debate about the optimal number to reduce the risk of cognitive impairment and Alzheimer's.

For example, in 2019, the SPRINT MIND study suggested that a target of less than 120 millimeters of mercury (mm Hg) for systolic blood pressure (the top number) is better for brain health than 120 to 140 mm Hg. "Work with your doctor to find an optimal number that is good for both your heart and brain," says Dr. Gale.

Hearing and vision. A study published in 2023 by *The Lancet Public Health* found that, among people with hearing loss, those who did not use hearing aids had a 42% higher risk for dementia compared with those who used hearing aids. The possible connection? Wearing a hearing aid might delay cognitive decline by preventing cognitive overload—that is, by keeping the brain from working too hard to process sounds and information.

Studies also have found that older adults with impaired vision—like declining eyesight, cataracts, glaucoma, and age-related macular degeneration—are at increased risk of developing cognitive problems.

As with hearing, correcting vision problems may lower a person's risk. A study published in 2022 in *JAMA Internal Medicine* found that those who had surgery to remove their cataracts were 30% less likely to be diagnosed with dementia in later years than those who didn't have the surgery.

The connection between vision problems and dementia might be indirect, says Dr. Gale: poor vision may promote inactivity, which is known to increase dementia risk. "It is also possible that poor vision leads directly to the breakdown of brain processes that rely on vision. This impairs overall brain networks and could increase the risk of losing more brain cells," he says.

Stimulation. While the science linking brain-engaging activities with a lower risk for Alzheimer's is ongoing, experts recommend stimulating the mind as much as possible. This can include joining social clubs, learning new skills, reading, doing puzzles, and playing games. ▼

IN THE JOURNALS

Managing stress and eating leafy vegetables may protect the brain

Scientists continue to examine what causes people's brain health to decline. While natural aging and genetics are part of the equation, lifestyle factors can also play a significant role. Two recent studies looked at how stress and diet affect cognitive function and protect against Alzheimer's disease.

In a 2023 study published by *JAMA Network Open*, perceived stress—the degree of stress people feel about their life—was linked to poor cognitive health among older adults. Researchers recruited more than 24,000 people (average age 64), then measured their stress and cognitive function with the Perceived Stress Scale and the Mini-Mental State Examination. The results? People who scored highest on the stress-level scale were more likely to have lower cognitive test scores. The reverse was also true—lower stress levels went hand in hand with higher test scores.

In a second 2023 study published in *Neurology,* researchers explored whether certain dietary habits lower the risk of Alzheimer's. The researchers analyzed data on 581 people from the Rush Memory and Aging Project cohort, a prospective study of older adults who agreed to undergo annual evaluations and to donate their brain at death. Participants reported on their dietary habits and completed annual food questionnaires.

The researchers found that people who regularly followed plant-based diets had lower amounts of beta-amyloid buildup in their brains, a marker for Alzheimer's. Among this group, people with the highest intake of green leafy vegetables—seven or more weekly servings—had less buildup than those who ate only one or two servings a week.

Drugs for Alzheimer's disease

Here are the available medications and how they can help.

While there is no cure for Alzheimer's disease, medication can help manage the condition. Currently, the main drugs used to treat Alzheimer's are what's known as symptomatic therapies, meaning they ease symptoms but don't address the cause of the disease. These include cholinesterase inhibitors and memantine. A more recent entry into the field, lecanemab, may help slow the progression of the disease. Here's a look at how these medications work.

Cholinesterase inhibitors

One way Alzheimer's harms the brain is by decreasing levels of a chemical messenger called acetylcholine, which helps with alertness, memory, and thought processing. Cholinesterase inhibitors boost the amount of acetylcholine available to nerve cells by preventing its breakdown in the brain.

Three drugs in this category are approved by the FDA: donepezil (Aricept), galantamine (generic), and rivastigmine (Exelon). They can be prescribed at any stage of Alzheimer's, from mild to severe. The drugs are taken daily in pill form. Rivastigmine is also available as a skin patch.

These drugs can turn back the clock on memory loss, but only so far. "They can restore your memory to like it was six to 12 months before, but the drugs can't slow the disease's progression," says Dr. Andrew Budson, chief of cognitive behavioral neurology at Harvard-affiliated VA Boston Healthcare System. "And you have to keep taking the drug to maintain that advantage." People generally show the effects of the drug within one to two months.

Dr. Budson says that most people do well with any of the cholinesterase inhibitors. "However, we have the most experience with donepezil, so we usually try that one first," he says. "Galantamine is generally second-line." The drugs are covered by Medicare and well tolerated by most people. Still, common side effects include upset stomach, nausea, vivid dreams, and loose stools.

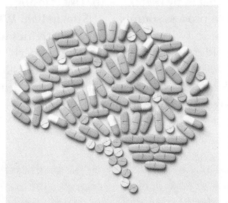

© Hiroshi Watanabe | Getty Images

Alzheimer's medications may help manage symptoms and slow the disease's progress.

Since rivastigmine comes in a patch, it is often used for people who can't tolerate the pills. Also, people with certain types of cardiac arrhythmias shouldn't take cholinesterase inhibitors, as they can slow the heart rate.

Memantine

Another symptomatic drug approved for moderate-to-severe Alzheimer's is memantine (Namenda). It works by modulating the effects of both glutamate and dopamine, two chemicals that send messages between nerve cells in the brain and are widely involved in brain functions, including memory.

Typically, doctors prescribe memantine when a person with Alzheimer's begins showing difficulty performing activities of daily living, like dressing and bathing. "It is prescribed to help slow down the progression of symptoms, which could enable some people to maintain some daily functions a little longer than they would without the medication," says Dr. Budson.

The drug is taken as a pill or liquid once or twice a day. It may take as long as three months, or even longer, to see any improvement. Common side effects include dizziness, headache, drowsiness, confusion, and agitation.

Lecanemab

This new drug, approved by the FDA in 2023, works differently from other Alzheimer's drugs, as it helps to slow the progression of the disease.

Lecanemab (Leqembi) is an immunotherapy that targets the protein beta-amyloid to slow the buildup of amyloid plaques in the brain. Plaques make it difficult for brain cells to communicate with one another, impeding memory and other mental functions. "The drug doesn't stop new plaque from forming, but slows the speed at which it can accumulate," says Dr. Budson.

The drug works only in people with early-stage Alzheimer's, which means they are showing mild cognitive impairment or mild dementia. "These are individuals who have trouble with thinking and memory and struggle with completing complicated tasks like paying bills and grocery shopping—but don't have problems with daily living," says Dr. Budson.

A 2023 study published in *The New England Journal of Medicine* looked at 1,795 people who had amyloid plaques in their brains (as confirmed by MRI) and mild memory problems. The researchers found that compared with people taking an inactive treatment, those who took lecanemab for 18 months had a slower rate of cognitive decline (as measured by cognitive tests) and less amyloid in their brains.

Lecanemab is administered every other week via an hourlong infusion. It is currently unknown whether a person must take it indefinitely. The drug's main risks are brain swelling and brain bleeding, so people who take powerful blood thinners are advised against taking lecanemab. Genetic testing for an Alzheimer's risk factor gene is recommended for candidates for lecanemab, as those who have two copies of the gene may have between three and 10 times the likelihood of side effects. 🛡

by **ANTHONY L. KOMAROFF, M.D.,** Editor in Chief, *Harvard Health Letter*

More evidence suggests multivitamins slow cognitive decline

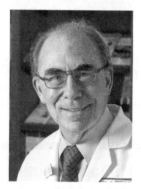

Q *I hear a new study shows that a daily multivitamin pill may help the brain. Any truth to that?*

A The new study you're referring to is probably one organized here at Harvard, involving medical centers around the country. It was the best type of study for determining if a treatment is effective: a randomized controlled trial. In it, some people were assigned at random to take the multivitamin pill, and others were assigned to take an identical-looking placebo (inactive pill). And neither the study participants nor the research team knew, until the end of the study, who had taken the multivitamins.

The study was published in 2024 in *The American Journal of Clinical Nutrition* and involved people ages 60 or older. It is better in many respects than past studies have been. It included more people (over 5,000), followed participants longer (more than two years), and more precisely measured cognitive abilities—both before and two years after starting on multivitamins. Two aspects of cognition known to predict the later development of Alzheimer's disease and related kinds of dementia were measured: global cognition and episodic memory. Since there is a slight natural decline in both of these measures with aging, the study was asking if the people taking multivitamins had a slower decline than those taking the placebo.

Indeed, both of these cognitive measures declined less over two years in those taking multivitamins than in those taking the placebo. This was seen consistently in all groups of people, regardless of age, sex, race or ethnic group, weight, diet, or their level of cognitive ability before the study began. And no adverse effects from taking multivitamins were noted.

Based on the results of this study, I think it is likely that a daily multivitamin pill slows age-related cognitive decline, at least for two years, in people ages 60 or older. But that leaves many important questions unanswered. Would this benefit persist if people took multivitamins for more than two years? Do daily multivitamins also reduce the risk that a person will develop dementia? How do multivitamins produce their positive effects? The pill used in this study contained over 20 vitamins and minerals: are only some of them responsible for the positive effect? These questions can only be answered by research. We need those answers.

When to worry about your memory

How can you tell whether memory lapses are part of normal aging or early signs of cognitive impairment?

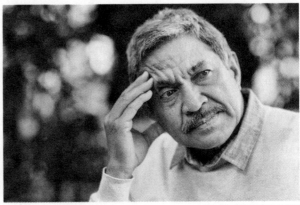
© LaylaBird | Getty Images

Memory issues that become worse or more frequent should be checked out.

Ever had those "senior moments"? You misplace your phone (which was just in your hand). You lose your train of thought during a conversation. You forget directions five minutes after being told. You can't remember the day, but then it pops into your head.

These memory slips can be embarrassing and stressful, but are they normal mental lapses—or early signs of dementia?

"The brain is like any other part of the body, and over time, it may not function as well," says Ana Trueba Yepez, a psychologist with the Division of Geriatric Psychiatry at Harvard-affiliated McLean Hospital. "Brain regions involved with memory—like the hippocampus and prefrontal cortex—can shrink, which makes it more difficult to multitask, stay focused, and hold on to information."

The good news is that these kinds of memory lapses are not automatic red flags for dementia. "These episodes can be alarming, but for the most part, they are not something to worry about," says Trueba Yepez.

Look for warning signs

Senior moments may come and go. It's when they become more frequent or severe, or if new cognitive issues emerge, that they may signal a problem.

For example, during conversations, you now have difficulty following conversations. Or you cut off people when they talk or begin discussing something unrelated to the conversation. Another warning sign is when memory lapses begin to interfere with daily life. For instance, you miss scheduled appointments, forget to pay bills, or fail to take regular medication. You may also have difficulty making decisions and forget regular grooming.

"Many times, people are not aware that memory issues have worsened," says Trueba Yepez. "If you suspect any changes, no matter how innocent, it's best to ask family or friends to look for and point out changes in your memory, with examples."

Still, even these changes are not an automatic indicator of dementia. Sometimes, other factors like diet, alcohol use, medication, and mental problems (such as depression and anxiety) affect your memory. "Many times, these issues show up in other ways besides memory problems, such as eating more unhealthy foods, showing less interest in your favorite activities, and not keeping up with hygiene and personal appearance," says Trueba Yepez.

Manage your memory with DANCERS

Enhance your memory and protect against dementia with DANCERS:

D: **Disease management.** Control your weight, blood pressure, cholesterol, and blood sugar levels.

A: **Activity.** Cardio exercise improves oxygen and blood flow to the brain.

N: **Nutrition.** Poor nutrition leads to poor brain health. Adopt a plant-based diet.

C: **Cognitive stimulation.** The more you engage your brain, the more likely it is you'll retain memory.

E: **Engagement.** Social isolation is linked to lower cognitive function.

R: **Relaxation.** Your brain needs downtime. Do relaxing activities like yoga, meditation, or reading.

S: **Sleep.** Sleep is when your brain cleans out toxins. Get seven to nine hours of sleep per night.

Seeking help

A primary care doctor is your first point of contact if you, or someone else, suspects a problem. As scary as it may seem to confront changes in memory, there are many benefits to taking a proactive approach, including these:

Ruling out other causes. A medical evaluation can help determine if symptoms are related to a condition, like depression, anxiety, or insomnia. Other factors also can affect memory, such as an infection, a new medication, or an unintended interaction between a prescription drug and an over-the-counter product. Addressing the underlying problem may lead to improved memory.

Discovering a problem early. Memory issues could be related to tiny strokes that produce only subtle symptoms, such as short episodes of confusion. In these episodes, small arteries in the brain become narrowed or clogged with fatty deposits, decreasing blood flow. "The brain damage is often so small and subtle that most people don't notice it or shrug it off," says Trueba Yepez. It's important to spot this problem as early as possible to prevent it from progressing to a condition called vascular dementia. Certain medications, such as statins and low-dose aspirin, as well as lifestyle changes may help prevent further cognitive decline.

Getting help sooner. Your doctor may refer you for a neuropsychological evaluation to assess other cognitive skills, such as attention, executive function, and language. If you're diagnosed with dementia, it's best to catch it sooner than later so you can begin to manage the condition.

Extended sitting linked to higher dementia risk, despite exercise

Too much sitting is not good for the brain. But how much sedentary time is too much? According to a study published in 2023 by *JAMA*, remaining physically inactive for 10 or more hours per day is linked to a higher risk of later developing dementia.

For the study, 50,000 people (average age 67) who were free of dementia wore a wrist accelerometer 24 hours a day for one week to track their daily moving time. After the average of six years of follow up, the researchers checked to see which participants had been diagnosed with dementia and correlated that information with the activity readings from the start of the study. They found that people who had been inactive for at least 10 hours per day had a higher risk of dementia than those who spent more time moving.

The risk drastically increased the longer people were sedentary. For instance, compared with 10

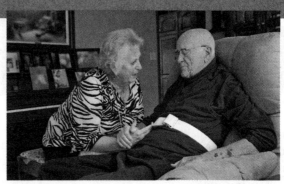
© wanderluster | Getty Images

Sitting for less time during the day is linked with lower dementia risk.

hours of sitting, dementia risk rose 50% at 12 hours and almost tripled at 15 hours. The risk was also consistent whether the sedentary time occurred in extended continuous periods or was spread intermittently throughout the day. And exercise didn't seem to change those odds. Among people who sat for 10 hours or more daily, those who worked out were as prone to dementia as those who exercised very little.

Blasting through mental health misperceptions

Fight back against pervasive stereotypes with these liberating strategies.

For all its downsides, the pandemic helped us to do a better job of openly discussing mental health. But that doesn't mean everyone is up to speed on how strikingly common mental illness is—or immune to stubborn stereotypes that label people struggling with mental health challenges as somehow defective.

An estimated 58 million American adults—more than one in five—live with a mental illness such as anxiety, depression, bipolar disorder, post-traumatic stress disorder, or obsessive-compulsive disorder, among others. More women than men receive treatment, such as medication or counseling, for these issues, according to the National Institute of Mental Health.

But, despite its pervasiveness, mental illness remains largely stigmatized, says Dr. Arthur Barsky, a psychiatrist at Harvard-affiliated Brigham and Women's Hospital.

"It still has that implication, I think, that it's somehow a failure of one's inner resources—a weakness," Dr. Barsky says. "Those with mental illness aren't viewed as winners on top of their game."

Damaging effects

Perhaps predictably, such stigma can prove quite damaging to people who cope with mental health problems, affecting their morale and even their recovery. Feeling labeled and marginalized by their condition can worsen people's depression or anxiety—for instance, by pushing them toward substance abuse or promoting secrecy or social withdrawal.

"It's got to worsen the underlying disorder, because you're feeling blamed for it," Dr. Barsky says. "Unfortunately, you may buy in to this thinking to some degree—thinking if you were stronger, you could beat

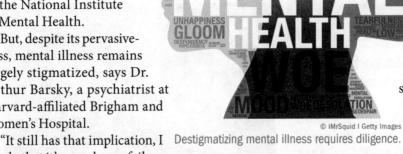

© iMrSquid I Getty Images

Destigmatizing mental illness requires diligence.

this. I think the stigma changes your view of yourself and also creates more isolation."

Changing minds

Fortunately, scientific advances are helping to dismantle long-held attitudes about mental illness. "One thing turning the tide is brain imaging that clearly shows structural changes to the brain in people with certain mental disorders," Dr. Barsky says. "That's probably eroded some of the stigma."

For example, more people now understand that someone with depression can't "snap out of it" any more than someone with liver disease, heart failure, or another physical ailment can simply decide not to have that condition.

"More recently, there's also some acknowledgment of anxiety disorders as being valid illnesses rather than part of the imagination," he says. "The pandemic accelerated that, but the trend has been to legitimize the fact that psychiatric illnesses are not a personal failing."

Turning the tide

If you deal with mental health challenges, Dr. Barsky suggests these strategies to help blast through any lingering stigma.

Embrace treatment. Don't let labels stop you from getting the treatment you need, whether it's therapy, medication, or both. (See "Tips to get the most out of therapy," page 44.) "While they're not miracle cures, we've got a repertoire of effective treatments," Dr. Barsky says. "Don't suffer needlessly."

Don't believe you are your illness. Remember that you need not be defined by your condition. For example, say "I have bipolar disorder," instead of "I'm bipolar."

Don't take offhand comments personally. Even well-meaning people say the wrong things occasionally, while others can be careless, cutting, or simply unconscious regarding word choices. "Think about why someone would say that and what it says about them rather than about you," Dr. Barsky says.

Share your story, if inclined. When you hear false or misleading information, you can help set the record straight by choosing to reveal details about your situation. "It can be terribly hard to do, but it's very beneficial," Dr. Barsky says. "It can take a tremendous load off your mind." ♥

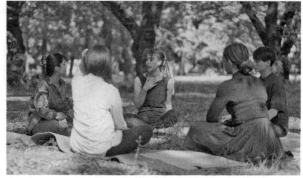
© credit | Getty Images

Sharing with others can ease the burden.

Too much TV might be bad for your brain

Excessive TV-watching—defined as four or more hours daily—is associated with a greater risk of developing brain-based disorders such as dementia, depression, and Parkinson's disease, a recent analysis suggests.

The study, published in 2023 by the *International Journal of Behavioral Nutrition and Physical Activity*, looked at data on more than 473,000 adults ages 39 to 72 enrolled in the UK Biobank. Researchers tracked participants until either they died; they were diagnosed with dementia, Parkinson's, or depression; or the study ended (2018 for some participants, 2021 for others). Participants reported how many hours they spent aside from work either exercising, using a computer, or watching TV.

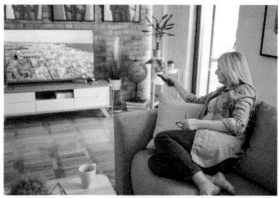
© Drazen_ | Getty Images

Excessive TV time may raise the odds of dementia, depression, and Parkinson's disease.

Compared with people who watched TV for less than an hour each day, participants who reported watching four or more hours of TV daily had a 28% higher risk of dementia, a 35% greater risk of depression, and a 16% higher risk of Parkinson's disease. But people who reported a moderate amount of computer use—30 to 60 minutes per day—appeared to have lower risks of those three conditions compared with participants who reported the lowest levels of computer use (see "Enjoy time online? It may be linked to lower dementia risk," page 43). The study was observational, meaning it couldn't prove that excessive TV watching in itself causes or contributes to these problems.

How to recognize the signs of mental health issues

Men are vulnerable to depression, phobias, and alcohol use disorder— and may be less likely to seek help than women. Here's what to look for.

People too often don't recognize that an underlying mental health problem is why they feel unwell.

A study published in a 2023 issue of *The Lancet Psychiatry* analyzed data collected over 20-plus years from more than 150,000 adults across 29 countries. The results showed that about half of people will develop at least one mental disorder by age 75. Among men, the most common disorders were depression, phobias, and alcohol use disorder.

Why may this be the case? "Older adults are vulnerable to mental disorders because they are exposed to many life-changing and traumatic events like health issues, the death of loved ones, and physical limitations," says Dr. Ronald Kessler, a professor of health care policy at Harvard Medical School and one of the study's co-leaders. "Many also don't recognize the signs of a mental disorder and thus don't seek medical help, which can make the disorder worse."

Here are the warning signs and symptoms for depression, phobias, and alcohol use disorder to look out for, no matter your gender. "People should find comfort in knowing that they are not alone when dealing with a mental disorder," says Dr. Kessler. "Effective treatments are available, so they don't have to spend their life in pain."

Depression

A depressed person may gain or lose weight, eat more or less than usual, have difficulty concentrating, and have trouble sleeping or sleep more than usual. They may also battle fatigue and low energy, so even small tasks may appear impossible to manage. Other symptoms of depression include one or more of the following:

- persistent sad or "empty" mood
- loss of enjoyment in favorite activities
- feelings of hopelessness or pessimism
- feelings of worthlessness and guilt about a specific life experience or in general
- increased boredom and apathy

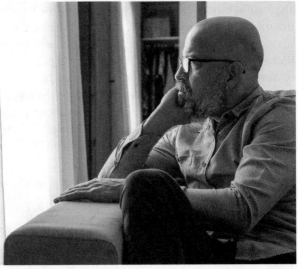

© Kar3k4 I Getty Images

Ignoring the symptoms of a mental health problem can delay helpful treatment.

- trouble concentrating or making decisions
- restlessness or irritability.

Get help. Speak with your doctor if you experience any of these symptoms most days for two weeks or longer. The doctor can refer you for counseling, prescribe an antidepressant, or both.

Phobias

A phobia is a persistent, excessive, unrealistic fear of an object, person, animal, activity, or situation. Phobias are a type of anxiety disorder.

Someone with a phobia either tries to avoid the object or situation that triggers the fear or endures it with great anxiety and distress. They also may overreact to a potential threat. Some examples of common phobias are fear of heights, public places, social situations, or closed spaces.

Physical symptoms may include rapid heartbeat, shallow or rapid breathing, sweating, dizziness, upset stomach (cramps, nausea, diarrhea), headaches, and general pains. Symptoms such as these also may lead to a diagnosis of panic disorder. It's also common for people with an anxiety disorder to suffer from depression and struggle with low self-esteem.

Get help. The first step to dealing with a phobia is to try to identify the underlying cause and possible stressors. You may be referred to a mental health professional for evaluation and treatment. Treatment for an anxiety disorder often includes a combination of medication and psychotherapy.

Alcohol use disorder

Today many experts recommend that people limit their alcohol use to no more than a single standard drink per day. In the United States, a standard drink is approximately 12 ounces of regular beer (5% alcohol by volume, or ABV), 5 ounces of wine (12% ABV), or 1.5 ounces of 80-proof spirits (40% ABV).

Moderate drinking wanders into alcohol use disorder when someone regularly drinks more than they planned and continues to drink despite the concerns of others and frequent attempts to cut down or quit. They also may indulge in binge drinking (consuming five or more drinks on one occasion).

After a person becomes dependent on alcohol, they will usually develop withdrawal symptoms such as headache, nausea and vomiting, anxiety, and fatigue if they can't get a drink.

Get help. Your doctor can help diagnose alcohol use disorder through a series of screening questions. Treatment consists of a combination of psychotherapy, and medication, and participation in self-help groups like Alcoholics Anonymous. ♥

Enjoy time online? It may be linked to lower dementia risk

Whiling away a few hours online by posting on social media, playing games, and surfing websites can certainly feel relaxing. But if you're wary that it's just a time sink, think again: using the Internet regularly may be linked to a lower risk of dementia, according to a recent observational study.

The 2023 study, published by the *Journal of the American Geriatrics Society*, tracked more than 18,000 people (average age 55) for an average of eight years. Every other year, researchers asked participants about their Internet use and administered cognitive testing. Nearly 65% of study participants reported being regular Internet users.

People who connected online for about two hours a day were about half as likely to develop dementia than those who didn't use the Internet regularly. The Internet users also maintained better verbal reasoning and memory. The benefits disappeared at high levels of Internet use—defined as six to eight hours a day.

The study authors speculated that online engagement could develop and maintain what's called cognitive reserve—the brain's ability to resist decline and find alternate ways to function efficiently. This could compensate for brain aging. But the study was observational, meaning it couldn't prove a cause-and-effect relationship between Internet use and dementia risk. Participants' Internet use was also self-reported.

"If we take the findings at face value, this would mean Internet use is another cognitive activity that can keep your brain active and healthy, which can potentially increase thinking and memory skills in the short term and reduce the risk of dementia over the long term," says Dr. Andrew Budson, a lecturer in neurology at Harvard Medical School. More study is needed to determine if specific types of online activity might be related to health outcomes.

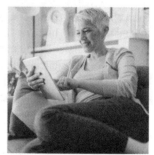

© vgajic | Getty Images

Online activities may help the brain resist cognitive decline.

Tips to get the most out of therapy

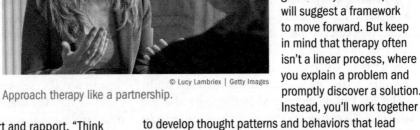

Embarking on therapy to tackle mental health troubles can feel like a leap of faith. But if you do it reluctantly, you're probably not poised to get the most out of the process, says Dr. Arthur Barsky, a psychiatrist at Brigham and Women's Hospital.

"People often resist getting help initially," Dr. Barsky says. "Some also have an inherent impulse to try to solve their problems themselves—to not ask for help or concede they're up against a problem they can't solve on their own."

Once you commit to therapy, however, you can maximize the results—and promote your own healing—by taking several key steps.

Choose your therapist carefully. Don't settle for someone who's merely convenient to your home or office; rather, look for a counselor who specializes in your particular problem. Once you meet her, get a sense of your mutual comfort and rapport. "Think about whether this person is someone you can spend time with and trust," Dr. Barsky says.

Treat therapy as teamwork. "Initially, you'll have to lead the show," he says. "But over time, as the therapist understands you and your situation, she's going to provide more insight and guidance and offer suggestions about how to tackle the problem. It's a collaboration, and it's not a cookie-cutter approach."

Be vulnerable. You can't benefit from therapy unless you're willing to fully open up about your experiences and feelings. And while it may be uncomfortable, you have to be willing to talk about things you'd often rather not discuss. "You need to share stuff that may be embarrassing, painful, or depressing," Dr. Barsky says. "Your therapist can't help you until she knows exactly what you're struggling with."

Take any prescribed medications. "It's pretty obvious, but if your therapist thinks you need medicine and you agree, then you need to take your pills," he says. "But don't agree and then go home and not take them." Many times, there are choices among medications. Ask about side effects, risks, and benefits, and work with your clinician to make the best choice.

Define success. Setting goals with your therapist will suggest a framework to move forward. But keep in mind that therapy often isn't a linear process, where you explain a problem and promptly discover a solution. Instead, you'll work together to develop thought patterns and behaviors that lead to healthier ways of living. "It's important to be able to think through where you'd like to be at the end of the therapeutic process and ask if the therapist thinks that's feasible or likely," Dr. Barsky says.

Be patient. Depending on your issue, effective therapy can take months or even years. "You can't expect you're going to walk out after a few sessions and the problem will disappear," Dr. Barsky says. "It may be a long process, but that doesn't mean it's not helpful."

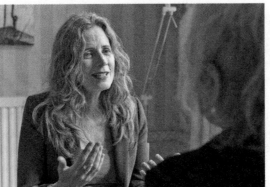

© Lucy Lambriex | Getty Images

Approach therapy like a partnership.

© Mekitik_Boy | Getty Images

Mood boosters

Feeling low? Here are some ways to clear your head and lift your spirits.

Everyone goes through periods of feeling low, lethargic, or stressed. These episodes usually pass after a while, but sometimes, you get stuck in a mental and emotional rut. When that happens, here are some strategies that can help pull you out.

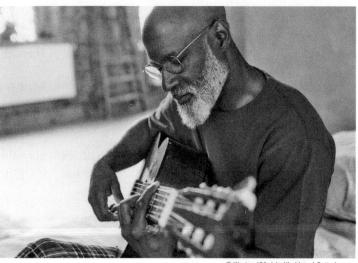

© Westend61 / Jo Kirchherr l Getty Images

Mentally stimulating activities improve mood by offering a feeling of accomplishment.

Get moving

Exercise stimulates your brain's production of endorphins—chemicals that create a sense of euphoria.

A review of more than 1,000 trials published in 2023 by the *British Journal of Sports Medicine* found that, compared with people who were sedentary, those who engaged in regular physical activity, like walking, resistance training, Pilates, and yoga, reduced their anxiety levels and improved mild depression-related symptoms.

Other research suggests aerobic exercise can have a powerful effect on mood. Any type of exercise is helpful, according to Dr. Darshan Mehta, medical director at the Benson-Henry Institute for Mind Body Medicine at Harvard-affiliated Massachusetts General Hospital. "Your exercise could be as simple as tending your garden or working on house projects," he says. "The point is to get moving, and move often."

Hang out with nature

Scientists believe spending time in a natural environment can calm neural activity in the prefrontal cortex, a brain region associated with negative emotions. Research also has found that interacting with nature can lower blood pressure and cortisol, the stress hormone. The type of setting doesn't matter as long as you find it soothing. "So, you walk a nature trail or sit in an urban green space," says Dr. Mehta. If you can't make it outside, looking at pictures of inspiring nature settings and listening to nature sounds on your smartphone or computer can have a similar effect.

Train your brain

"Engaging in mentally stimulating activities like painting and other art forms, learning to play a musical instrument, or learning a language can be a great mood booster, as they provide a sense of accomplishment," says Dr. Mehta.

Practice gratitude

Identifying and writing down things for which you are grateful can help offset feeling anxious or stressed. Begin a journal to record these examples of gratitude. Your entries might include big-picture items like your ability to exercise daily and enjoy a circle of close friends, or even satisfying occurrences like a friendly exchange at a store. "Try to provide details about why you are thankful and how these items improve your outlook," ▸▸

When to seek help

If your symptoms last for two weeks or longer or begin to interfere with daily life—for instance, if you're not sleeping well, becoming more isolated, or losing interest in favorite activities—you may be in the early stages of mild or moderate depression and should talk with your doctor. "Life changes like health issues or the loss of a spouse, family member, or friend can trigger depression symptoms, so be aware of any mood or lifestyle changes that occur after such events," says Dr. Darshan Mehta, medical director at the Benson-Henry Institute for Mind Body Medicine.

▸▸ says Dr. Mehta. You don't have to write every day—some studies have found that even just once a week is helpful.

Help others

You can reap many emotional rewards through volunteering. A study of 13,000 older adults, published in 2020 in the *American Journal of Preventive Medicine*, found that people who volunteered at least two hours per week felt happier and more optimistic than those who didn't. "Volunteering also can boost self-esteem by providing a sense of purpose," says Dr. Mehta. (See "Lending a helping hand" below.)

Make time to meditate

Practicing meditation can help you reduce stress by focusing on the present moment rather than ruminating about the past or future. You can learn the basics via online guided meditations at https://bensonhenry-institute.org/guided-relaxation-exercises. ▮

Lending a helping hand

Doing good deeds is good medicine for mood and memory.

The Greek philosopher Plato wrote, "Happiness springs from doing good and helping others." Almost 2,500 years later, research shows that Plato was correct—people who devote time to helping others are often happier than those who don't.

There are many ways lending a hand helps our minds and moods. One way is to turn our attention away from our own problems.

"Too much self-focused attention is linked with more negative thinking and a higher risk of anxiety and depression," says Robert Drozek, a psychotherapist with Harvard-affiliated McLean Hospital who specializes in the use of ethics in psychotherapy. "But serving redirects our energy and helps us realize that we have something to offer people, and they sometimes need our help."

Serving others helps brain health in other ways, too. It increases social connections, which can protect against loneliness and depression, and improves executive function skills like planning, attention, and

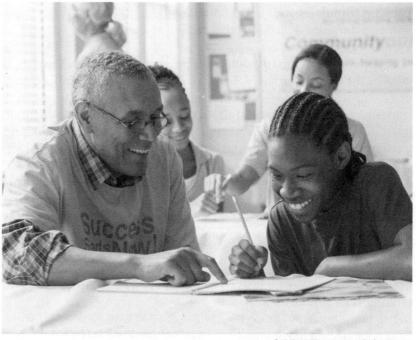
© KidStock/Blend Images LLC | Getty Images

Mentoring a youth offers the chance to share your knowledge, expertise, and life experience.

remembering tasks. And when you help others, your brain releases feel-good chemicals like serotonin and dopamine.

You don't need to devote much time to reap these benefits. A 2020 study published in the *American Journal of Preventive Medicine* found that older adults who did any kind of service work for two hours a week felt more optimistic and had a greater sense of purpose compared with those who performed no service.

How can you help yourself by helping others? Here are a few ways.

Volunteering

Volunteering provides a sense of purpose and an emotional boost as you support a cause or organization you believe in. You could also volunteer in professional fields or industries that match your life or work experience, like education, health care, or the arts.

"Volunteering in this way also offers opportunities to find structured and defined roles that fit your schedule, skills, and comfort levels," says Drozek.

You can even volunteer from home. For instance, thanks to computers, being a "virtual" volunteer is common. You can provide administrative, accounting, or marketing assistance via computer or video chat. Telephones are still crucial for volunteer work. For example, you can make calls to help raise money for nonprofits, answer a hotline, or make check-in calls to homebound adults.

Mentoring

Mentors share their knowledge, wisdom, and experience with people who need direction. Many times, this is a child or young adult.

A good place to begin is with a national program like Big Brothers, Big Sisters of America or the United Way. Also, many high schools, senior centers, churches, and faith-based organizations have mentoring opportunities. If you are more interested in sharing your professional expertise, contact your area Junior Achievement program, the local business community, or service clubs.

Random acts of kindness

Look for opportunities to serve others in daily life. For example, write to a friend saying you are thinking about them. Order takeout food for a neighbor. Send a gift in the mail. For an additional benefit, do the act anonymously, without telling anyone about it. "This further takes the focus away from you and your worries," says Drozek.

Different perspective

An indirect way to serve others is to see things from their point of view. When you interact with someone—whether a friend, acquaintance, or stranger—focus the interaction entirely on the other person. What is going on with them? What issues do they face? Are they in pain or feeling conflict?

Avoid injecting yourself—for instance, by describing how the same situation happened to you (unless they ask for feedback or advice).

"By lending an ear, you can provide emotional support they may need in that moment," says Drozek. "Even if the exchange is generic and friendly, placing emphasis on the other person can boost their mood, and in the process, yours, too."

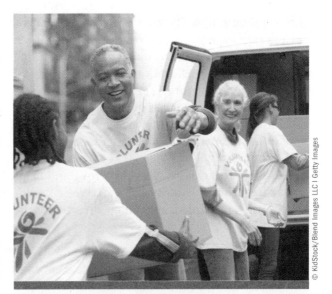

© KidStock/Blend Images LLC | Getty Images

Finding opportunities

Search online for volunteering opportunities in your ZIP code on websites such as Volunteer Match (www.volunteermatch.org) or Idealist (www.idealist.org). You can look for local mentoring programs at the website of the National Mentoring Partnership (www.mentoring.org).

Not just good for the soul

Science is pinpointing how forgiveness also benefits our brains and bodies.

When Oscar Wilde exhorted us (probably tongue-in-cheek) to "always forgive your enemies, because nothing annoys them so much," the Irish poet and playwright was focused on how others would respond.

But the real benefits of forgiveness might be better viewed with a more selfish eye. Whether we're bitter after an argument with a partner, a misunderstanding with a family member, or a spat with a friend, holding on to anger and resentment can do more than tax our souls—it can harm our health, Harvard experts say. And this is true even when it comes to weightier offenders, such as a sabotaging colleague or an unfaithful spouse.

A new Harvard-led study builds on earlier research that teases out the effects of this most human of actions, suggesting forgiveness boosts our mental well-being by reducing anxiety and depression. The results add to other recent evidence that it can also ease stress, improve sleep, and lower blood pressure and heart rate.

"Forgiveness acknowledges the wrong and helps you be free from it," says Tyler VanderWeele, co-author of the Harvard study and co-director of the

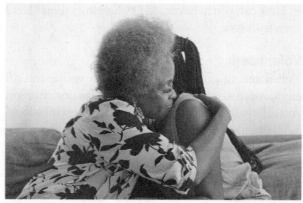
© LaylaBird | Getty Images

Forgiveness can reduce stress, improve sleep, and lower blood pressure and heart rate.

Initiative on Health, Spirituality, and Religion at the Harvard T.H. Chan School of Public Health. "It frees you from the offender as well. When appropriate, forgiveness can lead to restored relationships, bringing happiness, satisfaction, and social support—which evidence also links to better health."

Simple and complicated

For such a challenging undertaking, the definition of forgiveness is surprisingly basic. "It's simply replacing ill will toward an offender with goodwill," says VanderWeele, also director of Harvard's Human Flourishing Program.

Mindfulness can change the brain

Being mindful has a number of benefits: it makes it easier to savor the pleasures in life as they occur, helps you become fully engaged in activities, and multiplies gratitude. But it can also change the brain in ways that correlate with reduced stress and a better mood. In one study, researchers used brain imaging to identify a link between the practice of mindfulness and positive emotion in the brain. In people who were anxious, depressed, or hypervigilant, the right prefrontal cortex was active. In people who practiced mindfulness meditation, the left prefrontal cortex was more active. This side of the cortex is typically more active in people who have fewer negative moods. For improved moods, consider taking five minutes to give mindfulness a try.

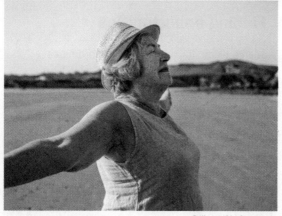
© Westend61 | Getty Images

Mindfulness activates the left prefrontal cortex, which is tied to reduced stress and improved mood.

But what forgiveness *doesn't* mean is a bit more nuanced: it doesn't condone the harm you've suffered—and it definitely doesn't mean you're expected to forget it, says Craig Malkin, a lecturer in psychology at Harvard Medical School.

"It's not excusing, explaining, or exonerating," he says. "Saying you forgive is easy, but doesn't change the feelings inside. We can be sad for what we experienced and angry about what happened. But above all, a state of forgiveness is accepting that what happened is over."

Unquestionably, the bigger the offense, the tougher it is to forgive. Emotional or physical abuse—or violence—are far harder to move past than smaller insults. It's a tall order for survivors of abusive relationships, for example, to be asked to forgive the person who hurt them, Malkin says.

That's why it's important to recognize that forgiveness doesn't always include reconciling with the wrongdoer.

"One can forgive and want what's ultimately good for the other person without the relationship being restored," VanderWeele says. "Likewise, one can forgive an offender while pursuing justice. So forgiveness can be compatible with a just anger."

Mental health advantages

In VanderWeele's study, which was presented at a Harvard conference in April 2023, he and colleagues randomly assigned nearly 4,600 adults from five countries—all of whom had experienced an "interpersonal transgression"—into two groups.

The people in one group received a self-guided forgiveness workbook filled with written exercises. Individual exercises sought to teach users techniques such as recalling hurt feelings and empathizing with the offender. For example, participants were asked to describe a person who'd hurt them and their offense. Participants then needed to write the story from the perspective of an observer without vilifying the wrongdoer or underscoring how the participant felt victimized.

This type of "switching seats" to adopt the mindset of both the offended and the offender is "difficult to do, but can be quite an insightful part of the process," VanderWeele says.

Two weeks later, those participants reported fewer symptoms of depression and anxiety than their counterparts in the other group, who had not yet received workbooks.

"We thought if we were able with a simple, self-directed workbook to improve people's capacity to forgive, it would probably have effects on their mental health as well," he says. "We found the effects were pretty substantial."

Learning to forgive

On the flip side, being unable to forgive places a bigger burden on your body than you might realize. "We do know that when we're in that state of unforgiveness, our blood pressure rises," Malkin says. "Logically, if that doesn't resolve, over time that affects our heart health in a very basic way. It can wreak havoc."

Feeling stuck in hostility can torment us mentally, too. This conundrum is marked by vengeful fantasies and intense rumination—looping negative thoughts that Malkin describes as "a churning."

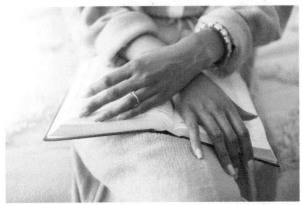
© Jacob Wackerhausen | Getty Images
Stories of forgiveness can help us cultivate it with others.

"If you're just unforgiving," he says, "you lose out on the opportunity for repair and the deeper closeness that comes from that repair."

For some people, however, the act of forgiving just seems to come more easily. People with certain temperaments and personality types are innately better at it, and evidence suggests that over all, women are more forgiving than men, VanderWeele says. That said, "it's an option open to everyone," he notes. "I don't think there's anyone who cannot forgive."

It's also a skill that can be learned, Harvard experts agree. The simplest way to approach it, Malkin says—though not with a violent or abusive person—is by sharing what hurt you. This requires a vulnerability ▸▸

▸▸ that can be hard to summon, but is far more productive than being angry, sad, or brittle.

"Always lead with the vulnerable feeling," Malkin says. "If you just blast them and say, 'I can't believe you did that,' they're going to be on the defensive and they can't open their heart. If you withdraw, there's no opportunity for repair."

Forgiveness strategies

Looking for ways to incorporate forgiveness into your life? Malkin and VanderWeele suggest these strategies:

Process your pain. Take some time to describe what happened to you and its aftermath in writing—but not to share with your offender. The document is just for you, to process your vulnerable feelings. "Don't censor or shortcut it," Malkin says. "It's an opportunity to take a more compassionate view of what you went through. This helps move you to a different place."

Seek stories of forgiveness. The gesture is as old as time, so find examples you can draw from. "I do think reading these stories can be very inspiring, as well as challenging," VanderWeele says. "Turning to those models can be quite helpful."

Reflect on the advantages. If you're the analytical type, weighing the cost and benefits of forgiveness may prod you forward. "As the writer Malachy McCourt once said, holding a grudge is like taking poison and hoping the other person dies," VanderWeele says. ▐

What does it take to forgive yourself?

Forgiving others is challenging enough. But what if you're the one who's done something wrong?

"It can feel a little odd to say, 'I'm going to pardon myself,'" says Tyler VanderWeele, co-director of the Initiative on Health, Spirituality, and Religion at the Harvard T.H. Chan School of Public Health.

But it's a worthwhile effort: as with forgiving others, self-forgiveness is linked with less psychological distress, including fewer symptoms of depression, according to a 2020 study VanderWeele co-authored in *Frontiers in Psychology*.

Getting started requires recognizing that no matter how badly you've behaved, you're in a relationship with yourself—one that deserves respect and compassion. Calling self-forgiveness a "second dimension" of the concept of forgiveness, a 2022 study published in the journal *Spiritual Care* pointed out that any genuine effort to self-forgive must include three

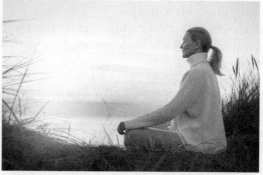
© Henrik Sorensen | Getty Images
Self-forgiveness often involves changing your ways.

components: remorse, apology, and the making of amends. Only then can you restore your self-esteem.

"Genuine self-forgiveness needs to acknowledge the wrong, but in spite of the bad, you should want what's good for you," VanderWeele says. "And that may involve changing."

Guilt and self-recrimination will only take you so far, says Craig Malkin, a lecturer in psychology at Harvard Medical School. But ultimately, forgiving ourselves liberates us to ask the same from others.

"You can't take action in a relationship if you're in that spin cycle of beating yourself up," Malkin says. "If we're riddled with guilt or shame, those feelings shut us down. From a self-forgiving stance, we can take action, even corrective action—but we can't do that if we're stuck in that loop."

Break the cycle

The circular thinking that characterizes rumination can harm your health. Take these steps to stop it.

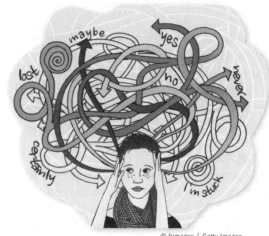

© frimages | Getty Images

Rumination can take a toll both physically and psychologically.

If you've ever gone through your day with a song running through your head, you know those "earworms" can be either amusing or annoying. But when a single intrusive thought is circling round and round, that's called rumination—and it's seldom pleasant.

An endless repetition of a negative thought or theme that spirals downward, tanking your mood, rumination often involves replaying a past scenario or conversation in your head or trying to solve a maddening problem. "I think it's quite common, and some people do it all the time—like picking a scab," says Dr. Jacqueline Olds, a psychiatrist at Harvard-affiliated Massachusetts General Hospital.

But rumination isn't harmless. It can disrupt your ability to get things done and can even damage your psychological or physical health. "Rumination is like getting stuck in a conversation with yourself," Dr. Olds says.

Triggers and consequences

Almost no issue, large or small, is off-limits for rumination. We might go in a mental circle if we believe we've made a mistake, looked foolish, said something wrong, or been responsible for a bad outcome.

"Maybe you have a conversation where everything seems to be going well, but when you go home, you think, 'Why did I say that?' You go over and over some minute incident that no one else probably even noticed, and blow it all out of proportion," Dr. Olds says.

Those feelings then dig in deeper. "You start thinking, 'I have no social sense. I'm always putting my foot in my mouth, and now I've probably alienated people for life.' Basically, you feel horrible about yourself," she adds.

However, people who ruminate continue to do so because they feel they'll gain hoped-for insight into a vexing problem. In essence, your brain is tricking you into believing you're figuring out something useful. But it's usually a trap: thinking endlessly about a problem often doesn't solve anything—it just proves exhausting, stealing your focus from things you'd rather be doing.

"It's just harder to navigate your way through life," Dr. Olds says. "Every day we have about a hundred decisions thrown at us. If someone is ruminating too much about every single thing, it slows them down and makes them have trouble with life's ordinary problems."

Mental and physical ramifications

Rumination isn't a psychological disorder in itself, but it can pose or be linked with mental and physical threats. An April 2020 study in *Behavior Research and Therapy* highlighted how rumination heightens our vulnerability to anxiety, depression, insomnia, and impulsive behaviors; interferes with psychotherapy and limits its effectiveness; and worsens and sustains the body's stress responses, such as inflammation.

"It can definitely get in the way of sleep," Dr. Olds says. "If you're in bed for seven-and-a-half hours and spend two-and-a-half of it ruminating and only five hours sleeping, that's a problem."

Often a major symptom of obsessive-compulsive disorder (OCD), rumination becomes an unseen compulsion that may feel productive in the moment but sustains the condition over the long term.

"People have the faulty assumption that there's a right way and a wrong way to do things, and they have to get it right," she says. "It leads people with OCD to think there's also a right way to think."

Rumination can also create an insidious loop that ropes in both depression and anxiety, Dr. Olds says. A 2020 study of nearly 6,000 adults published in the *Journal of Affective Disorders* enhances that perspective, suggesting rumination both increases the risk of ▸▸

▶▶ developing depressive symptoms and results from those same symptoms.

"The isolation depressed people experience often leads to more rumination, and then ruminating makes people feel anxious," she says. "It's a loop of its own."

Seeking help

Unlike some mental challenges that are evident to others, rumination largely happens in the shadows. No one can watch you do it, and they may never know you're prone to it if you don't tell anyone what you're going through. This "invisibility cloak" can pose barriers to seeking help, since you may be the only person who knows the true toll rumination is taking on your well-being.

When is it time to seek professional advice? If you feel your looping thoughts are blocking out everything else and you can't function normally, Dr. Olds recommends psychodynamic therapy or cognitive behavioral therapy (CBT). Psychodynamic therapy focuses on developing insights into the roots of your behavior, while CBT emphasizes behavioral change.

"How much does rumination slow your forward progress?" she asks. "How carried away are you getting? How much sleep are you losing, and how weary and depressed have you become?"

A therapist can help you identify why you ruminate, as well as address the underlying issues and help break the cycle. With therapy, Dr. Olds says, "you'll gradually start correcting your self-destructive assumptions."

Self-talk your way to calm

Rumination is essentially negative self-talk—a drag on your self-esteem shaped by constantly feeding yourself negative messages about your life and your ability to cope.

Want to flip the script? Try positive self-talk. It's a way of speaking to yourself like your best friend would—with optimism and encouragement. You affirm that you're capable and ready for any task at hand.

As basic as it sounds, positive self-talk can indeed prove motivational and reassuring, and keeping at it can crowd out the negative filter in your head, easing your anxiety. It can also help you reframe your fears as opportunities, says Dr. Jacqueline Olds, a psychiatrist at Massachusetts General Hospital. "Self-talk can help you coach yourself into a calmer space," she says.

Getting there requires asking yourself if an anxiety-provoking situation truly warrants an anxious response. "You have to figure out the probability of something being a catastrophe—to put your own anxiety system at arm's length," Dr. Olds says.

Therapy can help, since you'll gradually internalize your therapist's perspective that lays out problems in calmer, more logical ways. In the meantime, it may help to press the reset button on anxious thoughts by replacing them with affirmations or mantras that can change your mindset.

Try mentally repeating these messages to yourself instead:

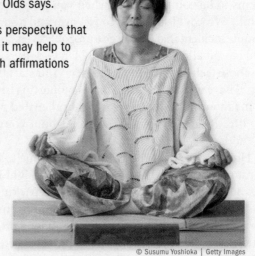

- ▶ I can overcome this challenge.
- ▶ I'm safe and in control.
- ▶ This feeling is only temporary.
- ▶ My best is good enough.
- ▶ I can move past this difficult moment.
- ▶ I can handle whatever happens.

© Susumu Yoshioka | Getty Images

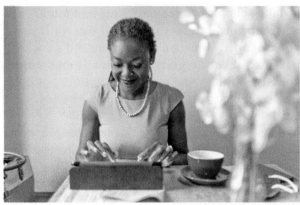

© Luis Alvarez | Getty Images

You can disrupt circular thoughts by heading to your "happy place."

Disrupt the cycle

But even before therapy—or alongside it—you have the power to disrupt your thought cycle and thwart rumination. Dr. Olds suggests these tactics:

Find a distraction. You're less apt to ruminate if you're busy doing something else. Try exercising, calling a friend or family member, cleaning out a drawer or closet, listening to music, watching a movie, or reading a book.

Change locations. Do you have a "happy place," such as a park, the beach, a book store, or a favorite coffee shop? If you can, head there to occupy a new headspace. ▶▶

Be cautious about herbal remedies for anxiety

Throughout the years, many different herbal remedies—including passionflower, St. John's wort, kava, valerian root, and chamomile—have been touted as natural alternatives to anxiety treatments. Although some studies have suggested that these preparations can relieve anxiety symptoms, it's important to remember that the FDA does not regulate supplements, and they can cause side effects. In addition, some supplements, such as over-the-counter weight-loss drugs, can actually increase anxiety. If you're thinking about taking a supplement for anxiety or any other condition, talk with your doctor first to see whether it's safe for you. And if you want to try an herbal preparation, herbal teas are typically safer than supplements.

TRY THIS — Four steps to changing negative thoughts

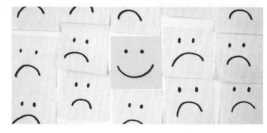

You can't control the outside world, but you can try to control your reactions to it. One way to do this is with a technique called cognitive restructuring. It helps change your negative thinking and stressful reactions to daily life. Here is the four-step process:

1. Stop. Consciously call a mental time-out when undesirable thoughts take over. By saying "Stop," you can halt the negative response cycle.

2. Breathe. Take a few deep breaths to reduce physical tension and step back from the stressor before you react.

3. Reflect. Ask yourself the following questions: Is this thought or belief true? Did I jump to a conclusion? What evidence do I actually have? Is there another way that I could view the situation? What's the worst that could happen? Does it help me to think this way?

4. Choose. Decide how to deal with the source of your stress. For example, challenge distorted, irrational thinking and adjust your view of reality. Remember, many things we worry about never come to fruition. Ask yourself, How else can I think about this? How can I deal with this in a positive way?

Here's an example of how this approach might work. If you get stuck in traffic on the way to meet a friend and feel agitated, stop and notice signs of stress in your body, such as a tight neck and shoulders. Try to relax and take a few deep breaths. Reflect: "It's just traffic. It's not worth getting upset." Now, choose how to deal with it. Don't assume your friend will be angry. Tell yourself, "I'll just be a few minutes late. I'm doing the best I can. I can manage this. It will be okay."

▸▸ **Rely on relaxation techniques.** Mindfulness meditation and deep breathing can help clear your mind, which may derail rumination. Find a quiet space, breathe deeply, and notice your surroundings.

Confide in a friend. A pal can offer a sanity check on runaway thoughts, helping put your worries in perspective. But choose wisely, veering away from dramatic personalities. "You want to choose a person who can talk you down," Dr. Olds says.

Take action. Do one small thing that might push you past your circular thoughts. If you really think you offended someone at last weekend's cocktail party, send your regrets in an email—but temper yourself. "Take some reasonable action, but don't prostrate yourself on someone's doorstep," Dr. Olds says.

Be patient. Expect to revisit some looping thoughts before you're able to break the cycle completely. ▾

IN THE JOURNALS

Regular physical activity can boost mood

Exercising regularly can improve symptoms of mild to moderate depression as well as anxiety and psychological distress, a review of many prior published studies suggests.

The analysis, published in 2023 by the *British Journal of Sports Medicine,* used 97 earlier research reviews involving more than 1,000 trials with a total of 128,119 people. Researchers compared the effects of exercise to standard care across a wide range of adults, including healthy people, those with diagnosed mental health disorders, and people with chronic diseases.

When compared with people who were sedentary, those who engaged in all types of physical activity and exercise, including walking, resistance training, Pilates, and yoga, showed greater improvements in symptoms of mild to moderate depression. Yoga and other mind-body exercises helped reduce anxiety the most, while resistance exercise appeared to help the most with depression.

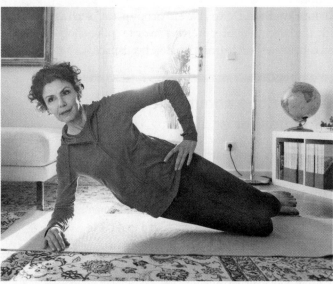
© Silke Woweries I Getty Images

Mind-body exercise, such as yoga, helps reduce anxiety.

The review findings don't mean that people with mental health conditions should sidestep standard care, such as medication and counseling. Rather, the results suggest that regular exercise is also an important approach and deserves renewed focus.

Best (health) friends

Want to improve your mental and physical health? Get a dog.

The saying goes that you can't teach an old dog new tricks. But a new dog can teach older adults how to stay active and healthy.

"Owning a dog can be one of the best ways to manage many health issues older adults face," says Dr. Beth Frates, director of lifestyle medicine and wellness in the Department of Surgery at Harvard-affiliated Massachusetts General Hospital. "It can be a real team effort, too. You take care of the dog, and the dog takes care of you."

How can a dog be your health's best friend? Here are a few examples.

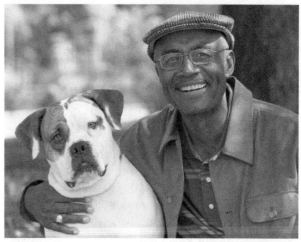

© Ariel Skelley | Getty Images

Research shows that dog ownership can help people stay active and live longer.

Healthier heart

Research has consistently found that dog owners tend to have a lower risk of cardiovascular disease than non-owners. A 2022 study published in *Current Hypertension Reports* suggested that having a canine companion helps prevent high blood pressure and may improve blood pressure control for those with the condition.

And 2019 research from the journal *Circulation: Cardiovascular Quality and Outcomes* reported that dog owners were 31% less likely to die from a heart attack or stroke than non-owners.

Having a dog may help you live longer if you suffer a heart attack or stroke. In the same issue of *Circulation*, another study found that, among people who had a heart attack or stroke, those who owned a dog had a 33% lower death rate in the 12 years after a heart attack and a 27% lower death rate after a stroke than people without a dog.

One way dogs may improve heart health is that they make their owners more active, thanks in part to the ritual of daily walks. In fact, research has found that, on average, people with dogs walk about 20 minutes more per day than those without dogs. ▶▶

The dogma of dog ownership

Before you adopt a dog, there are certain aspects to consider, like the dog's size, strength, and energy levels. "Larger dogs may require more exercise and be more difficult to handle than smaller dogs," says Dr. Beth Frates, director of lifestyle medicine and wellness at Harvard's Massachusetts General Hospital. "But smaller dogs can be tripping hazards." Dogs also require an ongoing financial commitment. Besides food, dogs need routine vaccinations, regular medical check-ups, flea and tick prevention, grooming, and often training. If you're not ready for dog ownership, you can still increase your interactions with dogs. For example, offer to walk a friend's dog or to dog-sit. You can also volunteer at an animal shelter or spend time at a dog park.

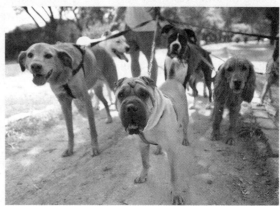

© Pamela Palma | Getty Images

Caring for a dog requires commitment and responsibility, but the mental and physical benefits are worth it.

Stress relief

Ever wonder why petting a dog is so pleasant? A study published in 2022 by *PLOS One* found that interacting with a dog, especially petting, stimulates the human brain's prefrontal cortex, which helps regulate emotions. Petting also lowers cortisol, the stress hormone, and raises oxytocin, the feel-good hormone, according to Dr. Frates. "The effect can continue long after the dog is no longer present," she says.

Dogs also can teach us to relieve stress by practicing mindfulness. During walks, dogs are engaged in the moment and focus on the various smells, sights, and sounds of their environment. "Following their lead can help people to 'stop and smell the flowers' more often," says Dr. Frates.

Dogs even play the role of therapists. "Dogs are great listeners," says Dr. Frates. "There's always someone to talk to when you have a dog. Plus, most dogs also are good at reading body language and sensing your emotions. Sometimes a dog will know you are upset and instinctively sit next to you or jump onto your lap."

And, of course, never underestimate the mood-boosting power of dogs' unconditional love. "No matter what is going on with your life, dogs are always so happy to see you," says Dr. Frates.

Social companions

Loneliness and social isolation are among the biggest health threats facing older adults, and dogs can help with both. "Dogs offer everyday companionship, and they depend on you for food and care, which creates a family-like bond," says Dr. Frates. (For more on these benefits, see "Pets may help fend off cognitive decline in single seniors," below.)

Dogs can also help expand your social circle. When you're out with your dog, whether walking in your neighborhood or visiting a dog park, you have the chance to converse with neighbors, fellow dog owners, and even people you don't know. "People are drawn to dogs and want to interact with them and pet them, and in the process engage with you," says Dr. Frates.

IN THE JOURNALS

Pets may help fend off cognitive decline in single seniors

If you live alone, having a furry, four-legged companion may help slow some measures of cognitive decline, research suggests. A 2023 study published in *JAMA Network Open* focused on 7,900 people (average age 66) living in the United Kingdom from 2010 to 2019. Researchers tested the participants' verbal memory, verbal fluency, and verbal cognition (all key indicators of cognitive health) over time. They also compared the test results based on the participants' living situations. About 35% owned pets, and 27% lived alone. People who lived alone and had pets showed slower rates of decline on the test results compared with people who lived alone without any pets. In fact, pet owners who lived alone had results equivalent to those of people who lived with other people. Living with a dog or cat may help ease loneliness—an important risk factor for cognitive decline, the study authors say.

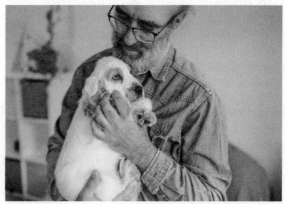

© bojanstory | Getty Images

Dog or cat? No need to play favorites: they're tied for health benefits.

Life can be challenging: Build your own resilience plan

Three strategies to help you find a way forward when you're feeling stressed, burned out, anxious, or sad.

Nantucket, a beautiful, 14-mile-long island off the coast of Massachusetts, has a 40-point resiliency plan to help withstand the buffeting seas surrounding it as climate change takes a toll. Perhaps we can all benefit from creating individual resilience plans to help handle the big and small issues that erode our sense of well-being. But what is resilience and how do you cultivate it?

What is resilience?

Resilience is a psychological response that helps you adapt to life's difficulties and seek a path forward through challenges.

"It's a flexible mindset that helps you adapt, think critically, and stay focused on your values and what matters most," says Luana Marques, an associate professor of psychiatry at Harvard Medical School.

While everyone has the ability to be resilient, your capacity for resilience can take a beating over time from chronic stress, perhaps from financial instability or staying in a job you dislike. The longer you're in that situation, the harder it becomes to cope with it.

Fortunately, it's possible to cultivate resilience. To do so, it helps to exercise resiliency skills as often as possible, even for minor stressors. Marques recommends the following strategies.

Shift your thoughts

In stressful situations, try to balance out your thoughts by adopting a broader perspective. "This will help you stop using the emotional part of your brain and start using the thinking part of your brain. For example, if you're asking for a raise and your brain says you won't get it, think about the things you've done in your job that are worthy of a raise. You'll slow down the emotional response and shift your mindset from anxious to action," Marques says.

Approach what you want

"When you're anxious, stressed, or burned out, you tend to avoid things that make you uncomfortable.

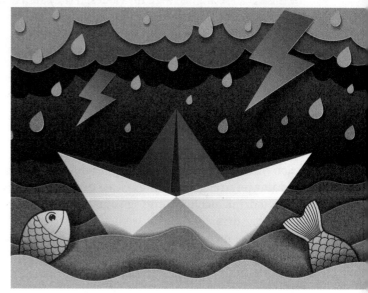

© Sylverarts | Getty Images

Resilience practices help cultivate responses to stress that support your well-being.

That can make you feel stuck," Marques says. "What you need to do is get out of your comfort zone and take a step toward the thing you want, in spite of fear."

For example: If you're afraid of giving a presentation, create a PowerPoint and practice it with colleagues. If you're having conflict at home, don't walk away from your partner—schedule time to talk about what's making you upset.

Align actions with your values

"Stress happens when your actions are not aligned with your values—the things that matter most to you or bring you joy. For example, you might feel stressed if you care most about your family but can't be there for dinner, or care most about your health but drink a lot," Marques says.

She suggests that you identify your top three values and make sure your daily actions align with them. If being with family is one of the three, make your time with them a priority—perhaps find a way to join them for a daily meal. If you get joy from a clean house, make daily tidying a priority.

Tips for success

Practice the shift, approach, and align strategies throughout the week. "One trick I use is looking at ▸▸

▸▸ my calendar on Sunday and checking if my actions for the week are aligned with my values. If they aren't, I try to change things around," Marques says.

It's also important to live as healthy a lifestyle as possible, which will help keep your brain functioning at its best.

Healthy lifestyle habits include:

▸ getting seven to nine hours of sleep per night
▸ following a healthy diet, such as a Mediterranean-style diet
▸ aiming for at least 150 minutes of moderate-intensity activities (such as brisk walking) each week—and adding on strength training at least twice a week
▸ if you drink alcohol, limiting yourself to no more than one drink per day for women and two drinks per day for men
▸ not smoking

▸ staying socially connected, whether in person, by phone or video calls, social media, or even text messages.

Need resilience training?

Even the best athletes have coaches, and you might benefit from resilience training.

Consider taking an online course, such as one developed by Marques (go to www.health.harvard.edu/learn/mentalhealth). Or maybe turn to a therapist online or in person for help. Look for someone who specializes in cognitive behavioral therapy, which guides you to redirect negative thoughts to positive or productive ones.

Just don't put off building resilience. Practicing as you face day-to-day stresses will help you learn skills to help navigate when dark clouds roll in and seas get rough. ▾

IN THE JOURNALS

Loneliness vs. isolation: Which one is worse?

Loneliness and isolation both contribute to adverse health consequences. Research has shown that people who are lonely or feel isolated have increased risks for chronic disease, cognitive decline, an inability to perform daily living tasks, as well as an earlier death. But loneliness and isolation are two distinct problems—and it's possible to have one and not the other. An observational study from Harvard published in 2023 in *SSM–Population Health* sought to find out if one problem might be more dangerous than the other. Researchers analyzed the health data of almost 14,000 people (ages 50 or older) who were followed for four years. Both loneliness and isolation were associated with poor health outcomes. But social isolation (living alone or not spending time with family and friends) was a stronger predictor of physical decline and early death. Loneliness was more predictive of mental health issues, such as depression or feeling that life had no meaning. The bottom line: Both loneliness

and isolation matter and fuel each other. You can fight them by making an effort to stay connected to others. And if you feel lonely, whether or not it's because you're isolated, it might be time to seek guidance from your doctor.

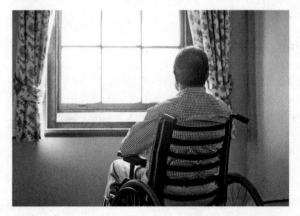

© shapecharge | Getty Images

Social connections are an important contributor to overall health.

Chapter 3

Blood Pressure and Cholesterol

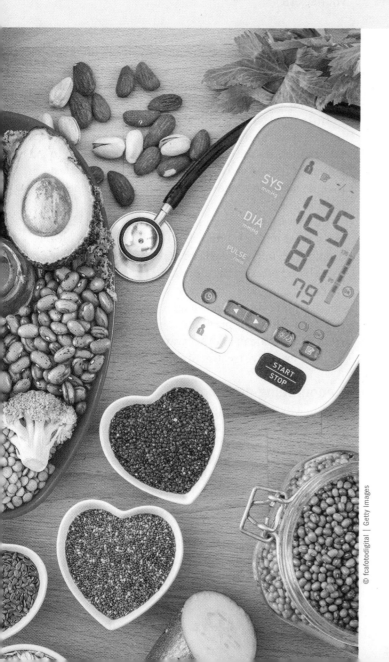

© fcafotodigital | Getty Images

Healthy Habits!
5 Things You Can Do Now

1 Breathe deeply. Slowing the breath can measurably improve blood pressure and overall health. (page 63)

2 Learn how to take your blood pressure. You're likely to get more accurate measurements than at the doctor's office. (page 64)

3 Eat more plant-based foods. Vegan and plant-based diets lower cholesterol and inflammation. (page 68)

4 Lower your sodium intake. Doing so can benefit most people, regardless of initial blood pressure levels. (page 71)

5 Try isometric exercise, such as planks and wall squats. Evidence suggests it has powerful benefits for lowering blood pressure. (page 77)

Is your home blood pressure monitor accurate?

Here's how to tell and what to do if the device might be wrong.

An inexpensive, easy-to-use blood pressure monitor that you use at home is a powerful tool to protect your health. It can help you see if your blood pressure is under control and how it responds to new medications or exercise. It may even provide a more realistic picture of your blood pressure than measurements taken in a doctor's office, which can vary for many reasons. But home monitoring can have problems, too—namely, the equipment.

In a letter published in *JAMA* in 2023, an international team of researchers reported findings indicating that the vast majority of top-selling blood pressure monitors sold on a popular website are not validated for accuracy. That's an issue, because using a nonvalidated device might threaten your health.

More about the study

The researchers identified the top-selling home blood pressure monitors available on Amazon.com in 2020 in 10 countries, including the United States. Then they checked to see how many of the devices were validated for accuracy.

Most of the devices—79% of those with an upper arm cuff and 83% of those with a wrist cuff—were not validated. Most of the nonvalidated arm cuff devices were sold in India or Australia. Most of the nonvalidated wrist devices were sold in the United States or Mexico. Meanwhile, other studies have suggested that 85% to 94% of all available blood pressure devices are not validated. This poses a risk.

What's the harm?

Using a nonvalidated device to measure your blood pressure means there's no way to know if the information it provides is correct—and relying on inaccurate measurements could then affect decisions you and your doctor make about treatment. For example, says Dr. Christopher Cannon, a cardiologist and editor in chief of the *Harvard Heart Letter*, "Inaccurate measurements that appear too high or low might warrant trips to the doctor's office unnecessarily. The measurements might also lead your doctor to start you on a blood pressure drug or adjust your current blood pressure medications, even though they might not need to be changed. Taking too much or too little of the drugs might harm your health."

Validation is tricky

Why are so many blood pressure monitors nonvalidated? It's hard to standardize and enforce rules for manufacturers based in different countries around the world. There's no global institution that does this.

Instead, we have medical organizations in varying countries or international groups that set validation guidelines for clinical accuracy. It's then up to manufacturers to pay independent investigators to test their devices and make sure they follow at least one set of guidelines.

But device makers aren't always required to have their products validated. In the United States, for example, manufacturers need to prove to the FDA only that a blood pressure monitor is safe to get it cleared for marketing. By "safe," the law means that the machine doesn't injure you when you take your blood pressure. But a machine that provides you with an inaccurate reading is unsafe in another way: it can lead to inadequate or excessive treatment.

Encouraging developments

Fortunately, reliable organizations have developed lists of blood pressure monitors that have demonstrated clinical accuracy based on a formalized set of criteria. The lists enable you to look up blood pressure monitors by brand name, device name, model number, or other details.

For blood pressure monitors available in the United States, with validation criteria set by the American Medical Association and other U.S. groups and experts, consult the U.S. Blood Pressure Validated Device Listing, or VDL (https://validatebp.org).

For blood pressure monitors that meet validation criteria set by organizations outside the United States, check out STRIDE BP (https://stridebp.org/bp-monitors).

How to verify your device is accurate

If you have a blood pressure monitor, look it up on one of the device lists to see if it's validated for accuracy. If it doesn't show up, it's probably not validated. But there's still a chance it's accurate.

"To find out, bring the monitor to your next doctor appointment and ask a nurse to take one measurement with your monitor and another with a monitor there in the office," Dr. Cannon says. "If your monitor isn't accurate, it's time to invest in a new one."

What to look for in a device

A blood pressure monitor shouldn't cost more than about $50 to $100. Just make sure it has several important features, including a large, easy-to-read display and a cuff that wraps around your upper arm, since finger or wrist monitors are not considered reliable. (See "Buying a blood pressure monitor.")

The blood pressure cuff needs to fit well: cuffs that are too small will give falsely elevated readings. "I have a patient who was getting very high readings that were different in both arms," Dr. Cannon says. "He brought his blood pressure monitor in, and sure enough, the reading on his home device was much higher than what our monitor in the clinic showed. His biceps were huge and the standard cuff size was too small for him." (See "Wrong-sized blood pressure cuff can throw off readings," page 62.)

It's also handy if the blood pressure monitor has a battery life indicator or, even better, if it can plug into an electrical outlet so you don't have to worry about replacing batteries.

The monitor should be approved by the FDA and validated by the VDL or STRIDE BP.

When to check pressure

When you first start measuring blood pressure at home, take it early in the morning, and again in the evening, every day for a week. If most readings fall within the goals recommended by your doctor, you can then check your blood pressure two or three times per week, and eventually shift to once a month. If you notice changes, report them to your doctor's office. ♥

Buying a blood pressure monitor

Of all the things you can measure to assess your cardiovascular health, blood pressure ranks at the very top. Follow this advice when selecting a device:

▸ Measure the circumference of the middle of your upper arm to ensure a proper fit. A cuff that's too small or too large won't give an accurate reading.

▸ Look for a device that has a large, easy-to-read display and a cuff that inflates automatically.

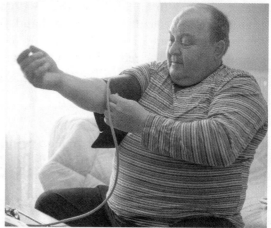

© Jakovo | Getty Images

Checking blood pressure at home can provide a more realistic picture than measurements taken at the doctor's office.

▸ Choose a monitor that appears on the U.S. Blood Pressure Validated Device Listing (https://validatebp.org). A 2023 report in JAMA found that 84% of the 100 best-selling home blood pressure devices sold on Amazon in the United States were not validated (that is, proven accurate).

Follow your doctor's advice about when and how often to check your blood pressure. For a video from the American Heart Association demonstrating the correct technique, visit https://targetbp.org/tools_downloads/self-measured-blood-pressure-video.

Wrong-sized blood pressure cuff can throw off readings

When it comes to measuring your blood pressure at home, cuff size matters. Using a "regular"-sized arm cuff with an automated device resulted in inaccurate blood pressure readings for people who needed a small, large, or extra-large-sized cuff, according to a study published in 2023 by *JAMA Internal Medicine.*

With individuals needing a small cuff, using a regular-sized cuff produced an average systolic reading (the top number) that was 3.6 millimeters of mercury (mm Hg) lower than with an appropriately sized cuff. On the other hand, for adults who needed a large or extra-large cuff size, using a regular-sized cuff resulted in higher systolic readings—an average of 4.8 mm Hg and 19.5 mm Hg, respectively. Smaller discrepancies also appeared in diastolic blood pressure readings (the bottom number) for adults who had cuffs that were either too large or too small. The researchers pointed out that most home blood pressure monitors come with a regular-sized cuff, which can accommodate arm circumferences of nine to 17 inches, but smaller and larger cuffs are available.

If you have questions about whether the size of your home blood pressure cuff is right for you, bring it with you to your next medical appointment and compare its results to those obtained by your doctor.

24-hour blood pressure monitoring outperforms clinic readings

Ambulatory blood pressure monitoring (ABPM) involves wearing a device that automatically records blood pressure every 30 to 60 minutes for 24 hours. New research suggests that ABPM—especially the nighttime readings—can better predict death from cardiovascular disease and other causes than conventional blood pressure readings done in a clinic.

The study included more than 59,000 people (average age 59) from 223 primary care practices in Spain. Most (59%) were being treated for high blood

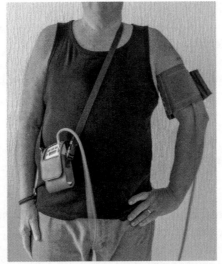

© clubfoto | Getty Images

Nighttime and continuous blood pressure monitoring may help save lives.

pressure. Researchers estimated the association between patients' clinic blood pressure and ABPM readings and deaths occurring during a median follow-up of nearly 10 years.

They found that ABPM was almost five times more informative for predicting death than clinic blood pressure measurements, and the nighttime readings were about six times more informative. The findings highlight the need to evaluate and control nighttime blood pressure, say the authors, whose study was published in 2023 by the journal *Lancet.*

Breathing exercises to lower your blood pressure

A regular breathing practice may reduce blood pressure as much as taking medication.

The average person breathes in and out some 22,000 times each day, usually with little effort or thought. But here's something worth pondering: practicing slow, deep breathing for just a few minutes a day can lower blood pressure, potentially reducing the first number in a reading (systolic blood pressure) by up to 10 points.

"Anyone with stage 1 hypertension, which is defined as a systolic reading of 130 to 139, should know that breathing exercises are an effective way to lower blood pressure without medication," says Dr. Kimberly Parks, a cardiologist at Harvard-affiliated Massachusetts General Hospital. For people with elevated blood pressure (a systolic reading of 120 to 129), deep breathing could help them avoid high blood pressure in the future, she adds.

Deep breathing benefits

For an adult at rest, a normal respiration rate ranges from 12 to 18 breaths per minute. Slow breathing, in contrast, is usually defined as anywhere from six to 10 breaths per minute and features a prolonged, slow exhalation period.

As you slowly inhale, your diaphragm (the strong sheet of muscle that separates your chest from your abdomen) contracts and pulls downward. Fully expanding your lungs stimulates the vagus nerve, which runs from the brain to the colon. This activates the "rest and digest" response of your nervous system. A larger volume of air in the lungs delivers extra oxygen to your body and brain, which increases the release of feel-good chemicals called endorphins and lowers levels of epinephrine, a stress hormone.

As you exhale, the diaphragm presses back upward against your lungs. As blood moves out of your lungs, your blood pressure rises slightly. To counteract that rise, your nervous system automatically lowers your heart rate and widens your blood vessels—another example of the "rest and digest" response. Prolonging your exhalation takes advantage of this reflex.

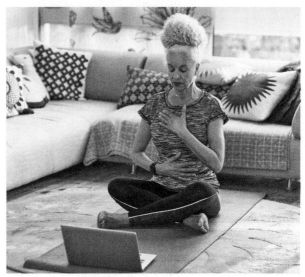

© Gary Burchell | Getty Images

Short stints of deep, slow breathing help calm your nervous system, lowering blood pressure.

What's the evidence?

A review article published in 2023 in *Frontiers in Physiology* looked at the effects of different breathing exercises in people with high blood pressure. Of the 20 studies included in the review, 17 documented declines in both systolic and diastolic blood pressure (diastolic is the second number in a reading). The studies varied widely in terms of how long, how often, and what type of breathing exercises the participants did, so it's hard to provide one specific prescription.

But it's likely that any type of breathing practice can be beneficial, says Dr. Parks. With her patients, she offers a menu of choices, she says: "I tell them, 'Here are several ways you can start a breathing practice. Which one seems best for you?'" The following are her suggestions.

For inspiration, count breaths

Try counting to five while breathing in through your nose, then exhaling for five counts. "Purse your lips, like you're blowing out candles on a birthday cake, which will help slow down your exhalation," says Dr. Parks. You can also try holding your breath after the inhalation period. One common pattern involves inhaling for four counts, holding for seven, and exhaling for eight, but you can vary the timing as you wish. Audio and visual prompts may be helpful. Look online for guided breathing exercises, or download one of the many free apps available for use on a smartphone or smart watch. ▶▶

Some people are drawn to the ancient technique of *pranayama* (*prana* is Sanskrit for breath; *ayama* means stretching or lengthening). This practice, often done as a part of yoga, comes in many different forms. Harvard Health Publishing's website has video demonstrations; see www.health.harvard.edu/alternate-nostril-breath for one example.

Device-guided breathing

For those who find meditation-focused practices too kooky, using a device might be more appealing, says Dr. Parks. Inspiratory muscle strength training (IMST) uses a small, handheld device that provides resistance as you inhale and exhale. You can buy the devices online for as little as $20. In 2021, a well-designed study in the *Journal of the American Heart Association* showed that doing IMST for just 30 breaths per day, six days per week, reduced systolic blood pressure by an average of nine points after six weeks.

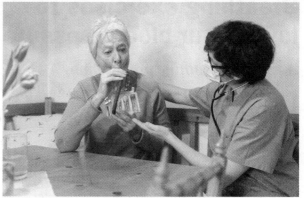

© Joos Mind | Getty Images

Inspiratory exercise devices help train breathing patterns, which can lower blood pressure.

A more elaborate option is an FDA-cleared device called Resperate, sold online for $350. It features a chest strap with a sensor to monitor your breathing pattern. You follow musical cues via headphones to gradually slow down your breathing.

IN THE JOURNALS

For controlling blood pressure, telemedicine may beat clinic visits

Telemedicine visits combined with self-measured blood pressure readings may help people control high blood pressure better than traditional office visits, according to a study published in 2024 in the journal *Hypertension*.

Researchers reviewed data from 31 trials lasting between six and 12 months that compared telemedicine to clinic visits for managing blood pressure. The telemedicine visits relied on blood pressure readings taken by patients at home, along with remote contact with health care providers via phone, video, or email.

In people using telemedicine, systolic blood pressure (the top number in a reading) dropped by an average of 7.3 points compared with office-based care. This advantage appeared more pronounced when the patients' medications were managed by pharmacists, who are well versed in drug interactions and dosing levels.

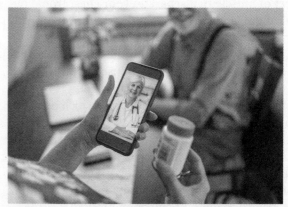

© PIKSEL | Getty Images

Virtual doctor appointments combined with home blood pressure monitoring may benefit heart health.

Blood pressure measurements vary widely at the doctor's office

About half of U.S. adults have high blood pressure, and only a quarter of them have it under control. Yet most people with high blood pressure don't monitor it at home; they rely only on measurements taken at health care visits. That's not going to give you an accurate picture, suggests a study published in 2023 by *Circulation: Cardiovascular Quality and Outcomes.*

In the study, researchers evaluated more than 7.7 million blood pressure measurements taken from more than 537,000 adults (average age 53) over more than two years. Each participant averaged 13 doctor visits during that time. The study found wide variations in blood pressure measurements from one visit to the next—especially in people with known high blood pressure. While a person's blood pressure can change substantially from hour to hour, the researchers say that faulty equipment or imprecise techniques used to measure blood pressure at the doctor's office may also explain the variability. Such wide variations in readings can make it hard to determine if blood pressure drugs are working or if someone should start taking medication. For more accurate measurements, take your blood pressure at home regularly, two or three times per week.

Eating more tomatoes may help lower high blood pressure

Can consuming more tomatoes help lower the risk of hypertension (high blood pressure)? A 2023 study published by the *European Journal of Preventive Cardiology* looked at about 7,000 people (ages 55 to 80) participating in the Spanish PREDIMED dietary study. About 83% of them had hypertension, and they all had one or more other cardiovascular risk factors, such as diabetes, smoking, high cholesterol, excess weight, or a family history of early-onset heart disease. Everyone filled out annual questionnaires on their food consumption, including raw tomatoes, tomato sauce, and gazpacho (a Spanish tomato soup). After three years,

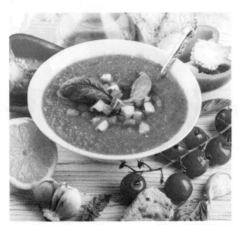
© Seqoya | Getty Images
A tomato a day keeps the cardiologist away?

researchers observed an association between eating more tomatoes and lower blood pressure. They also found that among participants who did not have hypertension at the start of the study, those who consumed the most tomatoes (more than 110 grams—about one large tomato—per day) reduced their overall risk for hypertension by 36%, compared with those who consumed the least (less than 44 grams). Researchers suggested that tomatoes' high amounts of lycopene are a possible reason. Lycopene, a plant chemical that gives tomatoes their red color, is a powerful antioxidant that helps fight inflammation and molecules that damage cells.

The new RNA-targeted drugs for heart disease

These cutting-edge therapies take aim at proteins that play a role in elevated cholesterol levels and high blood pressure.

Many people swallow two to three drugs daily to lower their cholesterol and blood pressure to healthy levels. What if they could achieve the same results with medications that require just a few injections per year—with no pills?

This isn't just a far-flung promise. Inclisiran (Leqvio), a long-lasting injectable drug that dramatically lowers LDL cholesterol, was approved in 2021. It's the first cholesterol-lowering medication that works through RNA interference, a technique that's the basis for an expanding class of novel therapies for treating a variety of diseases. Several additional RNA-targeted drugs for cardiovascular disease are currently in late-stage trials. How exactly do these drugs work, and who might benefit from them?

Harnessing the power of RNA

Found in all living cells, RNA is the molecule that copies and transfers genetic instructions from DNA (the cell's genetic blueprint) to create proteins. The human body contains tens of thousands of different proteins that provide countless functions, including supporting tissues and organs, carrying out biochemical reactions, and ferrying different molecules around the body. Many diseases, it turns out, result from problems with proteins.

For example, in people with very high cholesterol (hypercholesterolemia), the body produces too much low-density lipoprotein (LDL), one of the proteins that transports cholesterol. While cholesterol is vital for making cell membranes, many hormones, and vitamin D, excess cholesterol in the bloodstream contributes to artery-clogging plaque. Certain drugs for hypercholesterolemia use antibodies to block PCSK9, a protein made in the liver that regulates LDL. But inclisiran prevents PCSK9 from being made in the first place.

"Many of these therapies work by interfering with the strand of RNA before it has the opportunity to be synthesized into a protein," says cardiologist Dr. Michelle O'Donoghue, associate professor of medicine at Harvard Medical School. Some, known as small-interfering RNA (siRNA) drugs, have long-lasting effects. After being injected, the drug travels to the liver and, in the case of inclisiran, interferes with the

IN THE JOURNALS

Couples often share high blood pressure diagnoses

If your spouse has high blood pressure (hypertension), there's a fairly good chance that you do as well, new research suggests.

For the 2023 study, published in the *Journal of the American Heart Association,* researchers looked at the incidence of hypertension in nearly 34,000 middle-age and older heterosexual couples in India, China, the United States, and England. Women married to men with hypertension were more likely to have hypertension themselves than women whose husbands didn't have the condition. Likewise, hypertension rates were higher among men whose wives had hypertension compared to men whose wives did not. Rates of this so-called concordant hypertension ranged from 20% to 40% and were slightly higher in China and India.

Couple-focused strategies to address the problem together, such as exercise and other lifestyle changes, could be helpful, according to an editorial accompanying the study.

creation of PCSK9. Among people with stubbornly high cholesterol who are already taking the maximum dose of a statin, the drug reduces blood levels of LDL by about half.

Silencing Lp(a)

Other RNA-interfering drugs in development target a different particle called lipoprotein(a), or Lp(a). These particles feature an extra lipoprotein molecule that makes them "stickier," which appears to accelerate fatty plaque buildup inside arteries even more than regular LDL. High levels of Lp(a)—which affect about one in five people in the general population—have been linked to a higher risk of heart attack, stroke, and narrowing of the aortic valve (aortic stenosis).

Because Lp(a) levels are largely based on genetic factors, eating and exercise habits don't seem to affect the levels in your bloodstream. As yet, there are no FDA-approved drugs shown to effectively lower Lp(a), which is frustrating for patients and doctors alike. However, there are many promising drugs in the pipeline. Pelacarsen, olpasiran, zerlasiran, and lepodisiran are given by injection every one to six months and have been shown to lower Lp(a) levels between 70% and 100%. Larger, longer trials looking at whether these drugs will help prevent heart-related problems are currently under way, with results expected within the next few years, says Dr. O'Donoghue, who is a lead investigator on the clinical trials of olpasiran.

Decreasing blood pressure

Another siRNA drug, zilebesiran, interferes with the liver's production of angiotensinogen, a protein that plays a key role in blood pressure regulation. Nearly half of all adults have high blood pressure, defined as a reading at or above 130/80 mm Hg. And only about 22% of people with the condition have it under control, despite the availability of more than 200 different blood pressure medications.

In an early study, zilebesiran led to meaningful drops in blood pressure that persisted for six months; ongoing studies are testing it in combination with different blood pressure drugs. One concern about this particular drug, however, is that its effects can't be quickly reversed, which could pose problems for people who receive it and then later develop a serious infection or another condition that causes dangerously low blood pressure.

To date, side effects from all these medications are uncommon and include mild redness or pain at the injection site. "None have been studied on a large enough scale that we can be completely confident about their efficacy and safety. That's what the ongoing trials will answer. But so far, the evidence is encouraging," says Dr. O'Donoghue.

For heart-health benefits, add oats and barley to your diet

Rich in a type of fiber called beta glucans, barley has special heart-health benefits that help lower blood cholesterol levels. While barley is well known as an ingredient in soup, this chewy grain is equally delicious in casseroles, side dishes, and salads. Choose hulled barley (available as grains, grits, flakes, or flour) over pearl barley, which has been processed to remove the bran.

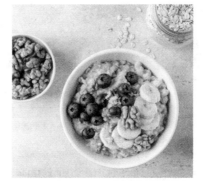

© ArxOnt I Getty Images

Oats and barley both contain beta glucans, a heart-healthy fiber.

Oats also help lower cholesterol levels. A humble bowl of oatmeal can be delicious (add heart-healthy nuts, cinnamon, and dried fruit). Like barley, oats are a source of the rare group of fibers called beta glucans, and (when eaten daily) have been linked with significantly lower blood cholesterol levels. Go beyond the breakfast table and add oats to dishes like veggie burgers, risotto, breads, and fruit-based desserts.

The portfolio diet to lower cholesterol: A smart investment for your heart

This eating pattern highlights a variety of plant-based foods that help lower cholesterol.

The portfolio diet, which emphasizes plant foods rich in fiber and healthy fats, was conceived some 20 years ago. Since then, many studies have documented the diet's ability to lower harmful LDL cholesterol. But because none of those trials lasted any longer than six months, the portfolio diet's long-term returns were unknown. Now, new research suggests that the more closely you follow a portfolio-style eating pattern, the greater your protection against heart disease and stroke.

Published in 2023 in *Circulation*, the study included more than 210,000 people who enrolled in three Harvard-led health studies in the 1980s and 1990s. Using data from diet questionnaires the participants filled out every four years, researchers scored each person's diet based on how well it complied with the portfolio eating pattern. After 30 years of follow-up, researchers compared the scores with the participants' health outcomes. People with higher scores (that is, those who followed the diet most closely) had a 14% lower risk of heart disease compared to those with lower scores.

"A lot of different foods can lower LDL cholesterol, but only by a little bit—about 5% to 10%. The idea behind the portfolio diet was to combine many of these foods together to get a larger reduction," says registered dietitian Andrea Glenn, a postdoctoral research fellow at the Harvard T.H. Chan School of Public Health and a co-author of the study.

Earlier studies found that the portfolio diet may lower LDL cholesterol by as much as 30%. In the new study, people with higher portfolio diet scores not only had better cholesterol profiles, they also had lower blood levels of C-reactive protein and other inflammatory substances compared to people with lower scores, says Glenn. Inflammation is a key player in the buildup of fatty plaque inside arteries—the root cause of most heart attacks.

What's in the portfolio diet?

The diet discourages foods from animal sources, particularly red and processed meat, high-fat dairy, and eggs, which means it's naturally low in saturated fat and dietary cholesterol, both of which raise LDL cholesterol in the body. The featured foods fall into five main categories. Here's a rundown, including ways to incorporate them into your meals.

Plant protein. This includes beans, lentils, and peas (collectively known as legumes), with a specific focus on foods made from soybeans, says Glenn. In 1999, the FDA authorized a health claim for soy protein, noting that consuming at least 25 grams daily as part of a diet low in cholesterol and saturated fat may lower the risk of heart disease. Soy protein comes in many different forms: edamame (whole, green soybeans often sold frozen in pods), soy milk, soy yogurt, tofu, or tempeh (fermented soybeans). But there are many other legumes to choose from, including black beans, pinto beans, chickpeas (garbanzo beans), lentils, and dried split green peas.

Nuts and seeds. All nuts—including almonds, cashews, hazelnuts, pecans, pistachios, walnuts—are included. So are

---

Try this plant protein

▶ Swap out some of the meat in homemade soups, stews, or casseroles with beans or tofu.

▶ Replace some dairy products (like milk and yogurt) with soy-based versions.

▶ Snack on edamame or hummus.

Try these nuts and seeds

▶ Add nuts or seeds to hot cereal, muffins or other baked goods, yogurt, and salads.

▶ Spread peanut butter or other nut butters on whole-grain crackers or sliced apples.

▶ Snack on mixed nuts.

Try this viscous fiber

▶ Build what Glenn calls a "super portfolio breakfast": oatmeal topped with soy milk, fruit, nuts, and seeds. Try combos such as raspberries, chopped walnuts, and chia seeds or diced apples, almonds, and sesame seeds.

▶ Swap regular bread for oat bran bread.

▶ Try different ways to prepare eggplant, such as a Chinese-style stir-fry or ratatouille, a French vegetable stew.

all sorts of seeds: chia, flax, hemp, pumpkin, sunflower, sesame.

Viscous fiber. Viscous fiber is a type of soluble fiber that has a somewhat sticky quality, says Glenn. "It's found in grains like oats and barley, certain vegetables such as eggplant and okra, and fruits like apples, oranges, berries, and persimmons," she says. One of the best sources is psyllium seed husks, which transform into a viscous gel when dissolved in water. People may be familiar with psyllium because the powdered husks are the key ingredient in Metamucil, which helps treat constipation, says Glenn. But you can buy plain psyllium seed husk in stores.

In the intestines, viscous fiber binds to bile acids, which carry fats from your small intestine into the large intestine for excretion. This triggers your liver to create more bile acids—a process that requires cholesterol. If the liver doesn't have enough cholesterol, it draws more from the bloodstream, in turn lowering your circulating LDL. In addition, viscous fiber is fermented in the gut into short-chain fatty acids, which may also inhibit cholesterol production.

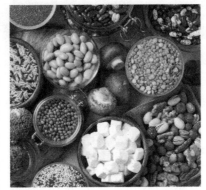
© Aamulya | Getty Images

The portfolio diet promotes consumption of plant-based sources of protein such as beans, lentils, peas, tofu, and nuts.

Plant sterols. Also known as phytosterols, these exist naturally in nuts, soybeans, peas, and canola oil. Plant sterols have a structure similar to cholesterol; eating them helps limit the amount of cholesterol your body can absorb. Margarine enriched with plant sterols, such as Benecol, provides a concentrated dose. But you have to eat quite a bit (about four tablespoons daily) to make a difference, says Glenn. It tastes similar to other types of margarine and can be used as a spread for toast and in sandwiches.

Monounsaturated fats. Used in place of saturated fats, these fats help lower cholesterol. Extra-virgin olive oil is the top recommendation; other good options include canola, soybean, or "high-oleic" sunflower or safflower oils. Stock a variety of these oils for use on salads and in cooking and baking. Avocados are also rich in monounsaturated fat.

You don't need to embrace every aspect of the diet to reap benefits, says Glenn. "But we saw a dose-related response in the study, which means that the more of these foods were added to the diet, the lower the risk of cardiovascular disease we observed," she says. ▼

IN THE JOURNALS

A vegan diet improves cholesterol versus an omnivore diet

Twins who ate a vegan diet for two months had better cardiometabolic health than their identical siblings who ate an omnivorous diet, a new study found.

The study, which appeared in 2023 in *JAMA Network Open*, included 22 pairs of identical twins. One twin from each pair was assigned a vegan diet, and the other an omnivore diet. Both diets contained fruits and vegetables, beans, and whole grains but limited sugars and refined starches. While the omnivore diet included animal-based foods such as chicken, fish, and dairy products, the vegan diet excluded all those foods and was entirely plant-based.

At the end of the study (after eight weeks on the diet), participants following the vegan diet had LDL cholesterol levels that were an average of 13.9 points lower than those on the omnivore diet. The vegans also had significantly lower insulin levels and lost an average of 4.2 pounds compared to the omnivores. The findings support what many earlier studies have shown: plant-based diets help improve heart health.

by **CHRISTOPHER CANNON, M.D.,** Editor in Chief, *Harvard Heart Letter*

Do I still need to keep taking a statin?

Q *I'm 81 years old, and I've been on a statin drug for 30 years because I'm at increased risk for heart disease. At my age, do I need to still keep taking it?*

A Statin drugs were introduced into medical practice in the 1980s. They are very effective at lowering LDL (bad) cholesterol and in reducing inflammation inside cholesterol-filled plaques of atherosclerosis. In people older than 75, are they still effective in lowering cholesterol and in reducing the risk of heart disease? In the last few years, we have started to get solid information that addresses your question.

A 2023 study from Denmark, published in *Annals of Internal Medicine*, included about 84,000 people—about 10,000 of whom were older than 75. Participants began taking one of two different statin drugs, simvastatin (Zocor) or atorvastatin (Lipitor), between 2008 and 2018. The study found that the people most likely to have their LDL cholesterol lowered by statin drugs were those older than 75.

So, statins remain effective at lowering cholesterol in people older than 75. But do they also reduce the risk of developing heart disease? Another observational study from Denmark, published in 2020 in *The Lancet,* identified more than 90,000 people not on statins who were free of heart disease or diabetes (a risk factor for heart disease)—and then started taking a statin drug. Over an average follow-up period of 7.7 years, the people who were most likely to benefit from statin drugs were those older than 75.

Randomized trials provide stronger evidence than observational studies. However, relatively few randomized trials of the ability of statins and other cholesterol-lowering drugs to reduce heart disease risk have included people older than 75. To overcome that problem, an international team based here at Harvard pooled the results for more than 21,000 people older than 75 (and even more who were younger than 75) from multiple different cholesterol-lowering drug trials. The study, published in 2020 in *The Lancet,* found that the older group benefited at least as much as the younger group.

In short, for people older than 75 who have heart disease already, or who, like you, are at increased risk of developing heart disease, I think there now is solid evidence that statins remain effective at lowering cholesterol and, more important, in reducing the risk of new or recurrent heart disease. For people older than 75 who have not been diagnosed with heart disease and are not at increased risk for developing it, I think the value of statins still is uncertain.

© Blend Images LWA/Dann Tardif | Getty Images

Work with your doctor to decide if taking a statin past age 75 is right for you.

Statin alternative lowers heart-related deaths

For people who can't take statin drugs, a cholesterol-lowering drug called bempedoic acid (Nexletol) can also lower the risk of heart attacks and related problems, a new study shows.

Published in *JAMA*, the 2023 study included about 4,200 people with high LDL (bad) cholesterol who experienced statin side effects. Their average age was 68, and two-thirds had diabetes. Participants took either bempedoic acid or a placebo. Over a follow-up period of 40 months, those taking the drug were 30% less likely to die of a heart-related condition, have a heart attack or stroke, or need an artery-opening stent compared with the placebo group. Bempedoic acid reduced LDL levels by 21%.

About 5% to 10% of people who try statins have to stop taking them, mostly because of muscle-related symptoms. This problem is less likely with bempedoic acid, although the drug has other side effects, including a slightly increased risk of gout and gallstones. Still, bempedoic acid can be a good alternative for people at high risk of heart disease who don't do well on statins.

Dietary salt and blood pressure: A complex connection

Genetic variations play a role in salt sensitivity, which affects your risk of heart disease.

One of the cardinal rules of heart-healthy eating is to avoid excess salt, which makes sense. The average American consumes the equivalent of about 1½ teaspoons of salt per day—about 50% more than the recommended amount. Getting too much sodium (a main component of salt) is closely linked to having high blood pressure (see "How sodium affects blood pressure").

But on an individual basis, people respond differently to sodium. About a third of healthy people—and about 60% of people with high blood pressure—are salt sensitive, meaning they have a strong response to dietary sodium. Their blood pressure rises by 5 points or more if they switch from a low-salt to a high-salt diet. However, an estimated one in 10 people have what's called inverse salt sensitivity: their blood pressure goes up when they eat less salt.

Unfortunately, there's no easy way to tell who is sensitive or insensitive to salt, and many people fall somewhere in the middle of those two extremes. But research is helping unravel the genetic basis of these differences, which

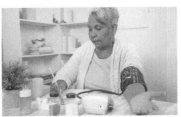
© LifestyleVisuals | Getty Images
Most people with high blood pressure are salt sensitive, meaning their blood pressure rises when they eat a high-sodium diet.

may one day improve how doctors treat high blood pressure, according to endocrinologist Dr. Gordon Williams, professor of medicine at Harvard Medical School.

The genetics of salt sensitivity

To date, there are 18 known genetic variants associated with salt sensitivity and blood pressure. Dr. Williams and colleagues recently discovered that one variant, which encodes a protein called striatin, leads to salt sensitivity by two distinct mechanisms that differ by sex. "In men, the striatin variant causes problems with blood flow through the kidneys. But in women, the variant causes an inappropriate rise in the hormone aldosterone," says Dr. Williams. Secreted by the adrenal glands, aldosterone helps the kidneys regulate water, sodium, and potassium.

Targeted treatment?

The 2024 findings, published in *Hypertension*, could have implications for treating high blood pressure. Men with the striatin variant would respond better ▸▸

to blood pressure drugs known as ACE inhibitors and angiotensin-receptor blockers,* whereas women would benefit more from drugs that target aldosterone and act as diuretics, called mineralocorticoid-receptor antagonists.*

In fact, giving the "wrong" drug (that is, a drug different than what the genetic findings suggest would be best) might even be detrimental, says Dr. Williams. Of note: This study included only white people. Black people may be more likely to have salt sensitivity than whites, possibly due to other genetic variants that predispose them to retain sodium.

Genetic differences related to how people's bodies handle salt help explain the longstanding observation that for some people, finding the best blood pressure drug is a matter of trial and error, Williams says. "If one drug doesn't work, we try other drugs from different classes until we find a combination that works," he says. Salt-sensitivity genes may also explain why some people have low blood pressure despite eating a high-salt diet.

How sodium affects blood pressure

Your body responds to excess sodium by holding on to water to dilute the sodium. As a result, the amount of fluid within your blood vessels increases. That raises the pressure inside your blood vessels and makes the heart work harder. In fact, excess sodium essentially counteracts the benefits of two types of blood pressure medications—namely, diuretics and vasodilators. Diuretics* help flush excess fluid and sodium from the body, while vasodilators* relax blood vessel walls. A high-sodium diet will cause the body to retain additional fluid and refill your relaxed arteries, putting you back where you started.

*The American Heart Association describes and lists examples of common heart medications, including blood pressure medications, here: health.harvard.edu/heartattacktreatment.

© DJClaassen I Getty Images

Using a person's genetic profile to optimize drug therapy—an approach known as precision medicine—is already used to treat many cancers and certain rare genetic diseases. One day, we may be able to apply this same precision to high blood pressure. "If future clinical trials confirm the most important variants, a simple blood test could reveal which blood pressure drugs would work best for you and how much salt is safe for you to consume," says Dr. Williams.

Reducing sodium can help most people lower their blood pressure

The degree to which sodium intake affects blood pressure varies. For many people with hypertension (high blood pressure), eating a high-sodium diet definitively increases blood pressure. But a 2023 study published by *JAMA* found that dramatically lowering sodium intake can potentially lead to lower readings for the great majority of people, even those with normal blood pressure.

Researchers recruited 213 adults, ages 50 to 75. Some had normal pressure, and some had hypertension. For one week, everyone was randomly assigned to follow either a high-sodium diet—an extra 2,200 milligrams (mg) of sodium per day above their usual intake—or a very low-sodium diet, at a total of 500 mg of sodium per day. They then switched to the opposite diet for another week.

When the researchers compared the results, they found that a very low-sodium diet could significantly reduce blood pressure in about 74% of the participants—regardless of their prior blood pressure status or whether they took blood pressure medication.

The findings suggest that more people than previously recognized have sodium-sensitive increases in their blood pressure, even if they don't have hypertension. While it's unrealistic to expect people to limit sodium intake to the extremely low levels used in this study, efforts to decrease the average American's consumption of 3,400 mg sodium per day can have major health benefits.

When high blood pressure affects the lungs

Pulmonary hypertension—a serious illness that affects the lungs and heart—is challenging to diagnose and treat.

High blood pressure (what doctors call hypertension) usually affects all the body's arteries, the vessels that carry blood from the heart to the rest of the body. But a separate condition, known as pulmonary hypertension, causes abnormally high blood pressure in the arteries that carry blood from the right side of the heart to the lungs (see illustration). This serious condition has many possible causes, including a range of diseases and underlying conditions as well as genetic mutations and exposure to certain drugs. Pulmonary hypertension and classic hypertension can occur together in the same person, but the two conditions are not related.

While there's no cure for pulmonary hypertension, various treatments can ease symptoms and slow the progression of the disease. Earlier this year, researchers reported promising results with an experimental drug called sotatercept in people with pulmonary arterial hypertension (PAH), one of the five main types of pulmonary hypertension (see "Types of pulmonary hypertension").

"The drug targets one of the dysregulated signaling pathways that causes PAH," says cardiologist Dr. Jane Leopold, associate professor of medicine at Harvard Medical School. In a study of people with PAH (most of whom were already taking two or three other medications), the drug improved their ability to exercise as measured by a six-minute walk test. The study was published in 2023 in *The New England Journal of Medicine*. Sotatercept, which is given by injection every three weeks, acts like a sponge, trapping specific molecules responsible for causing the pulmonary arteries to narrow and stiffen, says Dr. Leopold. While the drug was tested only in people with PAH, it might also prove beneficial for certain other types of pulmonary hypertension, she adds.

Diagnosis and treatment

Pulmonary hypertension doesn't have any distinct warning signs. Early in the disease, people feel fatigued and short of breath during physical activity. "But these vague symptoms are easy to attribute to being out of shape or simply growing older," says Dr. Leopold. As the disease advances, the most common symptoms, including dizziness, chest pressure, and palpitations, are similar to those of other heart and lung conditions. As a result, it takes an average of two years to correctly diagnose a person with pulmonary hypertension, Dr. Leopold says. ▶▶

Types of pulmonary hypertension

Experts classify pulmonary hypertension into five groups, based on the underlying cause, as follows:

1. Pulmonary arterial hypertension. This occurs when the pulmonary arteries become narrow, thick, or stiff, raising blood pressure inside the vessels. Causes include inborn heart problems or other genetic causes, use of certain drugs (including methamphetamine), and such diseases as HIV/AIDS, chronic liver disease, and connective tissue disorders.

2. Left-sided heart disease. This category includes mitral valve or aortic valve disease and problems with the heart's main pumping chamber (left ventricle). These conditions cause blood to back up in the heart, raising pressure in the pulmonary arteries.

3. Lung diseases. These include chronic obstructive pulmonary disease and scarring inside the lungs (pulmonary fibrosis). These disorders limit blood flow through the lungs, raising pulmonary blood pressure.

4. Blockages in the lungs. Blood clots and the scars caused by these clots prevent normal blood flow through the lungs. The resulting stress on the right side of the heart elevates blood pressure in the pulmonary circulation.

5. Other health conditions. Certain types of blood, metabolic, kidney, and inflammatory disorders are associated with pulmonary hypertension. But the underlying connections and triggers remain uncertain.

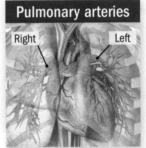

Pulmonary arteries

Right   Left

Pulmonary hypertension affects the artery that carries blood from the heart's right side to the lungs.

© Leonello Calvetti/Science Photo Library | Getty Images

▶▶ First, doctors rule out more common problems, including thyroid, liver, or heart problems, some of which may underlie pulmonary hypertension. But the only way to definitively diagnose pulmonary hypertension is a right heart catheterization, which directly measures the pressure inside the pulmonary arteries and checks how much blood your heart pumps per minute. Imaging tests (including ultrasounds and CT scans of the heart), lung function tests, blood tests, and other tests can help pinpoint the underlying cause.

In addition to addressing conditions that contribute to pulmonary hypertension, treatment may include medications that ease symptoms, slow the progression of the disease, and reduce its complications. People with pulmonary hypertension are now surviving longer than in the past, thanks to earlier diagnosis that enables treatment to start sooner, Dr. Leopold says. The Pulmonary Hypertension Association (www.phassociation.org) has additional information for patients, including resources for finding in-person, phone, and online support groups. ♥

Overcoming resistant hypertension

This condition is more common among older adults who battle high blood pressure.

Up to 70% of adults ages 65 and older have high blood pressure (hypertension). This is diagnosed when your systolic pressure (the top number on a blood pressure reading) measures 130 millimeters of mercury (mm Hg) or higher or your diastolic pressure (the bottom number) measures 80 mm Hg or higher.

Common drug treatments include calcium-channel blockers, ACE inhibitors, angiotensin-receptor blockers (ARBs), and diuretics, given either individually or in combination. Calcium-channel blockers help blood vessels relax, and ACE inhibitors and ARBs block a key hormone pathway involved in raising blood pressure, while diuretics eliminate excess sodium and water in the body. Adopting healthy habits that help lower high blood pressure is also an important part of the treatment strategy—like losing weight, quitting smoking, reducing salt in your diet, and being more active.

Extra help

However, some people do not respond to such therapies. If your blood pressure remains above 130/80 mm Hg despite following healthy habits and taking the best dosage you can tolerate of at least three different blood pressure medications (with one being a diuretic), you have what's called resistant hypertension.

"Resistant hypertension often takes longer to control and requires more intensive evaluation," says Dr. Naomi D.L. Fisher, director of the Hypertension Service at Harvard-affiliated Brigham and Women's Hospital. "We

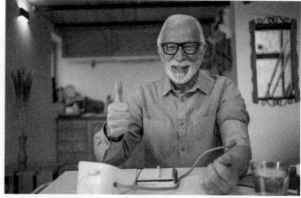
© Milan Markovic | Getty Images

Monitoring your blood pressure at home helps to ensure more accurate readings.

pay close and careful attention to patients with resistant hypertension, as it can significantly increase a person's risk for a heart attack or stroke."

About 20% of people with hypertension battle resistant hypertension, according to the most recent statistics from the American Heart Association. Still, some people may be classified as having resistant hypertension when other factors are keeping their blood pressure elevated. "These should be checked first before making changes to existing medication," says Dr. Fisher.

For instance, people might not be taking their blood pressure medication as prescribed. They may skip doses because they forget, fear possible side effects, don't think the problem is serious, or can't afford the pills. "Speak with your doctor if you're having trouble taking your medication," says Dr. Fisher. "The doctor may offer solutions, like finding more affordable medication, combining pills, or changing your dosage to make it easier to take."

Other problems

Another issue is white-coat syndrome. Blood pressure readings are often taken at a doctor's office or medical clinic. These environments can increase anxiety levels and temporarily spike blood pressure. There are a few ways around this problem.

For instance, after your first reading at the office, ask the nurse or medical assistant who took your blood pressure to repeat the measurement after several minutes to see if it has changed. You also can help ease anxiety by doing several minutes of deep breathing exercises before your reading.

Still another option is to take readings at home with a blood pressure machine. If you have hypertension, guidelines recommend you measure your blood pressure in the morning and evening for one week—always before taking your pill—and then share the information with your doctor.

What's next

Your doctor will also explore other underlying issues that can contribute to resistant hypertension. These may include the following:

Sleep apnea. This common condition is marked by repeated pauses in your breathing—lasting from a few seconds to a minute or so—while you sleep. Research has found that sleep apnea can quadruple the odds of having resistant hypertension among people at high risk for heart disease.

Alcohol. Excess drinking can elevate blood pressure. "Men should limit their intake to no more than two drinks daily," says Dr. Fisher.

NSAIDs. Nonsteroidal anti-inflammatory drugs (NSAIDs)—over-the-counter painkillers like ibuprofen (Advil, Motrin) and naproxen (Aleve)—can raise systolic blood pressure anywhere from 2 mm Hg to 5 mm Hg. "If you are taking more than occasional doses to control pain, you should discuss this with your doctor," says Dr. Fisher. Your doctor also may check for specific medical conditions that can affect blood pressure, such as kidney disease or a problem with one or both adrenal glands.

After all these boxes have been checked, there are other steps your doctor can take to treat resistant hypertension. These include re-examining your lifestyle habits, increasing your current medication dosage (if possible), or adding a fourth drug from another class, such as a mineralocorticoid-receptor antagonist like spironolactone (Aldactone) or eplerenone (Inspra), which inhibits harmful actions of the adrenal hormone aldosterone.

IN THE JOURNALS

Treating high blood pressure may lower dementia risk

Older adults who take medications to lower their blood pressure may reduce their risk of dementia, according to a 2023 study published in *JAMA Network Open*.

The report pooled findings from 17 separate observational studies that included a total of more than 34,000 adults ages 60 to 110. Their average age was 72, and they were followed for four years, on average. People with untreated high blood pressure were 42% more likely to develop dementia compared with healthy older adults. Those who were untreated had a 26% greater risk than people with treated high blood pressure. And when researchers compared people with treated high blood pressure to healthy older adults without high blood pressure, they found no meaningful difference in dementia risk between the two groups. The findings reinforce the connection between heart and brain health and suggest that treating high blood pressure in later life may benefit both organs.

When blood pressure falls after you stand up

Known as orthostatic hypotension, this condition becomes more common with age and frailty.

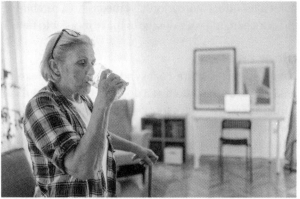

© supersizer | Getty Images

Drinking water throughout the day may help people deal with orthostatic hypotension, which causes blood pressure dips upon standing.

That odd sensation of feeling lightheaded or dizzy after standing up happens to most people at least once in a while. Caused by a temporary delay in blood flow to the brain, the feeling usually resolves within a few seconds. But in some people, blood pressure plummets and stays low for a minute or longer after they stand up from a seated position. The problem, known as orthostatic hypotension (hypotension means low blood pressure) can cause people to fall, possibly leading to injury and disability.

However, most people with orthostatic hypotension don't have any symptoms. Another complication: it affects about one in 10 people with high blood pressure, which is very common in older adults. In fact, nearly 75% of people ages 60 and older have blood pressure readings of 130/80 mm Hg or higher (the definition of high blood pressure). An optimal blood pressure level is less than 120/80 mm Hg.

"Current guidelines for treating high blood pressure encourage doctors to screen people for orthostatic hypotension," says Dr. Alyson Kelley-Hedgepeth, a cardiologist at Harvard-affiliated Brigham and Women's Hospital. It's defined as a decrease in systolic pressure (the first number of a blood pressure reading) of at least 20 points or a decrease in diastolic pressure (the second number) of at least 10 points when measured within three minutes after standing up from a seated position.

What causes orthostatic hypotension?

When you stand, gravity pulls blood downward, away from your brain and heart. Special receptors in your neck and above your heart activate nerve and hormonal signals that tell your heart to beat stronger and faster while narrowing your blood vessels. This temporarily raises blood pressure and restores normal blood flow to the brain and heart. But with age, those monitoring receptors can become less responsive and don't immediately notice the drop in blood pressure.

When treating people with high blood pressure, doctors sometimes worry that intensive treatment (that is, taking medications that drive blood pressure down

below 120/80) may worsen orthostatic hypotension. However, a 2020 study in *Annals of Internal Medicine* found that intensive blood pressure treatment actually lowered a person's risk of orthostatic hypotension.

Still, some blood pressure drugs (and certain other medications) can contribute to orthostatic hypotension, says Dr. Kelley-Hedgepeth. "If I find a person has orthostatic hypotension, the first thing I do is review their medications," she says. Diuretics, which flush extra fluid from the body, are a common culprit. Drugs that lower blood pressure by relaxing the blood vessels, such as beta blockers and calcium-channel blockers, can also be problematic. Because there are so many different blood pressure drugs, just changing from one class of drugs to another can help.

Aside from blood pressure drugs, other potentially problematic medications include those used to treat
- an enlarged prostate, such as alfuzosin (Uroxatral) and tamsulosin (Flomax)
- erectile dysfunction, such as sildenafil (Viagra)
- depression, such as paroxetine (Paxil) and amitriptyline (Elavil).

For people on these drugs, it's worth trying a different medication to see if it makes a difference. But the change won't happen overnight, and it may take a few months to find out, says Dr. Kelley-Hedgepeth.

Finally, several diseases, including diabetes and Parkinson's disease, can damage the nerves involved in blood pressure control, leading to orthostatic hypotension.

Coping with orthostatic hypotension

If you have symptoms of orthostatic hypotension, these strategies may help:

▸ **Don't forget fluids.** Drink water throughout the day; don't wait until you're thirsty. But avoid alcohol, which can cause you to become dehydrated.

▸ **Avoid big meals.** A related condition, called post-prandial hypotension, can cause blood pressure to drop after eating; it's also mostly seen in older people. It happens because of the increased blood flow to the intestines needed for digestion, which leads to reduced blood flow to other parts of the body.

▸ **Support your legs.** Compression stockings that squeeze the legs may help. Thigh-high or waist-high versions are much more effective than knee-high stockings.

▸ **Take care when rising.** Getting out of bed is a common trigger, so pump your legs up and down a few times while still sitting on the edge of your bed to get your blood flowing before you stand up. ▾

The best strength-building exercise to lower blood pressure?

Exercise that engages your muscles without movement—such as wall squats and planks—may help lower blood pressure. But traditional physical activity is important, too.

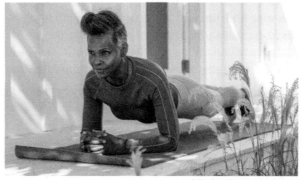

© The Good Brigade | Getty Images

Although a plank involves no movement, this isometric exercise uses muscles throughout most of your body.

Aerobic exercise involves moving the largest muscles of your body in a rhythmic, repetitive pattern—think brisk walking, running, cycling, and swimming. It's long been considered the best type of activity to lower blood pressure. But growing evidence shows that strength training can also reduce blood pressure. According to a new study, the most effective type involves contracting your muscles without any movement, which is known as isometric or static exercise (see "Muscle-strengthening activity: Types, terms, and examples," page 198).

Published in 2023 in the *British Journal of Sports Medicine*, the study pooled findings from 270 clinical trials involving a total of more than 15,000 people. All the trials lasted at least two weeks and reported the effects of exercise on blood pressure. As expected, most

To lower blood pressure, add exercise

One of the most rapid results of exercise is that it lowers your blood pressure. While you are actively exercising, blood pressure rises temporarily, as your body works harder to pump more blood. But afterward, it falls to levels lower than before you started. With regular exercise, many people reduce their average systolic pressure (the first number in a blood pressure reading) by 4 to 8 mm Hg. High blood pressure doubles or triples your risk for developing heart failure and can lead to other heart diseases, strokes, aortic aneurysms, kidney disease, and damage to other organs. By contrast, regular aerobic exercise can help bring down high blood pressure—or keep you from developing it in the first place.

▶▶ types of exercise helped lower blood pressure. But the most effective workout, especially in people who had high blood pressure, was isometric exercise training.

"It's an interesting and somewhat provocative finding because of the historic focus on aerobic exercise for reducing blood pressure," says Dr. Timothy Churchill, a cardiologist at the Cardiovascular Performance Program at Harvard-affiliated Massachusetts General Hospital. Aerobic (which means "with oxygen") exercise boosts your heart rate and increases blood circulation to deliver oxygen throughout the body. The blood pressure benefits appear to stem from improvements in heart and blood vessel health.

Adding isometric exercise

The new findings add to the evidence that strength-based exercises are also good for cardiovascular health. But rather than taking priority over all other types of exercise, strength training should be incorporated into your overall routine, says Dr. Churchill. While isometric exercise—especially wall squats—appeared to lower blood pressure the most, the study authors were somewhat cautious about overselling that finding, given that relatively few studies (18 of the 270) included isometric exercise, and none compared it directly against other forms of exercise.

Still, experts have speculated about a possible mechanism. During isometric exercise, clenched muscles temporarily constrain blood flow. The subsequent surge of blood may stimulate the release of factors that help relax the vessels and ultimately contribute to a reduction in blood pressure.

Isometric exercise has some additional advantages. Because you don't move your joints, isometrics can be easier and safer for people with joint injuries or diseases. Many of the exercises don't require any special equipment, and you can do them anywhere.

The physical activity guidelines don't specify how long to do muscle-building exercises. "But even just 10 to 15 minutes, two days a week, is a good place to start," says Dr. Churchill. Try doing some wall squats or a modified plank (see illustrations).

Remember to breathe!

During any type of strength training, be careful not to hold your breath. Some people do this unintentionally, although others have a misguided belief that breath holding increases their effort and power. But breath holding during exertion can cause blood pressure to spike to dangerous levels, says Dr. Churchill.

When you do dynamic strength training, exhale as you lift, push, or pull, and inhale as you release. When doing isometric strength training, take a big breath as you move into position. Then take shallow breaths as you hold the pose, and take regular full breaths during your rest and recovery phase. ◗

Wall squats

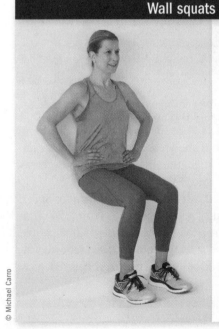

To do wall squats, stand with your back flat against a wall. Walk your feet about 18 inches from the wall, placing your feet shoulder-width apart. Tighten your abdominal muscles, then inhale and exhale as you slide your back down the wall until your thighs are as close to parallel as possible to the floor and your knees are above your ankles. Hold for 20 to 60 seconds. Slide slowly back up the wall to a standing position. Rest for 30 to 60 seconds, and repeat two times.

© Michael Carro

BLOOD PRESSURE AND CHOLESTEROL

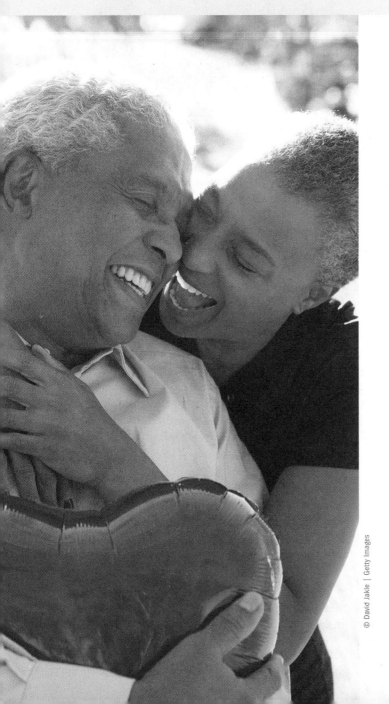

Chapter 4

Cardiovascular Health

Healthy Habits! 5 Things You Can Do Now

1 **Avoid unnecessary tests.** New guidelines recommend against some routine tests for people with heart disease. (page 83)

2 **Eat fatty fish—but stop taking fish oil.** Research has not borne out early hope for the supplement. (page 90)

3 **Replace sitting with standing and movement.** Moving around throughout the day can make a difference in overall health. (page 95)

4 **Try tai chi.** This gentle form of exercise has been shown to lower blood pressure. (page 97)

5 **Call an old friend.** Social connections are increasingly recognized as important to heart health. (page 98)

© David Jakle | Getty Images

Know your **Big 3** heart numbers

Healthy blood pressure, cholesterol, and blood sugar can lower your risk for cardiovascular disease.

Many tests and numbers can help you manage your overall health. But when it comes to heart health, you need to focus on the Big 3: blood pressure, cholesterol, and blood sugar.

"These best predict cardiovascular disease risks, including heart disease, heart attack, and stroke," says Dr. Howard LeWine, editor in chief of *Harvard Men's Health Watch*.

While there are standard guidelines for what is considered healthy for the Big 3, your ideal numbers may differ depending on your health and other risk factors. "Your doctor can direct you about which numbers and ranges you should aim for and the best ways to achieve them," says Dr. LeWine.

Here's a look at the Big 3, why they matter, and how to measure them.

1 Blood pressure

A blood pressure reading has two components: systolic pressure and diastolic pressure. Systolic pressure (the top number) represents the pressure in the blood vessels when the heart contracts to pump blood. Diastolic pressure (the bottom number) refers to the pressure in the vessels between heartbeats.

While both numbers are essential for diagnosing and treating high blood pressure, doctors primarily focus on systolic pressure. "Most studies show a greater risk of stroke and heart disease related to higher systolic pressures rather than elevated diastolic pressures," says Dr. LeWine. "That's especially true in people 50 and older." Blood pressure is measured in millimeters of mercury (mm Hg). Readings are categorized as follows:

▶ normal blood pressure: less than 120/80 mm Hg
▶ elevated blood pressure: 120/80 to 129/89 mm Hg
▶ Stage 1 hypertension: 130/80 to 139/89 mm Hg
▶ Stage 2 hypertension: 140/90 mm Hg and higher.

If either component of your blood pressure is above the normal range, your initial action should be lifestyle changes. This includes losing weight, if necessary; increasing daily physical activity; eating more fruits and vegetables; and limiting salt intake. "Many

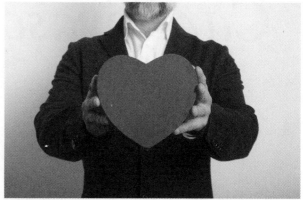

© Jordi Calvera Solé | Getty Images

Keeping tabs on key heart health numbers can help protect against heart attacks and strokes.

people don't need to have perfect blood pressure," says Dr. LeWine. "You and your doctor can decide on your personal goal numbers, which may be higher than the magical 120/80 mm Hg, or possibly lower if you have heart disease or other cardiovascular issues."

He adds that a home blood pressure monitor is the best way to regularly check your blood pressure. Look for a model with an upper arm cuff that automatically inflates. (Devices with a wrist cuff or fingertip sensors are less accurate.) Make sure the cuff is the proper size, as cuffs that are too small or large can give a false reading (see "Wrong-sized blood pressure cuff can throw off readings," page 62). Dr. LeWine suggests taking measurements twice daily—morning and evening—for several days to get a baseline reading. (Blood pressure should be lowest when you first wake up and typically rises in the late afternoon and evening.) After that, take readings daily or every other day for the next couple of weeks. In the long term, check your blood pressure two to three times a week or when you think it might be high (for example, if you feel stressed) or low (because you feel fatigued).

"You should alert your doctor to any changes outside your personal goal range that last longer than a few days," says Dr. LeWine.

2 Cholesterol

Cholesterol is a fatty substance that occurs naturally in the body. Different forms of cholesterol and other fats (lipids) circulate in the blood. A traditional blood lipid panel measures low-density lipoprotein (LDL) cholesterol, high-density lipoprotein (HDL) cholesterol, total cholesterol (both LDL and HDL), and triglycerides.

"Doctors primarily focus on 'bad' LDL cholesterol levels because of their close connection with the amount of fatty plaque buildup inside arteries, raising the risk of heart attack and stroke," says Dr. LeWine.

Your goal level for LDL depends on your risk factor profile. In general, the lower the number, the better. If you already have cardiovascular disease or are at high risk for it, you should aim for an LDL of less than 70 milligrams per deciliter (mg/dL).

Achieving less than 100 mg/dL with lifestyle changes is reasonable for people at average risk. You and your doctor can decide if you need to take a statin drug to lower your LDL. However, if you do not have cardiovascular disease and have no risk factors for it, an LDL level of 100 to 130 mg/dL may be acceptable. Levels higher than 130 mg/dL usually require drug therapy when lifestyle changes aren't enough.

A blood lipid panel also reveals your triglyceride level. Triglycerides are a type of fat in the blood that the body uses for energy. The combination of high levels of triglycerides with low HDL or high LDL can also increase your risk for heart attack and stroke.

In general, a triglyceride level of less than 150 mg/dL is a good goal. With levels between 150 and 500 mg/dL, the usual strategy to lower levels is by moderating alcohol intake, losing weight, and cutting back on carbs.

If you have elevated levels of LDL and triglycerides, a statin can lower both. Other drugs are available that target high triglycerides.

3 Blood sugar

Keeping track of your average blood sugar levels, even if you don't have diabetes, can also help assess your heart health. A blood test for hemoglobin A1c measures your average blood sugar (glucose) levels over the past three months. The test can be done anytime during the day and does not require fasting.

The results can determine if you have prediabetes or undiagnosed type 2 diabetes, either of which greatly increases your risk of cardiovascular disease. "If you fall into one of these categories, you will likely want lower goals for both blood pressure and LDL cholesterol," says Dr. LeWine.

A normal A1c reading is below 5.7%. A reading of 5.7% to 6.4% indicates prediabetes, and a reading of 6.5% or higher is classified as having diabetes. If your results are normal and your weight remains stable, you probably won't need another test for two to three years.

If you have prediabetes, your doctor will recommend that you try more intensive lifestyle changes and have another test in six months to a year. "Many older adults with prediabetes don't progress to full diabetes if they maintain a healthy weight, exercise regularly, and eat a healthy diet," says Dr. LeWine. "But prediabetes indicates a need to pay even more attention to all other cardiovascular risk factors." 🛡

When heart-related pain goes unrecognized

Silent heart attacks are surprisingly common. Make sure you're aware of the subtle and less common symptoms of coronary artery disease.

Most people don't know you can have a heart attack without realizing it. In fact, these so-called silent attacks account for an estimated 30% to 60% of all heart attacks. Recognizing and responding to a silent heart attack is important: they can be harbingers for a more serious, potentially deadly heart attack.

"Heart attacks can be silent for a variety of reasons," says cardiologist Dr. Peter Stone, professor of medicine at Harvard Medical School. Just like a regular heart attack, a silent one occurs when the heart muscle doesn't receive enough blood, usually when a clot blocks blood flow inside a narrowed heart artery.

The quality, duration, and intensity of the resulting pain can vary quite a bit. Some people describe the sensation as a dull ache or crushing pressure, ▶▶

▶▶ which may be mild or short-lived—and therefore unnoticed or ignored. Typically, the reduced blood flow must last about 15 to 30 minutes to result in a detectable heart attack (that is, part of the heart muscle becomes damaged or dies). Sometimes symptoms come and go, which doctors refer to as stuttering symptoms. "When a clot obstructs an artery, the body's natural clot-busting process is instantly set in motion," Dr. Stone explains. If the clot dissolves, symptoms may abate—but then return if the clot-forming forces win.

Radiating and referred pain

Various quirks related to pain perception may also play a role in a heart attack going unrecognized. "People often think the discomfort has to be on the left side of the chest, because that's where the heart is located," says Dr. Stone. But nerves within the heart can send signals to the surrounding nerves, causing pain that may radiate to the stomach, back, neck, arm, or jaw.

For example, if an artery blockage occurs near the bottom of the heart, it may affect nerves in the diaphragm, the muscular membrane that separates the chest from the abdominal cavity, Dr. Stone explains. This can be perceived as abdominal discomfort or nausea. Or people may experience shoulder pain, a classic example of referred pain. This phenomenon—when pain is felt in a location other than the actual source—happens because of overlap in the network of nerves in the spinal cord.

© DjelicS | Getty Images

Heart attack symptoms

During a heart attack, about three-quarters of both men and women experience the classic symptom of chest discomfort that spreads through the upper body. But some people experience other symptoms. These less common symptoms might be slightly more frequent in women and in older people, but they can also happen in men and younger people.

Classic symptoms

▶ Pressure, aching, or tightness in the center of the chest

▶ Pain or discomfort that radiates to the upper body, especially shoulders or neck and arms

▶ Sweating

Other symptoms

▶ Shortness of breath

▶ Weakness

▶ Nausea or vomiting

▶ Dizziness

▶ Back or jaw pain

▶ Unexplained fatigue

Mistaken attributions

Problems with the lungs and the esophagus (the tube connecting the throat to the stomach) are sometimes mistaken for a heart attack, but the opposite can also occur. Sometimes, people assume their chest pain is caused by a respiratory infection or other lung disease when they're actually having a heart attack. Another possible misattribution is heartburn, which happens when stomach acid rises up into the esophagus.

If you have diabetes, you're more likely to have a silent heart attack. Over time, high blood sugar can damage your nerves and the small blood vessels supplying those nerves—including those that transmit pain signals.

While pain tolerance may be physiological, emotional and cultural factors can come into play as well, says Dr. Stone. For instance, people may dismiss or ignore pain because they don't want to appear weak.

How are silent heart attacks detected?

Heart muscle damage from a heart attack creates a distinct signature on an electrocardiogram, or ECG, a recording of the heart's electrical activity. A heart ultrasound (echocardiogram) can also detect a prior heart attack. If either test suggests heart damage, it should be a wake-up call to prioritize efforts to avoid more damage. Follow healthy lifestyle habits (and take medications, if necessary) to make sure your weight, blood pressure, cholesterol, and blood sugar are within normal ranges. ▌

Living with heart disease? Avoid unnecessary testing

New guidelines recommend against certain routine tests and procedures for people without symptoms.

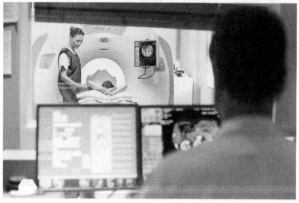

© Morsa Images | Getty Images

Diagnosing coronary artery disease may require a one-time special test like CT angiography.

Medical tests are an important part of managing chronic health problems such as cardiovascular disease. Some, like checking blood pressure or cholesterol levels, are fairly simple and straightforward. But others (especially those that use special equipment to visualize the heart) are time-consuming, stressful, and costly—and, in some cases, unnecessary.

It's not uncommon for people with known chronic coronary disease (see "What is chronic coronary disease?") to undergo such imaging tests on a routine basis, even when they don't have any symptoms to suggest that their condition is progressing or worsening. Now, new guidelines recommend against this practice.

"People with established coronary disease who don't have symptoms shouldn't be undergoing tests on a periodic basis," says Dr. Dhruv Kazi, who directs the Cardiac Critical Care Unit at Harvard-affiliated Beth Israel Deaconess Hospital. The guidelines, published in 2023 in the journal *Circulation*, say that for those people, there is no benefit for the following three tests:

Cardiac CT angiography uses a CT scanner to take multiple high-speed x-rays to create three-dimensional views of the blood vessels and other heart structures. It requires an injection of special dye into a vein in the arm or hand that "lights up" the blood vessels.

Echocardiography uses ultrasound to show how well the heart's muscles and valves are working and to measure ejection fraction, an assessment of the heart's pumping ability.

Stress testing monitors your blood pressure, your heart rate, and your heart's electrical activity to check for evidence of decreased blood flow to the heart, either during exercise or after an injection of a drug that mimics the effects of exercise. It may also involve getting an echocardiogram (a variation called stress echocardiography) or an injection of a small amount of a radioactive substance and a PET scan (a variation known as a nuclear stress test).

No help, possible harm

When people without symptoms get testing "just to be sure," the results are unhelpful—and in some cases harmful, says Dr. Kazi, who was on the writing committee for the new guidelines. For example, if test results aren't clear, that often generates additional testing or unnecessary procedures, including some that expose people to radiation for no reason. These tests add expense without any corresponding benefit, and the costs are increasingly being passed back to patients in the form of copayments or higher premiums, he adds.

For people with chronic coronary disease, the real bang for the buck lies elsewhere, says Dr. Kazi. "As the guidelines emphasize, people should focus on getting regular exercise, eating a healthy diet, and taking medications to control their blood pressure and cholesterol—all strategies that we know help people live longer, healthier lives," he says.

What is chronic coronary disease?

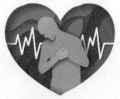

© SiberianArt | Getty Images

People are said to have chronic coronary disease if they

- have had a heart attack or stable angina (chest pain that occurs with activity or emotional stress)
- have had a procedure to restore blood flow to the heart (angioplasty with a stent or coronary artery bypass surgery)
- have a low ejection fraction from coronary blockages
- show evidence of coronary artery disease on an imaging test.

Seeking a second heart-health opinion: When, why, and how?

Another cardiologist's perspective may help in certain situations.

Maybe you're wondering if the heart procedure your doctor has recommended is really necessary. Or perhaps you're experiencing persistent heart-related symptoms despite treatment, but your physician has told you "There's nothing more we can do."

These scenarios are examples that often prompt people to seek a second opinion—an option that may be increasingly appropriate as new treatments for heart disease become more widely available and more specialized.

"In recent years, minimally invasive procedures for treating structural heart problems have become widespread," says cardiologist Dr. Dale Adler, executive vice chair of the Department of Medicine at Harvard-affiliated Brigham and Women's Hospital. Problems such as a leaky or narrowed heart valve (which once required open-heart surgery) can be addressed using a catheter that's inserted through a tiny incision in the upper thigh or wrist and passed up to the heart, he says. Catheter-based procedures are also used to close an opening between the heart's upper chambers (a patent foramen ovale) or to place a device inside the heart to inhibit formation of blood clots in its upper left chamber (a left atrial appendage closure device).

Delivery of energy via catheter tips is also used to treat heart rhythm disorders, especially atrial fibrillation. But variations in both the techniques and the recommended timing of these procedures may leave patients wondering which option they should choose and when to do it.

A general cardiologist is usually in the best position to decide if you need more focused expertise from a subspecialist (see "Heart disease specialists"). But even if you've been referred to one of these experts, it's reasonable to ask about possible drug therapies or to get a second opinion from another generalist.

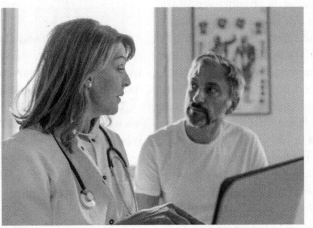

© RealPeopleGroup | Getty Images

A second opinion may be helpful before undergoing invasive cardiovascular procedures.

First doctor, second chance?

Before you undergo any surgery or procedure, be sure you fully understand the potential benefits and risks, which may vary depending on your age and any other health conditions you have. Most health care practices now let you send messages to your physician through a patient portal, which is a good first step if you have any questions, says Dr. Adler. You can send a note explaining your concerns and say you're thinking about getting another opinion, he says. "Often, your doctor will say, 'Oh, you're welcome to get a second opinion. But let's set up a video visit to discuss all your questions to make sure you're clear about the proposed treatment plan,'" says Dr. Adler. Not only are video visits more convenient, you can invite loved ones to join. Sometimes, people ask their spouse and one or more of their adult children to participate, both for emotional support and to address the family's questions, he adds.

Different treatment options

Because of the movement toward shared decision making in medicine, your doctor may offer two different treatment options and leave the decision to you. If you're not comfortable making that choice, a different doctor's advice may be welcome. In other cases, people feel frustrated with their current treatment plan. They don't feel well and aren't improving, so they hope to find a doctor who can offer other options. For instance, people with advanced heart failure may be candidates for more intensive treatments, including home infusion therapy (which delivers drugs that improve the heart's pumping ability), a left ventricular assist device (a small device implanted in the chest to support the heart's pumping function), or a heart transplant, Dr. Adler says.

Finding other experts

Your doctor, family members, or friends may be able to recommend an expert for a second opinion. Or contact a nearby medical center or hospital; they usually have online resources or call centers that can refer you to an appropriate physician for your particular problem. Check with your insurance provider to see whether the visit and any additional costs will be covered. ♥

Heart disease specialists

These are the three main types of heart specialists who perform procedures:

Cardiovascular surgeon. Performs open-heart surgery, such as coronary artery bypass grafting. Repairs or replaces poorly functioning heart valves, often together with an interventional cardiologist. May also place devices that assist heart function. Highly specialized surgeons perform heart transplants.

Interventional cardiologist. Diagnoses and treats narrowed arteries in the heart (and elsewhere in the body), thickened or leaky heart valves, and holes in the heart, using thin, flexible tubes (catheters) inserted through small incisions. Places some short-term heart assist devices.

Electrophysiologist. Diagnoses heart rhythm disorders such as atrial fibrillation, and treats them using specialized catheters to destroy tiny areas of abnormal heart tissue. Also implants pacemakers and cardioverter-defibrillators.

IN THE JOURNALS

Calcium score may foretell heart risk better than genetic test

Specialized tests may help doctors better determine a person's risk of developing heart disease. A new study suggests that one such test, a calcium score—which quantifies the plaque inside the heart's arteries—appears to improve risk assessment, while a gene-based risk score does not.

The 2023 study, published in *JAMA,* included 3,208 adults from two large studies; none had heart disease at the outset. For each participant, researchers calculated a traditional heart disease risk score based on factors such as body mass index, blood pressure, and cholesterol values. Participants got CT scans to determine their calcium scores. They also got a polygenic risk score, which relies on a blood test that detects multiple genetic variants associated with heart disease.

After a median follow-up of just over 14 years, researchers found that combining the calcium score with the traditional risk calculation provided a meaningful improvement in predicting heart disease risk. That was not the case for the polygenic risk score. However, the polygenic risk score may prove more useful in people who are younger than the study participants, who were, on average, in their mid-60s.

Race, racism, and heart disease: Why awareness matters

Discrimination and its downstream effects may underlie the survival gaps in cardiovascular disease between racial groups. The aftermath affects everyone.

In the United States, Black adults are more than twice as likely to die of cardiovascular disease than white adults. Growing evidence points to structural racism as a "fundamental driver" of this stark disparity, according to a 2020 presidential advisory from the American Heart Association (AHA).

Structural racism refers to the systems in a society that create and maintain racial inequality. But the damaging health effects of the underlying problem—racial discrimination—have been studied for decades. More than 25 years ago, sociologist David R. Williams, professor of public health at the Harvard T.H. Chan School of Public Health, developed the Everyday Discrimination Scale. It's designed to quantify the hassles and indignities people experience in daily life and whether they feel this unfair treatment is due to their race, gender, age, or other characteristics. A recent update reviewed some of the cardiovascular effects related to race (see "Racial discrimination and heart health: The evidence").

"While there's a great deal of literature on the health effects of stress, the traditional measures have not always fully captured the stressful effects of discrimination, which can extend beyond daily indignities to also include

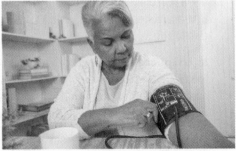

© LifestyleVisuals | Getty Images

Racial discrimination and heart health: The evidence

Cardiovascular disease and related health problems such as high blood pressure, diabetes, and obesity are often collectively referred to as cardiometabolic disease. Dozens of studies have explored how racial discrimination may worsen these common conditions. A 2023 review in the *Journal of Racial and Ethnic Health Disparities* synthesized the evidence to date.

The review assessed 123 peer-reviewed studies done in the United States and published from 1996 to 2022. All the studies included people with cardiometabolic diseases who belonged to racial or ethnic minorities. Blacks were the most frequently studied racial group, accounting for 53% of participants across all the studies. The Everyday Discrimination Scale (see main story) was the most commonly used measure of discrimination. About three-quarters of the studies found that racial or ethnic discrimination was significantly associated with an increased risk of cardiometabolic disease.

a higher frequency of traumatic experiences, such as being unfairly stopped by police and exposure to gun violence," says Williams.

Downstream effects

Discrimination can also affect employment opportunities and advancement, which has downstream effects that contribute to health disparities, according to Dr. Michelle Albert, president of the AHA. "If you can't get a well-paying job or develop wealth, these circumstances limit where you can afford to live. That, in turn, affects your access to healthy foods, safe places to exercise, and good medical care," she says. In addition, discrimination has been linked to other factors that are hard on the heart, including social isolation, depression, and unhealthy coping skills such as smoking and alcohol use.

Like other stressful experiences, the experience of discrimination can activate the fight-or-flight response, triggering a release of hormones that raise blood pressure. Over time, blood pressure spikes can damage the blood vessels, kidneys, and heart, says Dr. Albert, who is also director of the Center for the Study of Adversity and Cardiovascular Disease at the University of California, San Francisco.

The price we pay

Given that cardiovascular disease is a leading cause of disability and death in this country, the financial impact of race-based health disparities is substantial, says Williams. The cost to society at large includes not just higher health care spending but also productivity losses related to job absenteeism and premature death. While Blacks make up about 14% of the population, nearly 40% of people currently living in the United States belong to a racial or ethnic minority. People in other groups, which include Latinos, Asians, and Native Americans, also experience cardiovascular disease disparities to varying degrees.

The AHA's Office of Health Equity sponsors community and workplace programs to address discrimination and other barriers to equitable health care. But on a personal level, everyone can benefit from becoming more aware of their implicit biases—the unconscious assumptions people have about groups of people that may underlie some discriminatory behaviors. Project Implicit (see health.harvard.edu/bias) includes online tests to explore implicit bias.

"The data on the health effects of discrimination are a call to each one of us to treat each person we encounter every day with the dignity and respect that they deserve as a human being," says Williams.

Alert: This hidden condition increases heart attack and stroke risks

Find out if you have the components of metabolic syndrome.

It has an unfamiliar name, produces few symptoms, and involves a cluster of health problems. But metabolic syndrome is a common and dangerous condition that's steadily increasing in adults of all ages in the United States, largely as a result of the obesity epidemic. The syndrome significantly increases risk for heart attacks, strokes, diabetes, and more.

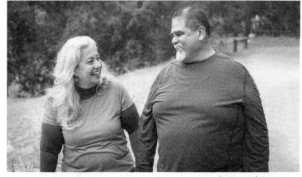

© adamkaz | Getty Images

A large waistline (more than 40 inches for men, and more than 35 for women) can signal metabolic syndrome.

What is it?

Metabolic syndrome is a constellation of interrelated conditions. A diagnosis requires at least three of the following cardiovascular risk factors:

Obesity. You have this risk factor if your waistline is greater than 40 inches for men or 35 inches for women, no matter your height, or if your body mass index is 30 or more.

High blood sugar. After you eat, your body converts carbohydrates into blood glucose, a type of sugar that the body uses for energy. Sugar in the blood then enters your cells, where it's needed to produce energy. In people with diabetes or prone to it, this process is impaired, raising sugar levels in the blood and damaging the cells and blood vessels. A fasting blood sugar level of 100 milligrams per deciliter of blood (mg/dL) or more is considered high. Having diabetes (a fasting blood sugar of 126 mg/dL or higher) also counts as a metabolic syndrome risk factor.

High triglycerides. Triglycerides are a type of fat in the blood. Having a high level—150 mg/dL or higher—increases your risk for heart disease and stroke. (You can find your triglyceride levels in your cholesterol test results.)

Low HDL (good) cholesterol. A low blood level of high density lipoprotein (HDL) cholesterol not only counts in deciding if you have metabolic syndrome, it's also linked to a greater risk of cardiovascular disease. If your HDL is below 40 mg/dL in men or 50 mg/dL in women, it's considered low. ▶▶

▶▶ **High blood pressure.** Blood pressure is considered high if your systolic pressure (the top number in a measurement) is 130 millimeters of mercury (mm Hg) or higher, or your diastolic pressure (the bottom number) is 80 mm Hg or higher. If you're already taking medication for high blood pressure, you should still count this condition as a metabolic risk factor.

What does it mean?

When three or more of these risk factors occur together, metabolic syndrome is present, and numerous studies have shown that means you have higher risks for heart disease and stroke.

"Having just one of the risk factors is bad enough. But having more makes the likelihood of bad health outcomes greater. That's why clinicians developed the term metabolic syndrome many years ago: it helped identify people at risk for cardiovascular disease and diabetes. Today we have even better risk calculators, which take other risk factors into account, such as age and activity levels. But you can still pay attention to metabolic syndrome as a way to recognize that trouble is brewing," says Dr. David M. Nathan, a Harvard Medical School professor and the director of the Diabetes Center and Clinical Research Center at Massachusetts General Hospital.

Metabolic syndrome also increases the risk for developing liver disease, kidney disease, and sleep apnea (a condition marked by pauses in breathing during sleep).

Diagnosis and treatment

You can measure your waist to see if you have at least one metabolic syndrome risk factor. But you can't see the others. So discuss it at your next doctor appointment, and double-check your annual blood work results.

The good news is that you can reverse metabolic syndrome. Losing weight is central to reducing many of its features. Lowering elevated blood pressure, blood sugar, and cholesterol levels also plays a major role in reducing your risk for heart disease and stroke.

If you can do that and live a healthy lifestyle—exercising daily, eating a healthy diet, getting enough sleep, not smoking, and limiting alcohol intake—you'll not only decrease your risks for heart disease and diabetes, but also increase your odds of living longer. ◆

What to eat when you have metabolic syndrome

Having metabolic syndrome means you're likely overweight or that you have another condition, such as high blood sugar, cholesterol, or blood pressure, that may be stoked by an unhealthy diet. One of the best antidotes is eating a healthy plant-based diet. Swap junk food for lots of vegetables, fruits, nuts, and whole grains; moderate amounts of fish and poultry; and limited portions of red or processed meats. And do one more thing: "Eat less. If you expend more calories than you're taking in, you'll lose weight," says Harvard Medical School diabetes expert Dr. David M. Nathan. His go-to tricks: eat smaller portions and focus on foods high in fiber (such as vegetables and legumes), which will keep you fuller longer.

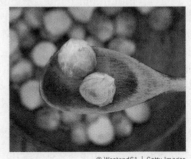

© Westend61 | Getty Images

High-fiber foods such as Brussels sprouts can aid weight loss.

by **ANTHONY L. KOMAROFF, M.D.**, Editor in Chief, *Harvard Health Letter*

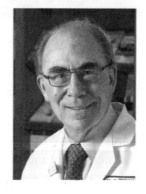

Does my daily aspirin therapy dose or pill coating matter?

Q *I have heart disease, and I take aspirin to reduce my risk of new heart problems. Does it matter how much aspirin I take, or whether the aspirin is the type that is "enteric-coated" to protect my stomach?*

A What we know for sure is that people who have heart disease reduce their risk of developing new heart problems by taking aspirin. So, I'm glad you're taking aspirin. But the best dose, and whether the enteric-coated form is better, remain uncertain.

People with heart disease benefit from taking aspirin because aspirin makes the blood a bit less likely to clot. It also reduces inflammation. Heart attacks typically happen because a blood clot has formed in one of the arteries of the heart, blocking the flow of blood to part of the heart muscle. Inflammation inside of plaque deposits in the walls of the arteries makes such clots more likely to happen. So, theoretically, aspirin should benefit people with heart disease—and studies definitively show that it does.

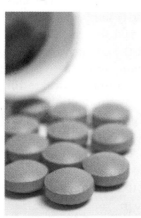

Enteric-coated aspirin vs. regular aspirin? No difference in benefits or risks.

© dlerick | Getty Imagess

However, aspirin also increases the risk of bleeding. The most common site of bleeding is the gastrointestinal tract, particularly the stomach and intestines. The enteric-coated form of aspirin was created to try to protect the stomach from bleeding. The most dangerous site of bleeding is inside the brain: when this occurs, it results in a hemorrhagic stroke. Fortunately, the studies that show aspirin benefits people with heart disease also show that these benefits are greater than the risks of bleeding.

So, to your question, what dose of aspirin is best, and should you take an enteric-coated or uncoated aspirin pill? A 2023 study in *JAMA Cardiology* provides some insight. Over 10,000 people with heart disease were assigned, at random, to take either a regular-dose aspirin (325 mg) or a low-dose aspirin (81 mg) every day for about two years. While the dose was assigned at random, the study participants were allowed to choose whether they would take enteric-coated or uncoated aspirin.

The study concluded that neither the dose nor the enteric coating affected either the benefit or the risk from aspirin: there was no statistically significant difference. However, in my opinion, the study does not really settle the question. As big as it was, it was not big enough to have the statistical power needed. Also, it would have been better if participants had been assigned at random to enteric-coated or uncoated aspirin, and followed for more than two years. In particular, the study did observe a greater tendency for gastrointestinal bleeding in the uncoated aspirin groups.

In my opinion, this study and others indicate that people with heart disease probably should take one low-dose, enteric-coated aspirin pill a day. Like you, I have heart disease, and that's what I do.

The false promise of fish oil supplements

Despite what the labels say, there's no evidence these amber capsules will improve your cardiovascular health—and they may even harm it.

© JW LTD | Getty Images

Millions of Americans—including one in five people over age 60—take fish oil supplements, often assuming the capsules help stave off heart disease. Who can blame them? After all, the product labels say things like "promotes heart health" and "supports healthy cholesterol and blood pressure levels."

"People will often say 'I don't like eating fish, but I know it's good for me. So I'm taking this supplement instead,'" says Preston Mason, a faculty member in the Cardiovascular Division at Harvard-affiliated Brigham and Women's Hospital who studies the unique fats found in fish oil, known as omega-3 fatty acids.

Here's the catch: Studies dating back more than a half-century find that people who eat fatty fish tend to have lower rates of heart disease. But over the past two decades, multiple randomized trials pitting fish oil against placebos show no evidence of heart-related benefits from fish oil supplements. While the supplements do provide omega-3 fatty acids, there are better ways to get these essential fats from your diet (see "Three key omega-3s").

Three key omega-3s

Omega-3 fatty acids are considered "essential," which means people must get them from their diet or other sources. Fatty fish such as salmon, tuna, sardines, and mackerel are good sources of two omega-3s: eicosapentaenoic acid (EPA) and docosahexaenoic acid (DHA).

Another omega-3, alpha-linolenic acid (ALA), is found in many plants, including seeds, nuts, and some green vegetables. Your body can convert a small amount—about 8%—of dietary ALA to EPA and DHA.

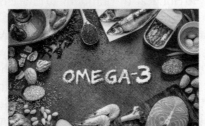

© carlosgaw | Getty Images
You're better off getting your omega-3 fats from fish or vegetarian sources than wasting money on fish oil supplements.

Nutrition experts suspect that one reason fish eaters have fewer heart attacks may be that they eat correspondingly less red meat or processed meats, both of which are associated with a higher risk of heart disease.

Vegetarians (who don't eat fish) and vegans (who avoid all animal-based foods) can meet their omega-3 requirements by eating plenty of ALA-rich foods, such as flaxseed, walnuts, pumpkin seeds, and soybean or canola oil. People who follow these plant-focused diets have lower rates of heart disease than omnivores, who include animal-sourced foods in their diets.

Confusing health claims

What's up with the misleading messaging? The FDA considers all dietary supplements, including fish oil, to be foods, not drugs. Unlike companies that make aspirin, antacids, and other over-the-counter drugs, supplement manufacturers aren't required to do any rigorous clinical testing or undergo any production oversight, Mason explains. Despite this, they're allowed to include limited health claims on their labels, and heart-related promises are common on fish oil supplements, according to a study published in 2023 in *JAMA Cardiology*.

Among the more than 2,800 different fish oil supplement labels the researchers checked, about 2,000 featured one or more heart-related statements. Most of these health claims (about 80%) featured general but vague descriptions of the role of omega-3 fatty acids in the body. Most (62%) were cardiovascular claims, such as "helps support a healthy heart."

In addition, the researchers analyzed 255 fish oil products from 16 major manufacturers and found a wide variability in the actual amounts of EPA and DHA (the two main omega-3 fatty acids) in the supplements. These findings confirm Mason's research.

What's more, many widely used fish oil supplements are produced through an industrial process that leaves the omega-3 fatty acids vulnerable to uncontrolled heat and oxygen, says Mason. "This results in the oxidation of these highly unsaturated fatty acids, with a consequent loss of any biological benefit," he says, adding that multiple laboratory tests on dozens of products have confirmed these findings. Consuming oxidized oil has been linked to vascular inflammation, a key cause of cardiovascular disease.

Prescription-strength EPA

If you have heart disease, you might ask your doctor about the prescription drug icosapent ethyl, a high-dose, purified EPA preparation that lowers cardiovascular risk when taken with a statin. "The unregulated fish oil supplements found in stores and online are not an effective substitute," Mason cautions. If you don't have heart disease, eating two servings of fatty fish weekly or following a vegetarian diet rich in healthy oils, nuts, and seeds is a far smarter strategy than buying fish oil supplements. ♥

How a healthy gut helps your heart

Both fiber-rich and fermented foods encourage a healthy gut microbiome, which may benefit cardiovascular health.

Your gut microbiome—a collection of trillions of microorganisms inhabiting your intestinal tract—has wide-ranging effects on your health. Your unique mix of bacteria, fungi, parasites, and viruses reflects your genes, your age, the medications you take—but most of all, what you eat.

Over the past two decades, numerous studies have explored how gut microbes and their breakdown products (metabolites) affect factors linked with heart disease. For the most part, the findings support the same basic advice health experts recommend: Follow a mostly plant-based eating pattern, and cut back on highly processed foods. Doing so can help promote a more diverse, healthier microbiome.

"The standard American diet—appropriately called SAD—features a lot of processed foods that are high in sugar, artificial sweeteners, and unhealthy fats," says Dr. Uma Naidoo, director of nutritional and metabolic psychiatry at Harvard-affiliated Massachusetts General Hospital. This nutrient-poor ▶▶

Fermented foods

Eating fermented foods may help dampen inflammation in the body. When shopping, look for the words "contains live cultures" when choosing yogurt or kefir, a yogurt-like drink with a tart flavor and a thinner consistency than yogurt. While both products are usually made with dairy milk, they also come in nondairy versions made from almond, coconut, or oat milk. Another beverage, kombucha, is a fizzy, tart, slightly sweet drink made from fermented tea that's often flavored with fruits and herbs. Look for brands without added sugar.

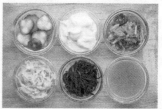

© marekuliasz | Getty Images

Naturally fermented pickles, yogurt, kimchi, sauerkraut, pickled beets, kombucha, and other fermented foods may benefit gut health.

For fermented products made from vegetables, look in the refrigerated section and check for the words "naturally fermented" on the label. When you open the jar, check for telltale bubbles in the liquid, which signal that live organisms are inside. Most supermarket pickles are preserved with vinegar and not made with a natural fermentation process using water and salt. For sauerkraut (pickled cabbage), choose raw or nonpasteurized products. If you're a fan of spicy food, try kimchi, a spicy, reddish fermented cabbage dish from Korea made with a mix of garlic, salt, vinegar, and chili peppers. From Japan, there's miso (a strong, salty paste made from soybeans fermented with brown rice) and tempeh (a firm, chewy product made from fermented soybeans).

diet can lead to dysbiosis, an overgrowth of harmful microbes. When bad microbes thrive in the gut, they form pro-inflammatory breakdown products and toxins, Dr. Naidoo explains. The resulting low-grade, bodywide inflammation contributes to obesity, poor mental health, diabetes, and cardiovascular disease.

Animal vs. plant-based foods

One metabolite of interest is trimethylamine (TMA), which is created when gut microbes feed on choline, a nutrient found in red meat, fish, poultry, and eggs. In the liver, TMA gets converted to trimethylamine N-oxide (TMAO). While some research suggests a link between TMAO and artery-clogging plaque, the evidence isn't consistent. Still, the advice to limit red meat consumption—the main source of TMA in the diet—makes sense.

But according to Dr. Naidoo, there's no need to avoid those animal-based foods, which most Americans aren't especially keen on doing. Instead, people should focus more on what they're not eating—namely, fruits, vegetables, and whole grains.

Diversify your diet

A woefully small percentage of adults—only about 10%—eats the recommended daily amount of fruit (one-and-a-half to two cups) or vegetables (two to three cups). Don't limit yourself to only a few favorites like apples or broccoli, says Dr. Naidoo. "Eat a wide variety of different fruits and vegetables on a regular basis to bring biodiversity to your microbiome," she says.

Despite a recent uptick, whole grains make up less than 16% of the average American's total grain intake. Whole grains such as oats, quinoa, spelt, and barley are healthier choices than most "whole-wheat" bread, which isn't always made with 100% whole grains. Other foods that promote gut health include beans, lentils, nuts, and seeds.

Fruits, vegetables, beans, and whole grains are good sources of fermentable or prebiotic fiber, which gets broken down by bacteria in your colon to form short-chain fatty acids. These compounds then circulate through the bloodstream and interact with receptors on cells that quell inflammation. These fatty acids also appear to play a role in keeping blood sugar, blood pressure, and cholesterol levels in check.

You can also increase good gut bacteria levels by consuming probiotics, which are found in fermented foods (see box, page 91). "Try adding a little bit of these foods to your meals and then grow from there," Dr. Naidoo suggests.

IN THE JOURNALS

Healthy, plant-based diet linked to better cardiovascular fitness

A heart-healthy diet that focuses on plant-based foods is closely tied to improved physical fitness, a new study finds.

The study included 2,380 middle-aged people in the Framingham Heart Study, a long-term, multigenerational study that seeks to uncover the underlying causes of cardiovascular disease. All participants underwent a cardiopulmonary exercise test, the gold standard for assessing fitness. They also completed questionnaires to assess the quality of their diets, noting how often they consumed 126 foods and drinks during the previous year. Higher-quality diets emphasized vegetables, fruits, whole grains, nuts, legumes, fish, and healthy fats, and limited red meat and alcohol.

Researchers adjusted for possible confounding factors that might affect the diet-fitness relationship, including how many calories the participants consumed, their body mass index, and their routine physical activity levels. They found that healthy dietary habits were strongly and positively linked with fitness. The improvement in fitness seen among those with the healthiest diets was similar to the effect of an additional 4,000 steps each day, say the authors. Their study was published in May 2023 in the *European Journal of Preventive Cardiology*.

Does coffee help or harm your heart?

Americans' favorite morning brew has gotten mixed reviews over the years. Here's a closer look at some of coffee's cardiovascular effects.

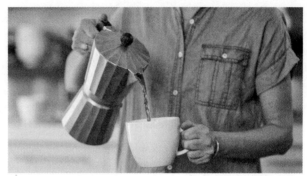

© PeopleImages | Getty Images

Drinking one to three cups of coffee daily doesn't appear to affect heart health.

Many people can't imagine starting their day without a cup or two of coffee. Despite its popularity, however, coffee has been a bit controversial when it comes to heart health.

"The thinking about coffee's effects on the heart has swung in both directions," says Dr. J. Michael Gaziano, professor of medicine at Harvard Medical School. In the 1960s, coffee was considered a risk factor for coronary artery disease, although later research suggested that only heavy coffee consumption (more than five or six cups a day) might harm the heart. But people who drink excessive amounts of coffee often differ in many other ways from those who enjoy modest amounts, Dr. Gaziano notes.

A java jolt?

Because coffee contains caffeine, a stimulant, people have long wondered whether drinking coffee might "jazz up" the heart, triggering palpitations (the odd sensation of a skipped, missed, or strong heartbeat) or atrial fibrillation (a heart rhythm problem marked by a rapid, irregular heartbeat).

However, people who drink moderate amounts of coffee (one to three cups per day) actually appear to have a lower risk of atrial fibrillation, according to a 2019 study co-authored by Dr. Gaziano. Those who drank either more or less coffee were no more or less likely to develop atrial fibrillation, the study found.

Like a lot of dietary research, that study was observational: people reported what they consumed and researchers tracked their health over many years. But a new study took a different approach—it directly measured the short-term effects of drinking coffee (see "The coffee connection: More steps, less sleep, possible palpitations?" on page 94).

Steps and sleep

"This new trial provides an important piece of the puzzle," says Dr. Gaziano. One finding—that people took more steps on coffee-drinking days—upholds other research showing that caffeine can slightly enhance physical performance. On the other hand, caffeine's adverse effects on sleep are also well known, and insufficient sleep is increasingly recognized as a risk to cardiovascular health.

It's hard to know whether the extra exercise balances out the decreased shut-eye people may get from drinking coffee. Most people know how they react to coffee and adjust their intake accordingly, says Dr. Gaziano, who enjoys a daily cup that contains half decaffeinated coffee.

Limitations of the study

But like all studies, the new study has limitations. For instance, it included only relatively young, healthy coffee drinkers. So the findings may not apply to older people, who tend to be more likely to have palpitations. In fact, people who avoid coffee (and so weren't part of the study) may avoid the beverage because they notice it triggers palpitations.

Other heart-related effects

The study also discovered that drinking coffee led to a slight increase in premature ventricular contractions. These brief rhythm disruptions (which can feel as though the heart is pounding or flip-flopping) are common and usually harmless, especially in healthy people. However, people with heart disease who notice persistent, odd heart rhythms should talk to their doctor.

Earlier research has investigated coffee's effects on other common heart-related risks. Although drinking coffee raises blood pressure, the effect is temporary and doesn't make you more likely to develop high blood pressure; it may even lower your risk. Unfiltered ▸▸

The coffee connection: More steps, less sleep, possible palpitations?

Many coffee drinkers appreciate the energizing buzz from a morning cup of joe. But does that boost have any short-term effects on the heart or other heart-related behaviors or risk factors—namely, exercise, sleep, and blood sugar levels?

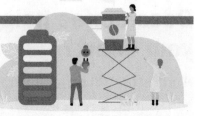
© PeopleImages | Getty Images

To find out, researchers put wearable sensors on volunteers for a two-week period. Their study, the Coffee and Real-time Atrial and Ventricular Ectopy, or CRAVE, trial, was published in 2023 in *The New England Journal of Medicine.* (Atrial and ventricular ectopy refers to premature contractions of the heart's upper or lower chambers. People typically experience these as strong, fast, or irregular heartbeats, known as palpitations.)

Who: 100 healthy men and women, average age 39.

What: Participants wore three separate devices: one that tracked activity levels and sleep, one that measured blood sugar, and one that monitored heart rhythm. They were also tested for common genetic variants that affect how quickly people metabolize caffeine.

How: Researchers directed participants to drink as much caffeinated coffee as they wanted for two days and to activate the heart monitor after every cup they drank. They were then to abstain from coffee for two days. They repeated this cycle for 14 days.

Key findings: On the days people drank coffee, they took an average of 1,000 extra steps per day. But they slept about 36 fewer minutes per night, on average. Coffee drinking had no apparent effect on blood sugar levels. And while coffee consumption did not increase premature atrial contractions, it did appear to slightly increase the incidence of premature ventricular contractions. Genetic differences in caffeine metabolism had no meaningful effects on any of these outcomes.

coffee, such as French press coffee and espresso, contains compounds that may raise harmful LDL cholesterol. But the effect is likely trivial compared with the rest of your diet, especially if you drink no more than two cups of unfiltered coffee daily.

"The question I have is, what is the overall impact on the outcome I care most about, which is cardiovascular disease?" asks Dr. Gaziano. When you look at the evidence as a whole, coffee doesn't seem to have a positive or negative effect, he says. If you like coffee, enjoy up to a few cups per day—as long as it's not interfering with your sleep. And don't dump a lot of cream and sugar into your coffee, he notes, since that adds saturated fat and empty calories.

IN THE JOURNALS

Seeing clogged arteries may inspire healthier habits

If people see evidence of plaque buildup inside their arteries, it may motivate them to take better care of their hearts, new research suggests.

The study, which pooled findings from six randomized trials, included more than 7,000 people in total. Most received scans to check for plaque in the arteries of their hearts or necks. Each of the studies randomly assigned people to two groups. Half were shown their scan results; the others were either not shown their results or were not scanned. The study follow-ups lasted one to four years.

Researchers found greater improvements among people who saw images of their plaque buildup. Compared with people who didn't see scans, those who did had lower cholesterol and blood pressure values at the end of the follow-up period, as well as lower overall risk of heart disease. The study was published in 2023 by *JACC: Cardiovascular Imaging.*

How much do you sit, stand, and move each day?

Swapping even just a few minutes of sitting with movement may lead to tangible improvements in heart health.

Let's say you sleep about eight hours a night. During the 16 hours you're awake, are you sitting for much of that time? If that's the case, you can improve your cardiovascular health by moving—or even simply standing—more during the day.

This advice is hardly new, as experts have been sounding the alarm about the health hazards of sedentary behavior for decades. Now, a new study sheds light on how different types and amounts of activity may affect indicators of heart health, such as body mass index (BMI), cholesterol values, and blood sugar levels.

"It's the first study to look at how different movement patterns over an entire 24-hour period may affect those factors," says Dr. Edward Phillips, associate professor of physical medicine and rehabilitation at Harvard Medical School. That's important because, whenever you make any type of lifestyle change, it's helpful to know not just what you're adding but also what you're subtracting. For example, when people eat more fruit, they may eat fewer cookies, and both shifts are beneficial. Likewise, people are better off when they move more and sit less, he says. The new findings include estimates about the potential advantages of choosing different activities—including sleeping—in place of sitting.

How was the study done?

Published in 2023 by the *European Heart Journal*, the article includes data from more than 15,000 people participating in six studies from five different countries. Their average age was 54, and nearly 55% were women. Most (88%) rated their health as good or better. Researchers assessed the participants' heart health based on their BMI (a measurement that incorporates both weight and height), waist circumference, cholesterol and triglyceride levels, and HbA1c (a measure of blood sugar used to assess diabetes risk). About a third were taking medication to control cholesterol, high blood pressure, or diabetes, and about 10% had been diagnosed with heart disease.

Participants wore special activity monitors that attach to the front of the thigh. These monitors are

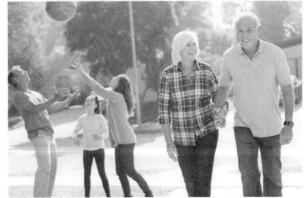

© Paul Bradbury | Getty Images

Every extra minute you spend walking—or even just strolling or standing—instead of sitting will benefit your cardiovascular health.

more accurate than those worn on the hip or the wrist for discerning between sitting and standing. Based on a week's worth of data, the average participant's day consisted of 7.7 hours sleeping, 10.4 hours sitting, 3.1 hours standing, 1.5 hours doing light physical activity, and 1.3 hours doing moderate-to-vigorous physical activity.

Note that the participants probably didn't do 1.3 hours of structured moderate- or vigorous-intensity exercise per day. Rather, the trackers recorded and added up all their short bouts of activity, such as walking up a flight of stairs or running to catch a bus, says Dr. Phillips.

What did the study find?

Not surprisingly, researchers found that moderate-to-vigorous activity proved most beneficial for heart health, while sitting was the worst. Next, they created statistical models to estimate what would happen if a person swapped one behavior for another. Replacing even just five minutes of sitting with moderate-to-vigorous activity (such as brisk walking, running, or cycling) could have a tangible effect on heart health, they reported.

Of course, extending that swap time to 30 minutes is even better. As an example, they estimated the potential change in BMI from doing moderate-to-vigorous activity instead of 30 minutes daily of each ▸▸

▶▶ of the four other activities. Routinely replacing light activity with moderate activity could nudge down BMI by about 0.15 points. Swapping standing or sleeping with moderate activity could lower BMI by 0.40 and 0.43 points, respectively. But replacing sitting with moderate activity could lower BMI by 0.63 points.

While adding longer, more intense bouts of exercise can reap greater rewards, even small, modest changes can make a difference. For instance, replacing sitting with standing led to positive changes across all the health parameters. "I tell my patients to take any opportunity to add more movement into their day, or even just standing instead of sitting all day," Dr. Phillips says.

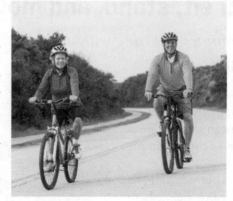

© kali9 | Getty Images

Moderate-to-vigorous activities include cycling, jogging, brisk walking, and swimming.

The sleep quotient

While the model suggests that even sleeping is better than sitting when it comes to heart health, it's not quite that simple. For example, indirect factors that lead to weight gain (for example, snacking while watching television) may explain why sitting appears worse than sleeping.

In addition, there's good evidence linking sleep deprivation with poor metabolic health. "When you're tired, you're less likely to exercise and won't eat as healthfully, and you feel more stressed," says Dr. Phillips. So if you're sleep deprived (that is, you routinely get less than six hours of sleep per night), you should prioritize getting at least seven hours of shut-eye every night rather doing more exercise.

Two workout strategies that reduce cardiovascular disease risk

Doing regular aerobic exercise—the kind that works your heart and lungs—is one of the best ways to reduce your risk of cardiovascular disease. Now, findings published in 2024 by the *European Heart Journal* suggest that doing a combination of aerobics and strength training might reduce cardiovascular risk factors just as effectively.

The study involved about 400 people (ages 35 to 70) classified as overweight or obese who also had high blood pressure. They were randomly assigned to one of four exercise programs: a 60-minute

© kali9 | Getty Images

aerobic workout three times a week, a 60-minute strength training workout three times a week, a 60-minute combination of aerobics and strength training (30 minutes of each) three times a week, or no exercise at all. After one year, people in both the aerobics-only group and the combination exercise group (but not the strength-training-only group) had a significant reduction in a combined measure of cardiovascular risk factors, compared with people who didn't exercise. These risk factors included blood pressure, LDL (bad) cholesterol, blood sugar, and body fat. People doing the combined workouts also improved their muscle strength. What this means: it might be equally healthful to replace half of your aerobic workout with strength training, without adding additional exercise time.

What else can you do?

One simple trick to make sure you get up out of your chair regularly? "Fill up a water bottle and drink it throughout the day, so you'll have to get up to use the bathroom," says Dr. Phillips. Another helpful habit: take a short stroll after lunch or dinner. "Using the large muscles in your legs helps absorb the glucose load from the meal, which helps regulate your blood sugar and insulin levels," he explains.

A fitness band or smart watch can help you keep tabs on your daily activity, including how much you exercise and sleep. Some models include default reminders to stand up at least once an hour for at least 12 hours per day. But don't feel you have to get one of these devices, says Dr. Phillips. A smartphone (which nearly everyone has these days) does a fine job tracking your daily steps, provided you remember to carry it with you most of the day. If you take about 500 steps during a five-minute walk, that counts as brisk walking. "Don't worry if you have a slower pace. Just get out of your chair and get moving as much and as often as you can," he says. 🛡

For mellow movement that helps your heart, try tai chi

Need a workout that's engaging but won't leave you feeling tired and sweaty? Tai chi may be just the ticket.

Most people recognize that exercise is one of the best ways to boost cardiovascular health. But what if traditional exercise seems either too challenging or otherwise inaccessible—or maybe even boring? Or perhaps you're recovering from a heart attack or other medical problem and need to ease back into activity. If so, tai chi might be worth a try.

"Tai chi is a gentle, adaptable practice that features flowing movements combined with breathing and cognitive focus," says Dr. Peter Wayne, associate professor of medicine at Harvard Medical School and medical editor of the Harvard Special Health Report *An Introduction to Tai Chi* (www.health.harvard.edu/TC). The cardiovascular benefits likely stem from a combination of the physical and mental aspects of this ancient Chinese practice.

Body and mind benefits

A tai chi session doesn't aim to dramatically raise your heart rate or build bulky muscles. But the slow, deliberate movements still help to tone your muscles. If you move more quickly from one position to the next and sink deeper into the postures, tai chi can even provide a moderate aerobic workout.

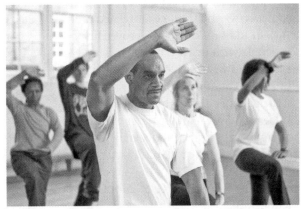

© Tim Platt | Getty Images

Tai chi requires focused attention that helps quiet distracting thoughts and promotes relaxation.

Conversely, you can dial down the intensity and even do certain movements while seated in a chair. Unlike yoga, tai chi doesn't require you to fully extend or stretch your joints, so it's fine for people who are not so flexible.

Like yoga, tai chi is a mind-body practice that requires focused attention as you move through a series of choreographed moves. Many have descriptive names that evoke scenes from nature, such as "wave hands like clouds" or "the white crane spreads its wings." Concentrating on that imagery, along with your breathing and movements, counteracts what Asian meditative traditions call "monkey mind"— the distracting mental chatter that often intrudes when people do traditional meditation. In this way, tai chi can foster relaxation and ease stress. Tai chi also teaches you to pay close attention to your ▸▸

▸▸ posture, breathing, and heart rate. "This increased body awareness can help prevent injury and overexertion," says Dr. Wayne.

Heartfelt effects

An article published in 2023 by *Cardiology in Review* considered the heart-related benefits of tai chi. Many studies have documented improvements in blood pressure after just eight to 12 weeks of practicing tai chi, including among older, sedentary adults and heart attack survivors. There's also good evidence that tai chi can be an effective alternative for people who don't want to do traditional cardiac rehabilitation (a structured program of exercise and education for people recovering from heart-related problems). In addition, tai chi has proved helpful for people with heart failure, who tend to be tired and weak as a result of the heart's diminished pumping ability.

The authors also point out that tai chi can be a gateway to other types of physical activity because the practice may improve balance, reduce the risk of falls, and even help ease lower back pain—a common reason for avoiding exercise. "More fundamentally, the fitness gains and self-awareness from tai chi training can give people the confidence to engage in other physical and social activities that can enhance health," says Dr. Wayne. ▼

Ready to try tai chi?

Tai chi classes are often offered at martial arts studios, but you can also find them at senior or community centers, health clubs, universities, or hospitals. Most facilities list class descriptions on their websites; if not, call to inquire which class would be best for you, based on your experience and fitness level.

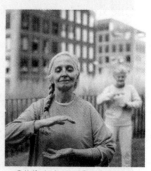
© Halfpoint Images | Getty Images

Many of the academic health centers throughout the United States with integrative health programs offer tai chi classes. Some cardiac rehabilitation programs, including those affiliated with several Harvard teaching hospitals, incorporate tai chi into their programs.

Hourlong classes usually cost around $15 to $25. Some centers allow you to pay by the week, month, or several months. Many places now offer online classes as well, and evidence shows that you can reap similar benefits from virtual instruction.

Wear loose, comfortable clothing and supportive shoes like sneakers (or no shoes, if you prefer). During the class, the instructor will demonstrate graceful, slow arm and leg movements, often done with a slight bend in the knees. The sequence of poses can be done standing or, in some cases, while seated in a chair.

You can also watch and follow along with the free videos that illustrate movements from the Harvard report on tai chi at www.health.harvard.edu/tai-chi-calisthenics and www.health.harvard.edu/tai-chi-elements.

Advice for the lonely hearts club

Loneliness and social isolation can leave you more vulnerable to cardiovascular disease. Making the effort to foster friendships, both new and old, can help.

That old Hank Williams song, "I'm So Lonesome I Could Cry," evokes the wistful sadness of loneliness that everyone feels at times. But this emotion is far more prevalent—and potentially detrimental to heart health—than most people recognize.

In 2023, U.S. Surgeon General Dr. Vivek Murthy released an 82-page advisory about the country's epidemic of loneliness, which he called an underappreciated health crisis. Even before the COVID-19 pandemic, about half of adults reported feeling lonely.

Being lonely or socially isolated has been linked to a 29% higher risk of heart disease and a 32% higher risk of stroke. In terms of mortality, the repercussions are similar to smoking up to 15 cigarettes per day—and are even greater than the risks associated with obesity and physical inactivity, according to the report.

The underlying mechanism is believed to be similar to what happens when people feel depressed or stressed. Nervous system changes activate hormones that boost blood pressure and trigger an outpouring of inflammatory substances in the blood that lead to a buildup of fatty plaque inside arteries.

Missing connections

Social isolation and loneliness certainly increased during the pandemic, but this trend had a small silver lining: a heightened awareness and appreciation of the importance of human connection. "COVID's consequences sharpened our focus on loneliness, and the isolation we felt was a reminder of how precious it is to see people in person," says Dr. Jacqueline Olds, a psychiatrist at Harvard-affiliated McLean Hospital and the co-author of two books on loneliness. Not only did people long to see their friends and families, but they also missed small everyday interactions with neighbors, their mail carrier, and people at their local coffee shop.

Loneliness tends to be more common in older people, especially those who are widowed or divorced. The winter holidays sometimes heighten feelings of loneliness, says Dr. Olds. "People often imagine idealized holiday scenes with lots of happy faces around the table," she says. Seeing photos on social media sites of people having fun can also exacerbate feelings of isolation. But keep in mind that these curated images aren't everyday reality for most people.

Initiating and keeping social plans can be challenging, especially if you live alone, Dr. Olds acknowledges. "It's true that it's much harder to do things by yourself, but it's not impossible," she says. Maybe you feel a little shy or anxious, or you're concerned about issues like coping with unpredictable weather, traffic, or staying out too late. Try to push yourself outside your comfort zone, she adds, and know that you'll be fine if you get a little wet in the rain or don't wear the right shoes.

Forging friendships

Start by reconnecting with an old friend or acquaintance, Dr. Olds suggests. Spending time with familiar

people can shore up your social skills, which can help you feel more confident about creating new connections. Say yes to social invitations, and make sure to take turns initiating and following through with plans to get together with people.

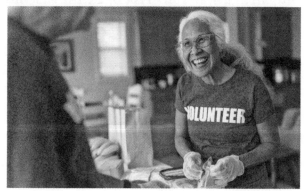

© Fly View Productions | Getty Images

Volunteering in your local community can be a good way to curb isolation and stave off loneliness.

Being around people who have similar interests is a good way to make new friends, since you already have something in common. Look online or at your local library for classes, in-person clubs, or volunteer opportunities that match your interests—or maybe something new you'd like to try. One helpful source is Meetup, an online social community that coordinates both in-person and virtual activities of all kinds, including many targeted to seniors (see www.meetup.com). There are hundreds of groups, including those focused on outdoor activities (for example, hiking, canoeing, or mini-golf) or hobbies (photography, Vietnamese cooking, motorcycle riding), as well as groups that meet to discuss books, movies, or just share a meal.

Volunteering in your local community is another nice way to connect with new people, with the added potential bonus of giving you a sense of purpose and satisfaction. Volunteer Match (www.volunteermatch.org) connects people with local volunteer opportunities that suit their interests and expertise, with such choices as fighting climate change, tutoring children, assisting immigrants and refugees, working with computers and technology, and numerous others.

Having a pet—especially a dog—can give you company at home and also help you meet people when you're out on walks or at the dog park. Animal lovers might also consider volunteering at an animal shelter or joining a bird watching group. 🛡

How positive psychology can help you cultivate better heart health

Expressing gratitude, focusing on your strengths, and performing kind acts may help lower your risk of cardiovascular disease.

Conversations about heart disease and mental health often dwell on the overlap between cardiovascular problems and negative emotions. It makes sense: People with depression face a heightened risk of heart problems. Also, it's common—and understandable—to feel moody, distressed, or irritable after a heart attack.

Increasingly, however, mental health experts are focusing on how optimism and other positive emotions can guard against serious heart-related events and death. Optimism is linked to a lower risk of cardiovascular disease, according to a 2022 review in *The American Journal of Medicine* that pooled findings from nearly 182,000 people from six separate studies. People who are happier or more optimistic may be more likely to exercise more, eat more healthfully, and sleep better, which might explain the link. But can people who aren't naturally cheerful actually improve their physical health by changing their mindset?

"There's good evidence that some simple exercises designed to enhance positive feelings can improve well-being and reduce depression," says Emily Feig, a clinical psychologist in the Cardiac Psychiatry Research Program at Harvard-affiliated Massachusetts General Hospital. Some of these interventions have been shown to encourage people—including those with heart-related issues such as heart attacks and heart failure—to exercise more and take their medications more consistently, she says.

Promoting positive feelings

One exercise, expressing gratitude, involves writing a letter to a person who did something in the past for

© SuslO | Getty Images
Focus on the positive to create momentum for healthy habits.

which you feel grateful. "Research shows that actually writing about your experience has a more beneficial effect than just thinking about it," says Feig.

In another exercise, people identify one of their own personal strengths from a list of different qualities, such as love, curiosity, persistence, or self-control. Then, they plan a new way to apply that strength to deal with a specific situation over the next week.

Performing an act of kindness for someone is another way people can cultivate positive feelings. For example, you might mow a neighbor's lawn or bring a meal to friend.

For each of these exercises, people are encouraged to pay attention to how they feel at each stage of the exercise—planning, execution, and response.

The upward spiral

Having a more positive outlook may help reinforce other positive behaviors, in what psychologists refer to as an "upward spiral." This momentum can help people start healthy habits like exercise, which then becomes self-reinforcing, says Feig. Practicing positive psychology also helps foster resilience, which can help you cope better during difficult times.

"We don't tell people to ignore or push away negative experiences or pretend they don't exist," says Feig. But your mood tends to mirror what you focus on. Even during a week that includes many difficult challenges, there are usually a few positive moments, she says. Focusing on those small, positive things may allow that emotion to broaden and help you feel more balanced. ▼

Chapter 5

Smart Eating

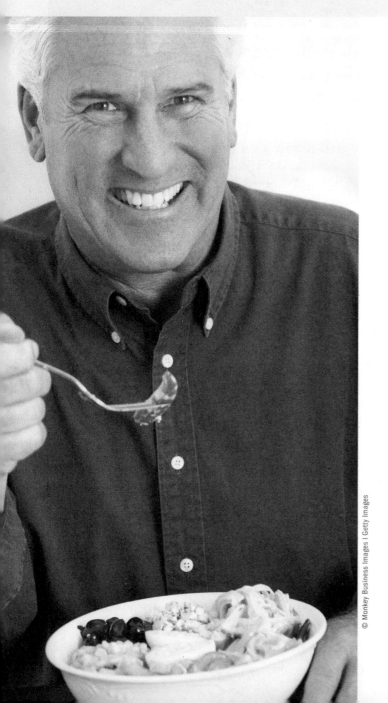

© Monkey Business Images | Getty Images

Healthy Habits!
5 Things You Can Do Now

1 **Try a new cuisine.** Asian- and Latin American–inspired meals that incorporate plenty of veggies provide substantial health benefits. (page 107)

2 **Stay hydrated.** Feelings of thirst can diminish with age, but everyone needs water to stay healthy. (page 119)

3 **Consider going alcohol-free.** Even a month away can bring surprising benefits. (page 120)

4 **Give intuitive eating a try.** This alternative to dieting encourages listening to your body. (page 121)

5 **Clean out old and expired foods.** Sources of food poisoning can lurk in your own kitchen. (page 124)

Healthy eating: How does your diet stack up?

The DASH diet—along with Mediterranean, pescatarian, and vegetarian eating patterns—received the highest marks in a recent ranking by the American Heart Association.

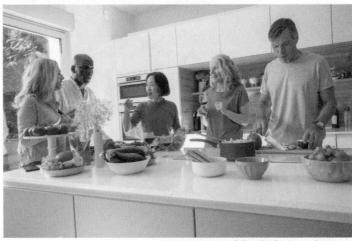

© PhotoAlto/Eric Audras | Getty Images

The common elements of all heart-healthy diets? Veggies, fruits, whole grains, and nuts.

When you consider that 80% of heart disease can be prevented by healthy lifestyle habits, it makes sense to prioritize the one habit you can't live without: eating. But many people—including doctors—aren't sure which diets are best for keeping your heart healthy.

This problem was the inspiration behind a 2023 scientific statement from the American Heart Association (AHA) published in *Circulation*, says Dr. Frank Hu, professor of nutrition and epidemiology at the Harvard T.H. Chan School of Public Health. "People hear about all sorts of popular diets in the news and on social media. But they don't have a good sense about which ones actually have scientific evidence behind them," he says. Neither do most doctors, as they receive very little nutrition training as part of their education. (Note that although the word "diet" is often associated with weight loss, it more generally refers to the kinds of foods people typically eat.)

Evidence-based ranking

The statement ranks 10 popular diets based on how well they align with the AHA's dietary guidelines, which recommend limiting saturated fat and excess carbohydrates, especially highly processed carbs and sugary drinks (see "Popular diets: Common names, key features, and rankings," page 103). The evidence comes from decades of randomized trials, population-based studies, and other research, says Dr. Hu, who served as a reviewer for the scientific statement.

"It's no surprise that all of the top-tier diets are mostly plant-based," says Kathy McManus, director of the Department of Nutrition at Harvard-affiliated Brigham and Women's Hospital. Vegetables, fruits, whole grains, beans, and nuts are all naturally low in saturated fat. They're also good sources of fiber and contain a variety of antioxidants. "What I like about the DASH and Mediterranean diets is that they include fish, which is a good source of both healthy fats and protein," she says. Canned fish, such as sardines, herring, and tuna, are affordable options, she adds. But these two diets can also include a range of other healthy proteins, like beans, nuts, poultry, dairy products, and eggs.

Another reason the top two diets get high marks is that they encourage people to limit refined grains and added sugars. "A healthy dietary pattern should focus on whole, real foods and limit processed foods, which tend to add extra salt, sugar, and fat into your diet," says McManus. Over all, vegetarian and pescatarian diets tend to be quite healthy, but not if people simply avoid meat and fill up on processed foods, she adds.

Be flexible

Don't feel you have to abandon the familiar foods you grew up eating. "Following cultural traditions and preferences is important for helping people stay with a diet over the long term," says Dr. Hu.

McManus agrees. "You might need to make some adjustments to how your traditional favorite foods are prepared by swapping in a healthier fat or using less sodium," she says. You'll be more likely to stick with healthy, lasting changes if you make small, gradual changes that are flexible, family-friendly, and realistic, she notes.

Popular diets: Common names, key features, and rankings

This table ranks popular diets based on how closely they align with heart-healthy guidelines. Those in tier 1 (green) adhere most closely. Tier 2 diets (light green) align well but may be harder to follow. Tier 3 diets (yellow) align somewhat but may restrict healthy foods such as nuts and plant oils. Tier 4 diets (red) align poorly, as they include too many animal-sourced foods high in unhealthy fats and restrict healthful plant-based foods.

DIET TYPE	OTHER NAMES AND VARIANTS	EMPHASIZE	INCLUDE	LIMIT/AVOID
DASH (Dietary Approaches to Stop Hypertension); see www.health.harvard.edu/DASH	Nordic, Baltic	Vegetables, fruits, whole grains, legumes, nuts, seeds, low-fat dairy	Lean meats and poultry, fish and shellfish, non-tropical oils	Limit saturated fat, sodium, fatty meats, refined grains, added sugars, alcohol.
Mediterranean; see www.health.harvard.edu/meddiet		Vegetables, fruits, whole grains, legumes, nuts, seeds, poultry, fish and seafood, extra-virgin olive oil	Red wine (in moderation)	Limit dairy, meat, sugar-sweetened beverages, commercial bakery goods, sweets.
Vegetarian plus fish	Pescatarian	Vegetables, fruits, whole grains, legumes, nuts, seeds	Fish and shellfish, dairy, eggs	Avoid meat and poultry.
Vegetarian, including eggs and dairy	Ovo-lacto-vegetarian		Eggs and dairy	Avoid meat, poultry, fish and shellfish.
Vegetarian, including dairy	Lacto-vegetarian		Dairy	Avoid meat, poultry, and eggs.
Vegan		(see above)		Avoid all products of animal origin.
Low-fat	Therapeutic Lifestyle Changes (TLC), Volumetrics	Vegetables, fruits, whole grains, legumes	Low-fat dairy, lean meats, poultry, fish	Limit fat (less than 30% of calories), nuts, oils, fatty meat, poultry, fish, alcohol.
Very low-fat	Ornish, Esselstyn, Pritikin, McDougal	Vegetables, fruits, whole grains, legumes		Limit fat (less than 10% of calories), sodium, refined grains, alcohol. Avoid oils, nuts, seeds, meats, poultry, fish, dairy, eggs.
Low-carb	Zone, South Beach, low glycemic load	Nonstarchy vegetables, fruits, nuts, seeds, fish and seafood, non-tropical oils		Limit carbohydrates (30% to 40% of calories), whole and refined grains, legumes, dairy, alcohol. Avoid added sugars, fatty meat.
Paleolithic	Paleo	Vegetables, fruits, nuts, lean meat, fish	Eggs	Limit sodium. Avoid added sugars, whole and refined grains, legumes, oils, dairy, alcohol.
Very low-carb	Atkins, ketogenic (keto)	Nuts, seeds, red meat, poultry, fish and seafood, eggs, full-fat dairy, oils	Nonstarchy vegetables, berries Ketogenic: 3000–5000 mg/day sodium	Limit carbohydrates (less than 10% of calories), alcohol. Avoid fruits (except berries), grains, legumes, added sugars.

Source: Adapted from American Heart Association Scientific Statement.

Focusing on six food groups may help prevent cardiovascular disease

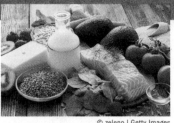

© zeleno | Getty Images

The staples of plant-based diets may offer the most heart benefits.

Plant-based diets like the Mediterranean and DASH diets are linked with better heart health. But do certain components of these diets stand out? A study published in 2023 by the *European Heart Journal* suggests that eating enough of six types of food common in these diets is associated with a lower risk of cardiovascular disease. The six food categories are fruits, vegetables, legumes, nuts, fish, and dairy products.

Researchers compiled a healthy diet score from 245,000 people from around the world. The score was determined by how much and how often people ate foods from these six categories. After more than nine years, the researchers found that people with the highest diet scores (meaning they regularly ate high quantities from the six categories) had fewer cases of cardiovascular disease, heart attacks, strokes, and death than people with lower scores. The researchers also determined that the following daily or weekly servings were linked to better health outcomes:

▶ two to three servings each of fruits and vegetables (a serving equals one apple or banana, 1 cup of leafy vegetables, or ½ cup of other vegetables)
▶ one serving of nuts (1 ounce per serving)
▶ two servings of dairy products (a serving equals 1 cup of milk or yogurt).

Weekly intake included
▶ three to four servings of legumes (a serving equals ½ cup beans or lentils)
▶ two to three servings of fish (3 ounces per serving).

Keto diet may harm the heart

The ketogenic (keto) diet—which is high in fat and protein and low in carbohydrates—doesn't meet standards for a healthy diet and may not be safe for some people with heart disease, according to a 2024 review in *Current Problems in Cardiology.*

The review summarized the current evidence on how keto diets may raise heart disease risk. While the diet may dramatically reduce fat mass and weight over the short term, there is scarce evidence for any long-term benefit. Ketogenic diets appear to lower blood levels of triglycerides but raise levels of

20% PROTEIN
5% CARBS
KETO DIET
75% FAT

© zeleno | Getty Images

artery-clogging LDL cholesterol. With respect to lowering blood sugar and blood pressure, the observed short-term benefits fade over time.

The diet's extreme carbohydrate restrictions may lead people to shun most vegetables and fruits and consume large amounts of leafy greens. However, the vitamin K in these foods may interfere with the anti-clotting drug warfarin taken by some heart patients. And drugs known as SGLT-2 inhibitors, which are used to treat diabetes and heart failure, may be incompatible with a keto diet, according to the review.

Eating for heart health

Dietary choices can raise or lower your heart disease risk. Here are the foods you should choose and those to avoid.

As the saying goes, you are what you eat, and that's especially true when it comes to heart health. Dietary choices can influence your weight, blood pressure, cholesterol levels, and blood sugar levels—all factors that can determine your risk for heart disease, heart attack, and stroke.

So when it comes to diet and heart health, what foods should you eat more of, less of, or not at all? Here's what a Harvard nutritionist and cardiologist suggest.

Eat less: Saturated fat

Saturated fat is found primarily in meats, such as beef, pork, and deli meat; dairy foods like milk, butter, cream, and cheese; and tropical oils like coconut oil and palm oil. High amounts of saturated fat also are found in many fast, processed, and baked foods like frozen pizza, desserts, hamburgers, and packaged sweets.

The main health issue with saturated fat is its impact on cholesterol levels. "Consuming high amounts of saturated fat produces more 'bad' LDL cholesterol, which can form plaque in the arteries that blocks blood flow and increases your risk for heart

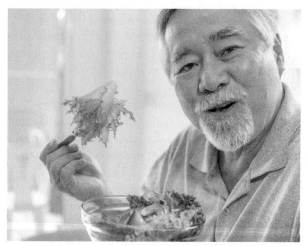
© lucky-sky | Getty Images

Focus on fruits and vegetables—and avoid saturated fats and refined sugars—to reduce your heart disease risk.

attack and stroke," says registered dietitian Marc O'Meara, an outpatient senior nutrition counselor at Harvard-affiliated Brigham and Women's Hospital.

Eat more: Healthy fats

"Besides avoiding saturated fat, you should increase your intake of healthy monounsaturated and polyunsaturated fat," says O'Meara. These "good" fats help lower LDL cholesterol and triglycerides.

Sources of monounsaturated fats are olive oil, peanut oil, canola oil, avocados, and most nuts. There are two main types of polyunsaturated fats: omega-3 fatty acids and omega-6 fatty acids. Sources of omega-3s include fatty fish, such as salmon, mackerel, and sardines; flaxseeds; walnuts; and soybean oil. Many vegetable oils—such as soybean, sunflower, walnut, and corn oils—are rich in omega-6s.

"For heart health, it's important to focus on eating omega-3 fats several times a week, since they are in limited foods," says O'Meara. "Omega-6 fats are easier to get as they are in a wider array of foods."

Eat less: Refined sugar

Refined sugar is what's added to food products to improve taste (which is why it's also known as "added" sugar). Refined sugar comes from cane, sugar beets, and corn, which are processed to isolate the sugar.

Refined sugar has several indirect connections with heart health. Consuming too much refined sugar contributes to weight gain, the leading cause of fatty liver disease and type 2 diabetes, both of

---

Follow the 80/20 rule

It's not realistic to refrain from all problem foods. It's fine to occasionally eat chips while watching the game, treat yourself to dessert, and dine out with friends. To ensure you consistently follow an overall heart-healthy diet, while allowing yourself to live a little, adopt the 80/20 rule: eat healthy 80% of the time, and save 20% of your meals and snack for fun foods. "This eliminates the stress of having to eat perfectly every day," says registered dietitian Marc O'Meara with Brigham and Women's Hospital. "Weekends count, so don't pile all your fun foods into a couple days. Instead, sprinkle them throughout the week for the best chance at weight control."

▶▶ which are closely linked to a higher risk of cardiovascular disease. Excess added sugar may also play a role in elevating blood pressure and stimulating chronic inflammation, two other factors related to heart disease.

The top food sources of refined sugar include soft drinks, energy drinks, fruit-flavored drinks, flavored yogurts, cereals, cookies, and cakes. But refined sugar is also found in many other processed foods, such as canned soups, cured meats, and ketchup.

Guidelines recommend men consume no more than 36 grams (about 9 teaspoons' worth) of refined sugar per day, about equal to what's in a 12-ounce can of soda. "The best way to control your intake of added sugar is to read food labels," says O'Meara. "To get an accurate amount, multiple the grams of sugar on the label by the total number of servings."

Eat more: Plant-based foods

Science has provided strong evidence of the heart-healthy benefits of plant-based diets like the Mediterranean and DASH (Dietary Approaches to Stop Hypertension) diets.

"These diets have consistently shown they help manage the main markers of heart disease: cholesterol, blood pressure, and blood sugar," says Dr. Ron Blankstein, a cardiologist with Brigham and Women's Hospital's Heart and Vascular Center.

Both diets emphasize high amounts of fruits and vegetables, whole grains, fatty fish, legumes, and nuts; olive oil as the principal source of fat; and minimal amounts of red meat, dairy, and alcohol. (While whole fruits and vegetables are ideal, low-sodium canned vegetables and frozen fruits and vegetables without added sauces and cream are just as nutritious.)

Here are three ways to get more plants in your diet

A plant-based diet can be as tasty as it is healthful. Here are three ways to give it a try:

1. Turn your favorite meat-based meals into plant-based ones. For example, if you like lasagna, try eliminating the ground beef and substituting mushrooms and spinach, or skip the beef in your burritos in favor of pinto beans.

2. Instead of animal protein, eat at least 3 cups a week of protein-rich legumes, such as beans, lentils, and peas. Try tossing chickpeas into a salad, adding beans to a stew, or including lentils in a vegetarian "meat" loaf.

3. Combine simmered whole grains, sautéed or raw vegetables, and cooked legumes on your plate. This age-old combination provides the perfect combination of proteins and nutrients to fuel your body.

"These diets offer nutrients your heart requires, like healthy mono-unsaturated and polyunsaturated fats and antioxidants that help fight inflammation," says Dr. Blankstein.

Perhaps best of all, following a plant-based diet also can steer you away from unhealthy eating habits.

"If you're eating more of these plant-based foods, that means you're eating less of processed and high-sugar foods," says Dr. Blankstein. "And always remember that it's never too late to begin paying more attention to your diet. Don't wait for some heart-related event to change how you eat." ⬤

To add a boost of vitamins and minerals, request extra vegetables when dining out

Many restaurant entrees don't come with a generous serving of vegetables. But you can easily remedy that by asking for more vegetables, ordering vegetables from the side dish selection, or substituting vegetables or a salad for a less healthful side dish, such as fries. Plus, you may find new-to-you vegetables that you enjoy, or discover new takes on old favorites.

Traditional Chinese diets:
A template for healthy eating habits

This popular cuisine highlights foods linked to cardiovascular health, such as vegetables, soy-based foods, pungent flavorings, and tea.

Chinese food has long ranked high on the list of Americans' favorite ethnic cuisines. Of course, restaurant offerings don't always reflect the traditional daily fare eaten in China. Some popular but less-healthful menu items—such as pork spare ribs and fried dough sticks—should be reserved for the occasional indulgence. Still, you can find lots of healthy options when dining out at a Chinese restaurant, and it's not hard to make your own healthy Chinese food at home, says Lilian Cheung, editorial director of the Nutrition Source at the Harvard T.H. Chan School of Public Health (www.hsph.harvard.edu/nutritionsource).

Chinese home cooking

"In general, traditional Chinese cooking has a lot of merit," says Cheung, a native of Hong Kong. Many staple foods, such as vegetables, tofu, and seafood, are all linked to a lower risk of cardiovascular disease. So are the unsaturated oils (such as canola, soy, or peanut oil) frequently used to prepare Chinese dishes.

Perhaps you're familiar with stir-fries made with broccoli or bok choy (Chinese cabbage). But you could also branch out and use snow pea leaves (also called pea shoots), which are delicate, slightly bitter greens. Bitter melon, which looks like a long, pale-green, rough-textured cucumber, is another option especially rich in vitamin A, potassium, and folate, says Cheung. You can find these vegetables in large Asian groceries.

Asian supermarkets also often have a large selection of whole fish, such as hake, grouper, or sea bass, which are often prepared steamed with ginger and scallions. Shellfish such as shrimp, clams, and mussels are good sources of protein and other nutrients; they're usually steamed or stir-fried, either alone or with vegetables.

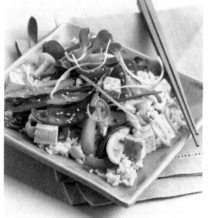

© Brian Hagiwara | Getty Images

A stir-fry made with tofu and vegetables served on brown rice is a heart-healthy Chinese dinner.

Shellfish are also far more environmentally friendly to farm than other animal-based protein sources such as beef, pork, and poultry.

Soybean curd (tofu) is another healthy, versatile protein common in the Chinese diet. Cheung likes to stir-fry soft tofu with green onions (scallions) and a little bit of oyster sauce and top it with a few drops of toasted sesame oil. "It takes just five minutes to make and is my favorite fast food," she says.

Healthy swaps and additions

Although white rice is embedded in Asian culture, nutrition experts urge people to opt for brown rice instead. Not only does brown rice offer more fiber and other nutrients, it's less likely than white rice to make blood sugar levels spike. Many Chinese restaurants now offer brown rice as an option on their menus, says Cheung.

Chinese cooking relies on soy sauce and other savory sauces (black bean, hoisin, and oyster), all of which are quite high in sodium. People with high blood pressure—about half of all Americans—should be careful not to consume too much sodium, which tends to raise blood pressure. When dining out at a Chinese restaurant, request that your food be prepared without monosodium glutamate (MSG), a flavor enhancer that also contains sodium, Cheung suggests.

For home cooking, you can buy soy sauce with 37% less sodium, which is marketed as "less sodium soy sauce." Adding a little lemon juice or vinegar allows you to use less soy sauce without sacrificing flavor. Also, aromatic roots like onions, garlic, and ginger can lend extra flavor to food.

Chili peppers, another classic ingredient in Chinese cooking, may also offer health benefits. Capsaicin, ▸▸

the chemical responsible for the spicy-hot flavor in chili peppers, may alter how the brain processes salty flavors, leading to lower sodium intake. Don't care for spicy food? You might enjoy the sweet but intense flavor of Chinese five-spice blend, which is a mix of star anise, fennel, Sichuan pepper, cinnamon, and cloves.

Drinks and desserts

In China, similar to many cultures throughout the world, tea is the beverage of choice. Both green and black tea are rich in compounds called flavonoids that help dampen inflammation, a culprit in heart disease. Tea drinking has also been linked to lower cholesterol and improved blood vessel function.

In China, fruit—especially sliced oranges—is a customary dessert. If you'd like to try something more exotic, seek out lychees, which are golf ball–sized tropical fruits native to Southern China. Also known as alligator strawberry, the fruit has a rough, pinkish-red skin and white flesh with a sweet, slightly floral flavor.

IN THE JOURNALS

Switching out just a serving of processed meats may boost cardiovascular health

Replacing one serving each day of processed meats with a serving of whole grains, nuts, or beans is linked with up to 36% lower odds of cardiovascular conditions such as heart attack or stroke, a 2023 study suggests.

For the analysis, published by *BMC Medicine*, researchers evaluated results from 32 earlier studies involving tens of thousands of healthy adults on three continents. Participants answered detailed questions about the foods they typically ate, and researchers followed them for an average of 19 years to assess any links between their diets and health outcomes, adjusting for other factors such as calorie intake, physical activity, and smoking and alcohol use.

Substituting a daily serving of processed meats—which include bacon, deli meats, hot dogs, and sausage—with nuts, beans, or whole grains was associated with 23% to 36% lower risk of cardiovascular disease. Replacing a serving of eggs each day with nuts was linked to 17% lower odds of cardiovascular problems. Meanwhile, participants were 10% less likely to develop diabetes if they substituted a serving of whole grains for red meat. The findings suggest that shifting from animal-based to plant-based foods can benefit cardiovascular health, the researchers said.

Do you know how much fiber you should be getting per day?

A high-fiber diet correlates with lower rates of heart disease, type 2 diabetes, and obesity, as well as better appetite control and digestive function—so it's important to get enough. For people up to age 50, the recommended intake for fiber is 38 grams for men and 25 grams for women (unless they are pregnant or breastfeeding, in which case the recommendations go up to 28 grams and 29 grams, respectively). Americans often fall short on fiber, consuming on average only about 15 grams of fiber a day. Aim to boost your intake by loading up on whole plant foods—especially legumes, whole grains, fruits, vegetables, seeds, and nuts. (For more about fiber, see "How to shop for healthier foods," page 127.)

Heart-healthy eating patterns inspired by Latin America

Adapt the Mediterranean diet to feature foods enjoyed in Mexico, the Caribbean, and Central and South America.

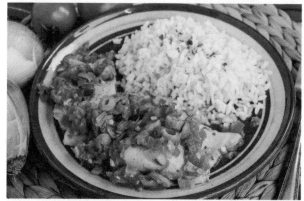

© Clara Murcia | Getty Images

Latin American cuisine includes many heart-healthy foods, such as fish and vegetables.

Long touted as one of the world's healthiest diets, the Mediterranean diet is backed by reputable evidence that this eating pattern protects against heart disease. But what if the foods and flavors of countries bordering the Mediterranean Sea simply aren't familiar or appealing to you? Or perhaps you just want to explore flavors from other parts of the world without abandoning healthful eating.

That's not a problem, says Josiemer Mattei, an associate professor of nutrition at the Harvard T.H. Chan School of Public Health, whose research focuses on links between nutrition and chronic disease with an emphasis on Latino and Hispanic culture. "You can adapt the basic guidelines of the Mediterranean diet to any cuisine you like. The key is choosing mostly plant-based foods and healthy fat sources that align with the different traditional cultures around the world," she says.

Almost 19% of people living in the United States are Hispanic or Latino, making them the second-largest racial or ethnic group. And Mexican food ranks among the most popular cuisines among Americans—although many restaurant offerings are a far cry from traditionally prepared dishes in Mexico, says Mattei. Following are suggestions for creating healthy meals inspired by fare found south of the border. Because Latin America includes about 35 countries, however, this is just a taste of this diverse cuisine.

Building a healthy, Latino-inspired plate

A Latino-inspired plate would align with the basic guidelines of the Mediterranean diet (see www.health.harvard.edu/meddiet) and Harvard's Healthy Eating Plate (www.health.harvard.edu/hp), featuring foods from these categories:

Plant-based protein. Latin American cuisine is known for its beans, which are good sources of both protein and fiber. Americans may be most familiar with pinto and black beans. But in Puerto Rico, Mattei's native country, pink beans and red beans are more common, along with pigeon peas. Different bean varieties have slightly different nutrient profiles, Mattei points out. For example, some have more folate (vitamin B9), while others contain more iron. "That's why I advocate eating a variety of beans, as well as nuts for the added benefit of healthy fats," says Mattei. Several nuts, including peanuts, cashews, and Brazil nuts, are native to South America.

Animal-based protein. Fish and seafood are popular in Mexico and other Latin American countries, especially near the seacoast. One popular preparation method is Veracruz style: white fish fillets cooked in a mixture of tomato, onion, garlic, olives, and capers (see photo, this page). Another animal-based specialty, chicken with mole poblano, features a savory sauce made with chocolate, chili peppers, and other spices. Some restaurants prepare alleged Mexican or Latino food with gooey, processed cheese, but that's not a part of traditional dishes, says Mattei. Instead, use sparing amounts of queso blanco or queso fresco, a soft, crumbly, white cheese that's similar to feta cheese but has a milder, less-salty flavor.

Carbohydrates. Whole or minimally processed grains or other starchy plants are some of the healthiest sources of carbohydrates. In Latin America, as in many cultures around the world, white rice is a staple. White rice is often eaten with fiber-rich beans, so it's best to serve at least as much beans as white rice on your plate for a healthier ratio, says Mattei. Swapping white rice for brown rice or corn, which is also commonly ground into corn flour (masa ▸▸

harina) to make tortillas or tamales, can provide added nutritional benefits. Plantains (starchy fruits related to bananas) are especially popular in Caribbean cuisine. One of Mattei's favorite meals features

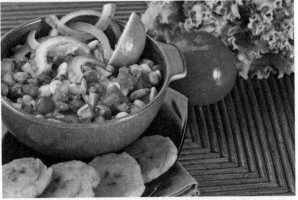

© Juan Gabriel Ortiz | Getty Images

A mixed bean dish (ceviche de legumbres) is a healthy option.

green plantains fried in plant-based oil (tostones) and mixed-beans stew.

Fruits and vegetables. Tropical fruits such as mango, pineapple, and papaya are found throughout Latin America and are also available in the United States. Those and more exotic options like açaí, guava, and passion fruit can be tasty, nutritious choices. Latino diets include many vegetables familiar to Americans, such as cabbage, carrots, tomatoes, and peppers. For variety, try jicama (a crunchy, mild-flavored root vegetable), chayote (similar to summer squash), or nopales (cactus paddles).

Healthy fats. Olive oil is available in Latin American countries, but other oils high in unsaturated fats, including soybean and canola oils, are just as healthy, says Mattei. Fish such as grouper and snapper, and avocados, which are native to the region, are also rich in healthy unsaturated fats.

The story on fish and heart health

Is eating fish healthy for the heart? Here's what the science says.

A diet that includes fatty fish (fish with more than 5% fat) has long been touted to support heart health. Population-based studies have found that people who regularly eat fatty fish have a lower risk of heart disease compared with those who don't eat fish.

While these were observational findings, when scientists looked closer, they found that the health benefit from fatty fish appears to arise from high levels of omega-3 fatty acids.

"The science linking fatty fish and heart health continues to evolve, but the evidence still points to omega-3s as a way to further protect against heart attacks and strokes," says Eric Rimm, a professor of epidemiology and nutrition at Harvard's T.H. Chan School of Public Health.

The three types

Omega-3s are essential fats, meaning the body can't make them and needs to get them from food. There are three main types of omega-3s: eicosapentaenoic acid (EPA), docosahexaenoic acid (DHA), and alpha-linolenic acid (ALA).

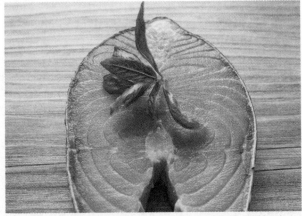

© Karl Tapales | Getty Images

Salmon contains some of the highest levels of heart-healthy omega-3 fatty acids among fatty fish.

EPA and DHA are found in seafood, especially fatty fish like salmon, mackerel, sardines, tuna, pollock, and cod. ALA is found mainly in nuts and seeds like flaxseed, chia seeds, pumpkin seeds, and walnuts, and in plant oils such as flaxseed, soybean, and canola oils.

"Your body can use ALA to make EPA and DHA, but the conversion is modest," says Rimm.

While all three omega-3s benefit the heart, EPA and DHA found in fatty fish have a more direct effect than ALA. Still, experts recommend that both fish and plant omega-3s be part of a healthy diet.

Why are omega-3s so helpful? They reduce triglycerides (a type of fat in the blood) and increase "good" HDL cholesterol. Omega-3s slow plaque buildup in arteries that can cause blood clots and trigger heart attacks and strokes. They help to ease inflammation and lower blood pressure. As a result, it's probably no surprise that fatty fish is a staple in most science-backed heart-healthy eating patterns, such as the Mediterranean and DASH diets.

Now serving fish

Eating two 3-ounce servings of fatty fish weekly is recommended by the American Heart Association. (There doesn't appear to be extra heart benefit from eating more than this amount.) Some fatty fish have higher amounts of omega-3s than others. (See "Top catches for omega-3s" below.)

Vegetarians (who avoid all types of meat) and vegans (who avoid all animal-based foods) can get enough omega-3s by increasing their intake of plant-based ALA, says Rimm. There also are algae-based EPA and DHA supplements available, and initial research shows their levels are comparable to fish oil.

However, relying on supplements probably shouldn't be your preferred strategy. Studies that have looked at omega-3 supplements' effect on heart health have shown mixed results. A 2021 analysis published in *Circulation* found that taking omega-3 supplements

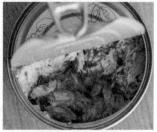

© Kinga Krzeminska | Getty Images
Canned fish packed in water contains similar amounts of omega-3s as wild fish.

may even slightly increase the risk of atrial fibrillation (an irregular heart rhythm).

"Based on the current evidence, there is little reason to take an omega-3 supplement if you already eat fatty fish," says Rimm. (For more on fish oil supplement safety, see "The false promise of fish oil supplements," page 90.)

Farmed or wild?

Most fatty fish that people buy is farmed, which is less expensive and more readily available than wild-caught fish. If people are worried about contamination, especially mercury, Rimm says that the overall risk is low whether fish is farmed or wild.

"The best advice is to eat a variety of fatty fish, but avoid frequently eating swordfish, which often have the highest levels of mercury," he says. "Overall, the benefits from eating fatty fish outweigh any possible risks from contamination."

Research has found that most farmed and wild fish have similar omega-3 amounts. The exception is farmed salmon, which actually has more omega-3s than wild. Canned fish is also on a par with wild fish in terms of omega-3s. Choose canned fish packed in water rather than oil. Some omega-3 fats are lost when the oil is drained.

How fatty fish is prepared usually doesn't matter, as cooking won't substantially change its omega-3 content, says Rimm. "However, you want to avoid fried and breaded fish, as they add extra unhealthy ingredients that your heart doesn't need." 🛡

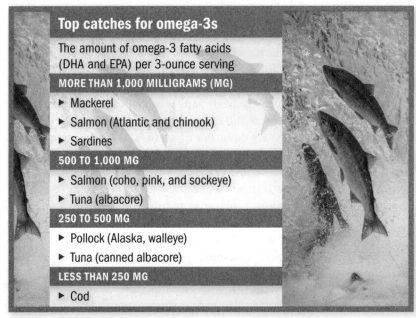

Top catches for omega-3s

The amount of omega-3 fatty acids (DHA and EPA) per 3-ounce serving

MORE THAN 1,000 MILLIGRAMS (MG)
- ▶ Mackerel
- ▶ Salmon (Atlantic and chinook)
- ▶ Sardines

500 TO 1,000 MG
- ▶ Salmon (coho, pink, and sockeye)
- ▶ Tuna (albacore)

250 TO 500 MG
- ▶ Pollock (Alaska, walleye)
- ▶ Tuna (canned albacore)

LESS THAN 250 MG
- ▶ Cod

Source: U.S. Department of Agriculture.

Practical pointers about protein

For optimal health, pay more attention to the quality of your protein sources rather than the quantity.

Popular diets often encourage people to cut back on carbs or eat less fat. When it comes to protein, however, advice about the ideal daily amount has been mixed. Does the average American eat too much protein—or not enough?

People who take weight-loss drugs and people with kidney disease—many of whom also have cardiovascular disease—may need to track their protein intake more closely. But in general, doctors say, it's more important to focus on the source of your protein than worry about the quantity.

"Almost all generally healthy diets will easily provide adequate amounts of protein," says Dr. Walter Willett, professor of epidemiology and nutrition at the Harvard T.H. Chan School of Public Health. That's even true for people who follow a plant-only (vegan) diet, he adds, provided they eat several servings of nuts, beans, or soy-based foods every day.

Why quality matters

Even if you include animal-based protein sources like meat, fish, eggs, and dairy products in your diet (as most Americans do), it's increasingly clear that an eating pattern that features plenty of plant-based protein (see table on page 113) is superior for cardiovascular health. That's because beans, nuts, and seeds are high in fiber, unsaturated fats, and other nutrients closely linked to a lower risk of heart disease.

To keep your heart healthy, experts recommend limiting protein sources that are high in saturated fat (such as processed and red meat), which raise harmful LDL cholesterol. Chicken and turkey are healthier choices. But fatty fish like salmon and tuna, which contain heart-protecting omega-3 fats, are an even better option. Eating an egg a day doesn't seem to affect heart disease risk. That's also the case for full-fat dairy products such as milk, yogurt, and cheese, although Dr. Willett suggests limiting yourself to one or two servings a day.

Protein requirements: Possibly misleading?

There's no firm consensus on the optimal amount of protein a person should eat each day, and it varies depending on your age, sex, and activity level (for more

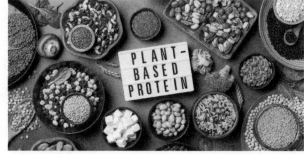

© Aamulya | Getty Images

Plant-based sources of protein like beans, nuts, and soy products contain heart-healthy nutrients, including fiber and unsaturated fats.

on protein needs for women and men through the lifespan, see pages 223 and 248). For the average adult, the Recommended Dietary Allowance—the amount you need to meet your basic nutritional requirements and avoid illness—is 0.8 grams per kilogram of body weight. According to this formula, you should multiply your weight in pounds by 0.36 to estimate the grams of protein to eat daily. The USDA calculator (www.health.harvard.edu/hnfscalc) uses that formula and also takes into account your age, sex, and activity level.

But this formula is based on older studies of protein requirements, says Dr. Willett. As such, it doesn't account for the fact that in the United States, the average body weight and fat mass have increased a great deal over the last 50 years, he notes. For gauging your protein intake, it may be reasonable to use your ideal body weight instead (see "Estimating your ideal body weight," page 113).

As an example, the average American woman is close to 5 feet, 4 inches tall and weighs about 170 pounds. If she's 65 years old and active, the calculator suggests 62 grams of protein daily. But if you instead use her ideal weight of 120, the estimate is far lower—just 44 grams per day.

"If you're overweight, which includes the majority of American adults, basing your protein requirement on your weight may give an estimate that's too high," says dietitian Marc O'Meara, an outpatient senior nutrition counselor at Harvard-affiliated Brigham and Women's Hospital. Consuming too much protein adds unneeded calories and contributes to weight gain, he says.

On the other hand, people who are taking the new weight-loss drugs semaglutide (Wegovy) or tirzepatide

(Zepbound) may actually eat too little protein. "Some of my clients who take these medications feel so full and satisfied from just small amounts of food that they barely eat," says O'Meara. They're losing lots of fat, but also some muscle mass—especially if they skimp on protein, he says.

This also may be an issue for certain older people (especially women) who don't eat enough protein due to a waning appetite. People with moderate to severe kidney disease also need to pay attention to their protein intake because eating too much may impair kidney function. If you fall into any of these groups, work with a dietician to ensure you're eating an appropriate amount of protein, O'Meara advises.

A simple take-home tip

O'Meara's advice—which makes sense for everyone—is to include some protein in every single meal and snack. Aim for roughly equal amounts of protein and carbohydrate, such as half an apple and a handful of mixed nuts, crackers and cheese, or hummus and carrots.

Wondering how to get more plant-based protein in your diet? Baked tofu (which is firmer and more flavorful than plain tofu) and tempeh (a fermented soy product) are easy to add to salads or stir-fries in place of meat, says O'Meara. Try different veggie burgers to find one you like. He also recommends trying nutritional yeast, which has a nutty, somewhat cheesy flavor, in place of Parmesan cheese.

Estimating your ideal body weight

The formula to estimate your ideal body weight differs depending on sex.

For a woman who is 5 feet tall, the ideal weight is 100 pounds. For every inch above 5 feet, add 5 pounds. For example, the ideal weight for a woman who is 5 feet, 4 inches tall would be 100 + (4 × 5) = 120 pounds.

For men, start at 106 pounds for the first 5 feet, then add 6 pounds for every additional inch. For example, the ideal body weight for a man who is 5 feet, 9 inches tall would be 106 + (9 × 6) = 160 pounds.

© Topuria Design | Getty Images

PROTEIN SOURCES

	Food	Serving Size	Protein (grams)
PLANT-BASED PROTEIN	Black beans	½ cup	7
	Nuts	¼ cup	7
	Nutritional yeast	3 tablespoons	8
	Quinoa	1 cup	8
	Lentils	½ cup	9
	Baked tofu	3 ounces	13
	Tempeh	3 ounces	18
ANIMAL-BASED PROTEIN	Egg	1 large	6
	Cheddar cheese	1 ounce	7
	2% milk	1 cup	8
	Greek yogurt, plain	6 ounces	17
	Salmon	3 ounces	19
	Canned albacore tuna	3 ounces	20
	Chicken or turkey breast	3 ounces	25

EXAMPLES OF PROTEIN ADDED THROUGHOUT THE DAY

EGGS AT BREAKFAST

QUINOA FOR LUNCH

PEANUT BUTTER SNACK

SALMON AT DINNER

Try to include some protein in every meal and snack you eat.

Getty Images: Egg breakfast: © Alexander Spatari; Quinoa lunch © Anchiy; Peanut butter snack: © David Montgomery; Salmon dinner: © Westend61

Putting processed foods into perspective

Processed foods—even some that are ultra-processed—can be part of a heart-healthy diet. But check the ingredient list, and choose wisely.

Make no mistake: Eating plenty of whole or minimally processed foods is considered the best strategy for keeping your heart—and the rest of your body—in good shape. We're talking about vegetables, fruits, whole grains, legumes, and nuts. But some processed foods definitely belong on your menu, too.

Anything that changes food from its natural state is considered processing. "For some foods, processing makes them safer—for example, pasteurizing raw milk," says Dr. Qi Sun, associate professor in the departments of nutrition and epidemiology at the Harvard T.H. Chan School of Public Health. This type of minimal processing doesn't substantially change the food's nutrient content. Other examples of minimal processing are chopping and freezing vegetables and fruits, and roasting chicken.

At the next level are processed foods, which have a few added ingredients. Examples of these foods are canned vegetables packed in water and salt, freshly baked bread, and peanut butter. Foods that are even more highly processed—so much that the original food often isn't recognizable—are "ultra-processed" foods (see table). They include additives such as preservatives, oil, sugar, salt, coloring, and flavoring. Examples include cheese puffs, doughnuts, breakfast cereals, frozen yogurt, packaged desserts, hot dogs, and microwavable dinners.

Calories—or something else?

The main problem with ultra-processed foods is that people simply eat far too many of them. More than half the calories in the average American's diet come from ultra-processed foods. Perhaps that's because many of them are sweet or salty carbs, like cookies and chips, that are easy to overeat. One small but carefully controlled study found that people tend to eat about 500 more calories per day when offered mainly ultra-processed foods versus mostly unprocessed foods, even when the meals contained equal amounts of major nutrients.

Processed foods: From minimal to ultra

Unprocessed and minimally processed foods retain their healthy nutrients, in contrast to many ultra-processed foods, such as those listed below.

Unprocessed foods	Minimally processed foods	Processed foods	Ultra-processed foods with low nutritional value
Whole apple	Prepackaged apple slices with no additives	Unsweetened applesauce made with apples, water, and ascorbic acid to prevent browning	Apple juice drink with high-fructose corn syrup and added coloring
Whole oat groats	Steel-cut or rolled oats	Instant oats with added sugar	Oatmeal cookie made mainly with white flour and sugar
Dried chickpeas	Canned chickpeas	Store-bought hummus made with chickpeas, spices, and oil, without preservatives	"Chickpea" chips made with mostly rice or potato flour with added salt, oil, and flavorings

Source: The Nutrition Source, Harvard T.H. Chan School of Public Health.

According to a 2024 review in *Advances in Nutrition*, ultra-processed foods are linked to a higher risk of diabetes, high blood pressure, unfavorable blood lipids, and obesity. Some research hints that certain additives used in processing, such as emulsifiers (which help fats and liquids blend together), play a role in raising cardiovascular risk. Another theory suggests that ultra-processed food may damage the microbiome (see "How a healthy gut helps your heart," page 91). But the evidence is still evolving, says Dr. Sun.

Is processing the problem?

Instead of focusing on how little or how much a food is processed, it still makes sense to pay attention to the food's basic ingredients. "For example, some ultra-processed foods made from whole grains and dairy, including breakfast cereals and fruit-flavored, sweetened yogurt, aren't necessarily unhealthy," says Dr. Sun. Yes, less-processed alternatives—such as rolled oats and plain yogurt with fresh fruit—are healthier. But in three large observational studies done in the United States, ultra-processed whole-grain bread, breakfast cereals, and yogurt were associated with a lower risk of type 2 diabetes and cardiovascular disease.

In contrast, artificially and sugar-sweetened beverages, processed meats, and ready-to-eat dishes were linked to higher risks of those conditions, Dr. Sun says. When it comes to cutting processed food from your diet, replacing soda with water and avoiding hot dogs, salami, bologna, and cured deli meats is a good first step. And don't forget that even some minimally processed foods, such as red meat and butter, aren't good for cardiovascular health, says Dr. Sun.

Ready-to-eat dishes or microwavable frozen meals come in handy for people who don't have the time or inclination to cook from scratch, and they're often a better option than a take-out hamburger and French fries. Look for choices that include whole grains and vegetables and healthy protein sources like beans,

Eat less salt by using more herbs and spices

Americans consume way too much sodium—more than 3,400 milligrams (mg) per day on average. While much of the sodium comes from prepared and processed foods, you can control your salt intake in all your other foods. Instead of reaching for the saltshaker, use herbs and spices to add flavor to your meals.

low-fat dairy, chicken, or fish. Make sure the meal contains no more than 500 milligrams of sodium and is low in saturated fat (less than 10% of the total calories).

There's no harm in having chips or candy as an occasional splurge. Just don't let these nutrient-poor treats crowd out more healthful foods.

Prebiotics in plant-based foods may help control unhealthy eating

Science has shown that a healthy gut can make beneficial changes in the brain, and vice versa, via a connection known as the gut-brain axis. A healthy gut requires good amounts of probiotics (beneficial bacteria), which grow by feeding off prebiotics, compounds found in plant fiber. A 2023 study published by the journal *Gut* suggests prebiotics have a role in the gut-brain axis beyond being a food source, and eating them might help people choose healthier foods.

Researchers recruited 59 overweight adults who regularly followed a Western diet (higher in red meat, saturated fat, and processed foods) and assigned them randomly to take either 30 grams of inulin (a prebiotic found in onions, leeks, artichokes, and bananas) or a

placebo supplement, every day for two weeks. Next, the participants had brain MRIs while they viewed pictures of various low-, medium-, and high-calorie foods and indicated how much they wanted them on a one to 10 scale. The MRIs measured how much of the brain's reward network was activated when the participants made their choices. Over a second two-week period, the process was repeated: everyone took the supplement they had not taken earlier, and then underwent the MRI session. The researchers found that after taking the prebiotic supplement, people were more likely to select medium- or low-calorie foods than high-calorie ones, and their MRIs showed less activation in their brain's reward network when shown high-calorie foods.

by **HOWARD LEWINE, M.D., EDITOR IN CHIEF,** *Harvard Men's Health Watch*

Should I take a daily multivitamin?

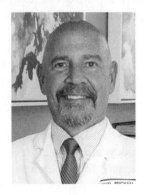

Q *I am in my late 60s, eat what I think is a well-balanced diet, and consider myself to be healthy. Should I take a daily multivitamin? What are the pros and cons? Are there individual supplements you recommend?*

A First, let's consider standard multivitamin-mineral (MVM) supplements. Standard MVMs contain the required daily minimum levels of the essential vitamins and minerals. In comparison, most individual supplements are loaded with much higher micronutrient doses. For example, a vitamin D supplement might contain two to five times the recommended dose. For vitamin B_{12} products, the typical daily dose is 1,000 micrograms, which is more than 400 times higher than the Recommended Dietary Allowance.

Most older studies have not shown a definitive health benefit of a daily MVM supplement for people like you. However, a clinical trial published in 2024 by *The American Journal of Clinical Nutrition* suggests taking MVMs may help delay cognitive decline in adults.

For the trial, 573 participants were given baseline cognitive and memory tests. Half were given one standard MVM daily, and the other half took a placebo. Both groups were unaware of which one they were given. The study participants were retested again after two years. The people who took the MVM scored slightly higher on the memory and cognitive tests than those who took the placebo.

Before this study, I supported anyone who wanted to take a standard daily MVM, although I did not promote its use for all my patients. Although most people with sufficient calorie and protein intake get enough micronutrients from their diet, an MVM provides some dietary insurance.

However, this new evidence has tilted my opinion in favor of a daily MVM for everyone. It's relatively inexpensive and quite safe.

Regarding other supplements, I recommend that adults, especially older adults, take an extra 1,000 international units (IU) of vitamin D daily or every other day (but avoid mega doses). The recommended daily intake of vitamin D for adults ages 50 to 70 is 600 IU and 800 IU for people older than age 70. Standard MVMs have only 400 IU, and getting enough vitamin D from foods can be challenging. Also, many people avoid vitamin D-producing sunlight to reduce their risk of skin cancer.

The grocery and drugstore shelves are full of other supplements, which are heavily promoted for all kinds of health benefits, most of which have no scientific evidence to support their use. It's always best to check with the pharmacist or doctor before taking any individual supplement. ◗

© D-Keine | Getty Images

For most people, a daily multivitamin offers dietary insurance with little downside.

Start vetting your supplements

Use these strategies and tools to uncover risks lurking in seemingly harmless supplements.

There are plenty of good reasons to take a dietary supplement. Maybe you're deficient in a particular vitamin or mineral, such as vitamin D or iron, or you have a poor diet and your doctor recommends a multivitamin. Or perhaps there aren't many ways to treat a health problem you have, such as osteoarthritis, and your doctor says it won't hurt to try a certain supplement that has a small chance of easing symptoms.

So there you are, standing in the supplement aisle of a drugstore, savvy enough to be wary of dietary supplements yet wondering how to recognize the bad ones. Fortunately, certain strategies and online tools can help.

Be cautious about quality

The supplement industry is notorious for producing products that don't contain what they claim. "The FDA leaves it up to companies to ensure the purity and safety of their products. But there's not much incentive. It rarely penalizes manufacturers for not having the right amount of ingredients in a product," says Dr. Pieter Cohen, an associate professor of medicine at Harvard Medical School who studies supplements.

For example, recent research by Dr. Cohen and his colleagues found that 25 brands of gummies contained dangerously high levels of melatonin (used to promote sleep)—up to 347% more melatonin than what was listed on labels. Some of the brands they tested also contained the marijuana derivative cannabidiol (better known as CBD), also at levels that exceeded label claims.

What you can do: Look for supplements with certification seals from vetted independent third parties. "Most seals of approval are meaningless. But the U.S. Department of Defense [DOD] has identified several certifying organizations that do a good job ensuring supplements are labeled accurately," Dr. Cohen says.

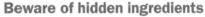

DOD-approved certifying organizations include the U.S. Pharmacopeia (www.quality-supplements.org) and NSF International's Certified for Sport program (www.health.harvard.edu/nsf/cps). Both test many types of supplements.

© guvendemir | Getty Images

Beware of hidden ingredients

The FDA is seeing an increase in supplements that contain hidden prescription drugs, controlled substances, or untested and unstudied components. If you use these products, there's a risk that they might cause serious side effects or interact with medications you're taking. The tainted supplements are widely available and sold online from sellers on eBay or Amazon and even through large retail stores.

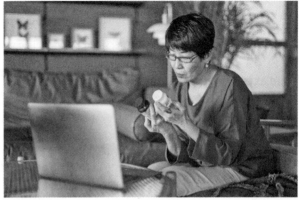

© AsiaVision | Getty Images

Online tools enable you to investigate the ingredients, safety, and effectiveness of dietary supplements.

What you can do: Look up ingredients you don't recognize on FDA websites that can help you identify potentially dangerous products or supplement ingredients.

One useful reference is the Dietary Supplement Ingredient Directory (www.health.harvard.edu/dsid), unveiled in 2023. It enables you to quickly look up dozens of different ingredients and get basic information as well as links to research and warnings about them.

The other is the Health Fraud Database (www.health.harvard.edu/hfpd), which lists some (but not all) products that have been subject to FDA-related violations.

Go over a checklist

The DOD has a resource anyone can use to check if a supplement seems safe. It's called the Operation Supplement Safety Scorecard (www.health.harvard.edu/opss/dietary). The scorecard provides a ▸▸

checklist of seven questions you can answer quickly to determine if a supplement seems safe. For example:

- ▸ Is there an approved third-party certification seal on the product label? (The scorecard displays images of the seals to look for.)
- ▸ Is the label free of claims or statements that seem questionable to you?
- ▸ Are there fewer than six ingredients on the label?

If you don't get at least four "yes" answers to the questions on the scorecard, the supplement is designated too risky to take.

Do some digging

Do a little detective work if your clinician suggests that you take a supplement, especially a botanical treatment (made of plants or plant extracts).

"Be skeptical: ask if there's a study about it," Dr. Cohen suggests. "It needs to be a large randomized controlled trial to be credible."

You can also look up medical studies on your own by going to a reliable search engine called PubMed (www.pubmed.ncbi.nlm.nih.gov) from the National Institutes of Health (NIH).

NIH also provides fact sheets on a wide variety of dietary supplements. Check them out (www.health.harvard.edu/dsfs) and see if there's a good reason to take the supplement you're considering. If not, it's probably safer to skip the risk. ▼

The lowdown on vitamins D, B$_{12}$, and B$_6$

Of the many micronutrients people need, older adults are more likely to have inadequate consumption of vitamin D, B$_{12}$, and B$_6$. Few foods are naturally high in vitamin D, and getting enough of the other natural source, sunlight, can be challenging since people try to protect their skin from sun exposure.

Vitamin B$_{12}$ deficiency can result from reduced stomach acid production caused by aging or from regularly taking proton-pump inhibitors or H2 blockers to manage heartburn or reflux. Without enough stomach acid, it's harder for the body to absorb vitamin B$_{12}$ from food.

Low levels of both B$_{12}$ and B$_6$ can stem from digestive disorders, such as Crohn's disease, celiac disease, and ulcerative colitis, as well as from procedures like gastric bypass surgery. A blood test can identify most deficiencies, and your doctor may then prescribe an individual vitamin or a multivitamin to help increase levels.

IN THE JOURNALS

Mindfulness may help people stick to a heart-healthy diet

© JLco - Julia Amaral | Getty Images

A mindfulness training program may help people with high blood pressure follow a heart-healthy diet, according to a 2023 study published in *JAMA Network Open.*

For the study, 101 people attended the eight-week program, which teaches people skills such as meditation, self-awareness, and emotional regulation. These skills are then directed toward behaviors known to lower blood pressure, including following the DASH diet (see www.health.harvard.edu/DASH). The 100 people in the control group received brochures about controlling high blood pressure.

Over six months, people in the mindfulness group began eating more in line with the DASH diet than those in the control group by making changes such as adding an extra daily serving of vegetables. They also showed improvements in their ability to sense and interpret hunger and satiety. Greater self-awareness may also help people to notice how different types of food make them feel and to be more cognizant of their eating habits, the authors note.

SMART EATING

The fountain of youth

Proper hydration is essential for optimal health, but many older adults still don't drink enough water.

When scientists search for life on other planets, they first look for the presence of water. After all, the laws of nature say that life as we know it needs water to exist and thrive.

Drinking water serves us earthlings in many ways. It helps deliver nutrients to cells, regulates body temperature and blood pressure, prevents infections, and keeps organs functioning correctly. It's probably no surprise, then, that adults who stay well hydrated appear to be healthier and develop fewer chronic conditions. Conversely, prolonged dehydration raises the risk of conditions like urinary tract infections, kidney stones, and constipation. Dehydration also can interfere with cognitive functions like attention and memory.

Are you dehydrated?

Even though water is the foundation of life, older adults have trouble drinking enough. "Part of the problem is that the sense of thirst diminishes with age, so many older adults can't always tell when they are dehydrated," says Dr. Qi Sun, associate professor in nutrition and epidemiology at Harvard's T.H. Chan School of Public Health. "And when they feel thirsty, odds are they are already dehydrated."

Signs of dehydration are fatigue, weakness, confusion, short-term memory loss, and increased irritability. One way to monitor hydration is by the color of

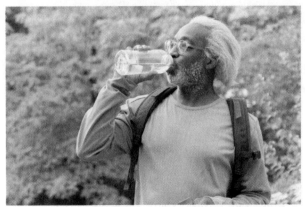

© PhotoAlto/Frederic Cirou I Getty Images

Staying properly hydrated helps to keep older adults healthier and more active.

your urine. When you're hydrated, your urine should be clear or a light straw color. A dark yellow or amber color is a sign to drink more water.

Going to the well

The best way to prevent dehydration is to consume enough water daily. The National Academy of Medicine suggests that men drink about 10 cups of water, expecting they will get another 3 cups from water-containing foods, while women should drink about 7 cups a day, assuming they'll get another 2 cups from food. This amount is not necessarily a daily target but a general guideline. "Still, for the average person, it's a good number to aim for," says Dr. Sun.

There are times when you need extra water, like when you sweat from exercise or when you're exposed to hot weather. (A rule of thumb is to drink two to three cups of water per hour in these situations, or more if you're sweating heavily.) People also need extra water when they lose bodily fluids from vomiting or diarrhea.

Dr. Sun says that plain water is the best fluid to drink. Still, all beverages that contain water, like coffee and tea, contribute toward your daily needs. It's a myth that caffeinated versions of these beverages increase dehydration because they make you urinate more. (It's their water content and not the caffeine that makes you need to use the bathroom after drinking two or three cups.)

"Still, too much caffeine can give you jitters or keep you from sleeping, so you should monitor your intake if you are caffeine sensitive," says Dr. Sun.

Drinking unsweetened carbonated water is also acceptable, but avoid sweetened beverages, energy drinks, sports drinks, and "vitamin waters" as your ▸▸

Watching the water

It's possible to consume too much daily water in some health situations. These include having problems with the thyroid, kidney, liver, or heart, or if you take medications that make you retain water, like nonsteroidal anti-inflammatory drugs, opiate pain medications, and some antidepressants. Other medications, like some blood pressure drugs and laxatives, can increase dehydration. If you are in any of these categories, check with your doctor to determine your daily water intake.

▶▶ primary fluid sources, as they can be high in sugar. Otherwise, here are some tips to stay hydrated:

Keep water handy. You are more likely to drink when you have water always within reach. Fill a 20-ounce water bottle four times daily and sip throughout the day.

Schedule regular drinking times. Set alarms on your phone or computer as a reminder to drink.

Drink when you eat. Drink a large glass of water with each meal and snack. In addition, drink room-temperature water. Research suggests that people drink the most water when it is served at room temperature.

Add some flavors. There are ways to make water more appealing. For example, perk up a pitcher of water with natural flavors like slices of citrus fruit (lemon, lime, orange, or grapefruit), ginger, cucumber, or crushed fresh mint. Another option is to add a splash of fruit juice to a glass of water.

Eat water-dense foods. Consuming foods with high water content also counts toward your daily amount. Examples include leafy green vegetables, cucumbers, bell peppers, celery, berries, and melons like watermelon and cantaloupe. These consist of about 90% water or even more. A general guideline is to count about half the serving as water. For example, one cup of watermelon contains about half a cup of water. ▮

Take the Dry January challenge

Why you should try abstaining from alcohol for a month.

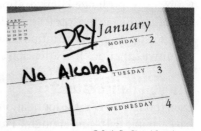

© OntheRunPhoto | Getty Images

People who quit drinking for a month often report they sleep better and feel more energetic.

Every January, millions of people commit to abstaining from drinking alcohol (beer, wine, and spirits) for one month. Known as "Dry January," the public health initiative was launched in 2013 by Alcohol Change UK to address the role alcohol plays in people's lives and health.

"Dry January can be a useful tool to help people change their relationships with alcohol," says Dr. Rocco Iannucci, director of the Fernside Residential Treatment Program at Harvard-affiliated McLean Hospital. "People take the Dry January challenge as a step toward changing their alcohol habits or to explore the effect a monthlong break can have on their health."

Several kinds of benefits

No matter their relationship with alcohol, many people see and feel some benefits after an alcohol-free month. "Some evidence has found that after 30 days of no drinking, people report they sleep better, have more energy, lost weight, and lowered their blood pressure," says Dr. Iannucci.

Even occasional drinkers can discover some benefits. "For some, Dry January offers a short-term challenge similar to other New Year health endeavors, like starting an exercise program and eating healthier," says Dr. Iannucci. "There's no downside to trying it."

He suggests approaching Dry January as a learning experience. Write down the reasons you want to do it. For example, do you want to achieve total abstinence? Reduce the amount and frequency you drink? Lose weight? Or simply change how you view alcohol, like not needing to drink during social activities?

After a month, reflect on your drinking patterns, how you feel, and how you want to move forward. Do you want to return to moderate drinking or cut back more? Or has the experience made you feel like quitting alcohol? Did you substitute another habit—like eating more snack foods—for drinking? How did you feel physically and mentally?

"You may decide to continue Dry January for another month and then evaluate again," says Dr. Iannucci.

Tips to staying dry

Here are some tips from Dr. Iannucci on how to do Dry January. One important caveat: daily drinkers should check with their physicians before they stop drinking. Abruptly quitting alcohol can lead to potentially dangerous withdrawal symptoms in people with an alcohol dependency.

Find a substitute nonalcoholic drink. For social situations, or when you crave a cocktail, reach for an alcohol-free beverage, like sparkling water, soda, or "virgin" drinks (nonalcoholic versions of alcoholic drinks). Nonalcoholic beer or wine are options, but some brands still contain up to 0.5% alcohol by volume, so check the label. Sugar is often added to these beverages to improve the taste, so choose low-sugar brands.

Avoid temptations. Keep alcohol out of your house. When you are invited to someone's home, bring nonalcoholic drinks with you.

Create a support group. Let friends and family know your intentions and encourage them to keep you accountable. Better yet, enlist someone to do the challenge with you.

Track your progress on your phone. One option is the Try Dry app (download it at www.health.harvard.edu/dryjanuary.) This free app tracks your drinking, helps you set personal goals, and offers motivational information like calorie counts and money saved from not drinking. You can use it for either cutting back or cutting out alcohol, depending on your goal.

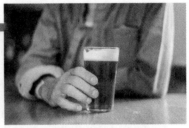
© Verity E. Milligan | Getty Images

Is alcohol healthy?

Some observational studies of moderate drinkers—no more than one to two standard drinks per day for men, and no more than one drink a day for women—have shown a link between alcohol intake and better heart health. However, results of more recent studies have suggested that alcohol doesn't offer heart protection and, in fact, may actually contribute to health problems. Still, none of these studies proves cause and effect. Researchers speculate that people's overall health habits may play a significant role in whether alcohol helps or hinders. Nowadays, the general consensus is that if you don't drink, there's no health-based reason to begin. If you drink only occasionally, don't increase your intake. The effects of alcohol also vary by gender. For more on alcohol's effects on women, see "The latest thinking on drinking," page 235, and for its effects on men, see "The (almost) last word on alcohol and health," page 250.

Don't give up. If you slip up, don't feel guilty. Just begin again the next day.

If you struggle during the month or give up after a week or so, you may need extra help cutting back. "The experience may reveal an underlying issue with alcohol you were unaware of that requires medical attention," says Dr. Iannucci. "You may not realize how much you drink regularly until you try to stop." 🛡

Feeding body and soul

Intuitive eating rejects a diet mentality and encourages us to pay attention to natural cues for hunger and fullness. How might you benefit?

Feeling battered by years of dieting? You've seemingly tried everything to lose weight: low-calorie, low-sugar, low-fat, low-carb—and frankly, low-satisfaction—regimens that left you worse off and worn out.

If the description fits, you may be drawn to an entirely different approach. Called intuitive eating, the decades-old concept is designed to help people stuck in the cycle of dieting build a better relationship with food. Fundamental is the notion that our bodies intrinsically know

what, when, and how much to eat to stay nourished. But a lifetime of relentless messaging—from orders to "clean your plate" to parades of stick-thin models—have stopped many of us from listening to that inner voice.

Intuitive eating rejects the rules and restrictions baked into a diet mentality, which often backfires, leading to yo-yo weight loss and gain. Indeed, evidence suggests about 80% of people who lose significant amounts of weight will regain some or all of it within ▸▸

a year. Instead, intuitive eating encourages us to simply eat when hungry and stop when full. It also takes into account your satisfaction—enjoying the foods you eat—which, ironically, may lead to weight loss.

"Gaining and losing weight for years and years can be counterproductive and is a hard way to live," says Emily Blake, a dietitian at Harvard-affiliated Brigham and Women's Hospital. "Intuitive eating is a framework that integrates mind and body and encourages you to trust in your own ability to feed yourself."

Balanced approach

Another key principle of intuitive eating is rejecting the idea that foods are inherently "good" or "bad." No longer are pizza, pasta, and burgers on the naughty list. Likewise, salads and fruit aren't "better."

"What people find over time is they end up craving a balance of foods," Blake says. "You'll start trusting yourself much more with the ability to eat what feels good to you physically without any emotional distress or guilt. Once you take the morality out of food, you start noticing that while you do crave less-nutritious foods at times, you also often crave fruits and vegetables."

On the flip side, some people misconstrue intuitive eating as a food free-for-all, says dietitian Nancy Oliveira, manager of the Nutrition and Wellness Service at Brigham and Women's Hospital.

"When people have food freedom, some may choose more ultra-processed, 'craveable' foods," Oliveira says. "It's a little tricky. It does help you have a better relationship with food over all, but you have to pair that with common sense and solid nutritional information. You have to know that eating potato chips all day long will not help you feel better in the long run."

Hungry vs. full

For many trying to adopt intuitive eating, a weighty challenge is reacquainting themselves with natural cues that signal hunger or fullness—and responding accordingly. "Most people recognize hunger pangs, but a lot of people struggle with fullness," Blake

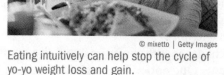
© mixetto | Getty Images

Eating intuitively can help stop the cycle of yo-yo weight loss and gain.

says. "It's not really the American way to recognize being full."

Maybe it's easy to pinpoint that your rumbling stomach or lightheadedness means you need to eat, pronto. But feeling full isn't the same as realizing you're bursting and queasy from overeating.

"Sometimes we use the term 'comfortably un-hungry,'" Oliveira says. "You feel mentally satisfied because you chose exactly what you wanted to eat, and you feel better afterward, with more energy."

To gauge your fullness, Blake suggests choosing a check-in point during your meal—for example, when you're halfway through—and taking a moment to assess your hunger and fullness levels. If you think you might be full, put your plate in the refrigerator. "If you're still hungry 20 minutes later, you can have more—it's not a big deal," she says. "This helps you become more comfortable with those cues. It's like building a muscle, but you're building a skill. It's going to take a while to get there."

Mind-body benefits

Intuitive eating might result in weight loss, especially if listening to hunger and fullness cues leads you to eat less. A 2019 research review in the journal *Obesity Reviews* incorporated 10 studies that tracked the eating habits of nearly 1,500 people. Participants who followed an intuitive eating plan lost about the same amount as those on conventional weight-loss diets, and lost more weight than those who didn't change their eating habits.

But Blake and Oliveira emphasize that weight loss isn't the goal of intuitive eating. Instead, learning to respect your body's "set point"—where your weight naturally falls when you're feeding it adequately and allowing for flexibility with food and movement—may be more realistic. A 2021 study in the *International Journal of Eating Disorders* suggests intuitive eating is linked with better self-esteem and body image.

"If people have a tough relationship with food stemming from a long history of dieting, they can feel better emotionally," Blake says. "This also makes it easier to accept where their body is in terms of weight."

Tips for success

Intrigued? Oliveira and Blake offer these tips to incorporate intuitive eating into your lifestyle.

Be mindful during meals. This means chewing slowly, pausing between bites, and avoiding distractions such as screens.

Stop feeling guilty. "I don't care if you eat pepperoni pizza for every meal for an entire week," Blake says. "Don't beat yourself up for any of your choices."

Keep a food journal, but skip the calorie counting. Track when you feel hungry and full, when and what you eat, and how you feel. "You're shifting focus from nutrient and calorie content to why and what you're eating, and that's useful self-reflection," Oliveira says.

Check your emotions. If you feel like eating shortly after your last meal, ask yourself if you're truly hungry, or if you're bored or stressed. This can stem from emotional eating. "Maybe you need a nice cup of tea, a warm bath, or a walk instead," Oliveira says.

Don't focus on weight loss. "If you're focused on the scale, you're not going to listen to your body," Oliveira says. "At least for a month, just focus on your body's signals."

Stay fueled. You're more likely to binge on cookies, for example, if you don't eat enough during the day and then come home to a waiting box of them. "Part of intuitive eating is making sure you're eating enough over all so you're not trying to practice these principles while starving," Blake says.

Seek support. Work with a registered dietitian or health coach for added insight.

Be patient. Learning to trust your body's signals again takes time. "There's going to be a lot of trial and error where you feel intuitive eating isn't working," Oliveira says. ▮

4 nutrition myths that can derail healthy eating

Despite an explosion of science-backed nutrition information in recent years, certain dietary myths just won't quit. But these misconceptions can stop us from incorporating necessary nutrients into our meals, derailing a healthy diet, says Nancy Oliveira, a dietitian at Brigham and Women's Hospital.

Social media is largely to blame, she says. Before the deluge of nutritional "advice" on Facebook, YouTube, and other platforms, people turned more readily to government guidelines and other trusted sources of health information. "Now all these voices are saying, 'You can't eat certain things.' It totally confuses people," Oliveira says. "It misleads and distracts them from what really matters."

Oliveira dishes on which myths seem most pervasive and why they're wrong:

Myth: *Plant-based milks are healthier than dairy.* Soy, oat, almond, and other plant milks are a great option if you're lactose-intolerant or don't like cow's milk. But a cup of the latter contains about 10 grams of protein and 25% of our recommended daily calcium, while plant milks tend to have far less protein. Oliveira recommends examining labels, since milk of any kind may be fortified with protein, calcium, and vitamin D. "If those nutrients are important to you, be sure to double-check, as amounts can vary among brands," she says.

Myth: *Avoid all carbs.* Carbohydrates are an important component of a healthy diet, but the type of carbs matters. Eat fewer refined carbs—such as those in cakes, cookies, chips, and white breads—which lead to blood sugar spikes. Complex carbs from whole grains, legumes, vegetables, and fruits keep us fuller longer and deliver a steadier fuel supply. "There are good carbs, and our bodies need them," Oliveira says.

Myth: *Fresh fruits and vegetables are healthier than frozen.* Produce starts losing nutrients at the moment it's harvested. But freezer versions are typically flash-frozen, preserving vitamin levels and preventing quick spoilage.

Myth: *Fat is bad.* Decades after a low-fat craze began in the '90s, some people still believe all types of fat are verboten. But saturated fat—which comes from animal products such as red meat—is the less-healthy, artery-clogging choice. Replacing saturated fats in your diet with unsaturated fats from foods such as avocados, nuts, seeds, olive oil, and fatty fish helps protect heart health by raising levels of HDL (good) cholesterol and lowering LDL (bad) cholesterol. Your body's cholesterol levels rise from eating a lot of fat, particularly saturated fat, but eating cholesterol itself doesn't have nearly the same impact. Beware of labels that say "no cholesterol"—this could signal a plant-based food that actually has a lot of saturated fat.

Spring cleaning? Prioritize your fridge and pantry

Avoiding food poisoning starts in your own kitchen.

With spring's arrival, maybe you're planning to attack those dusty baseboards, smeared windows, and cluttered closets. But if you've been neglecting your refrigerator and pantry, these hard-working storage areas should take priority—and they need far more than annual cleaning to help you avoid food-borne illnesses, Harvard experts say.

It's not a minor threat. Each year, an estimated one in six Americans—48 million people—get sick from germs in food, according to the CDC. About 128,000 of them are hospitalized, and 3,000 die as a result of food-borne illness.

Spring cleaning offers an opportunity not only to thoroughly scour your home, but also to give your fridge and pantry—which can harbor harmful bacteria—more than just a cursory swipe of a sponge. In the process, you can purge dated and possibly contaminated products from overlooked corners.

Think of it this way: these chambers don't just house your food; they also protect it—and you, by extension.

"It's tough to compare this to spring cleaning, because certainly I'd recommend cleaning out your refrigerator and pantry way more than once a year," says Cynthia Parenteau, associate director of public health in the Department of Environmental Health and Safety at Harvard University, who specializes in food safety. "Personally, I do it once a week. Every time new groceries go in, I make sure anything that's expired goes out, and I move older food to the front."

Dangerous complications

Food-borne illnesses result from microbes or toxins that contaminate foods or drinks. More than 30 pathogens (disease-causing agents), including *Salmonella*, norovirus, *Listeria*, *Escherichia coli*, and bacteria that cause botulism, are known to travel in food.

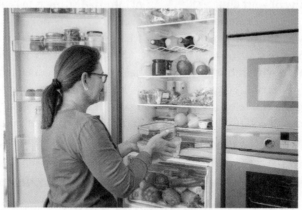

© fcafotodigital | Getty Images

To avoid food poisoning, purge your pantry and refrigerator of foods that are dated or possibly contaminated.

Raw or undercooked poultry or meat, raw eggs, unpasteurized milk or dairy products, raw fruits and vegetables, and foods prepared in large batches kept at unsafe temperatures are vehicles for these pathogens.

Some lucky folks manage to skirt the consequences of eating germ-laden foods, while others develop food poisoning and suffer through symptoms such as nausea, vomiting, diarrhea, intense stomach cramps, and fever.

"The majority of us eventually get a food-borne illness," says Parenteau's colleague Marykate Franks, a senior environmental public health officer. "Most people associate it with the last thing they ate, though that may not be the case. If we're lucky, we feel crummy for a day or two, rebound, and write it off."

While food poisoning symptoms often resolve without problem, infections spread by food can have lasting, dangerous consequences. They sometimes lead to conditions such as arthritis, meningitis, kidney damage, or brain and nerve damage. (See "When should you see a doctor for food poisoning?" on page 125.) Parenteau notes that certain people—including pregnant women, older adults, and those with weakened immune systems—are susceptible to worse cases and more serious outcomes.

Cleaning strategies

How can you better protect yourself? Parenteau and Franks recommend these tips to tackle your refrigerator and pantry:

Take everything out. Approach your food clean-out with the same commitment as you would a closet purge. Completely emptying your fridge and pantry allows you to appraise each item for safety as well as inspect the inside of each space. "Even with something as simple as cleaning out your pantry, you'll find a wayward cheese puff at the back or a pile of cracker crumbs," Franks says. "You also have to be alert for mice or flour weevils that might be really intrigued by what you have in your cabinets."

Wash everything thoroughly. Pull out all shelving and clean every surface with food-safe sanitizer spray. (For a homemade version, Harvard experts suggest blending one tablespoon of unscented liquid chlorine bleach with a gallon of water.) Pay particular attention to any spills or dried, sticky areas. Make sure surfaces are dry before putting anything back.

Check expiration dates. Toss all expired food or drink items, as well as those whose containers are rusted or leaking. If you don't know the expiration date, a rule of thumb suggests keeping opened refrigerated items for seven days or less. "This is a good opportunity to go through your refrigerator and pull out all the Tupperware and leftover restaurant containers and make way for new stuff," Parenteau says.

Use your senses. Expiration dates differ from sell-by or best-used-by dates, which only suggest freshness. This is often applicable to items such as condiments and salad dressings. If those dates have only recently passed, check the product's appearance and smell for signs of decay. "If something doesn't quite smell right or the color of the food is off, trust your instincts," Franks says. "Better safe than sorry."

Pay attention to packaging. Generally, unopened or vacuum-packed foods will stay fresher longer. But once they're opened, the clock starts. "The date to use a product by becomes pretty confusing when you see a freshness date a month or two down the road but you've already opened it," Parenteau says. She advises using a marker to note on the package the date you unsealed it. Then keep

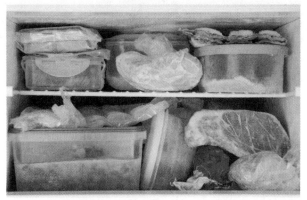
© hutchyb | Getty Images

Assess what's in your freezer every few weeks.

it for only another seven days—especially packaged deli meats or hot dogs.

Avoid cross-contamination. Keep raw meat, seafood, and eggs separate from ready-made foods so germs don't spread. Store these items in sealed containers so juices don't leak onto other foods. And if your refrigerator features dedicated meat and produce drawers, use them only for those items. "You don't want juices that leak from chicken or beef packages getting on produce or food items that are not going to be cooked," Parenteau says.

Don't forget your freezer. Since the whole purpose of freezing food is to keep it from spoiling, the freezer doesn't need as much attention as the refrigerator. But take a look at its contents every few weeks and weed items out. "Everyone is guilty of sticking something in the back of the freezer, saving it for a rainy day, and forgetting about it," Franks says. "It's good to pull that stuff out to check if it expired and assess if it's worth keeping." 🛡

When should you see a doctor for food poisoning?

In most cases, food poisoning symptoms are mild enough to ride out without medical attention. But certain symptoms should prompt a doctor's evaluation, according to the CDC. These include

- ▸ bloody diarrhea or diarrhea lasting longer than three days
- ▸ fever over 102°F
- ▸ vomiting so frequently you can't hold liquids down
- ▸ signs of dehydration, such as dry mouth and throat, scant urination, and dizziness upon standing.

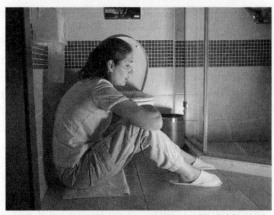
© Lenblr | Getty Images

by **HOPE RICCIOTTI, M.D., EDITOR IN CHIEF,** *Harvard Women's Health Watch*

Can apple cider vinegar curb appetite?

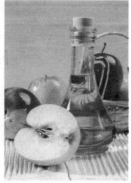

© Andrii Pohranychnyi | Getty Images

Q *My friend says she drinks apple cider vinegar at bedtime to help her eat less and lose weight. Could it work?*

A Scientific evidence doesn't support drinking apple cider vinegar to dampen appetite or help with weight loss. But even on a commonsense level, it's not likely. Here's why: changing only a single part of our routine—such as drinking a shot of apple cider vinegar each evening—can't help us shed excess pounds as effectively as broader efforts that include changing our overall diet and exercising more often.

Beyond that, apple cider vinegar's high acidity level makes bedtime a less-than-ideal time to drink it. Anyone prone to heartburn or gastroesophageal reflux disease (GERD) should avoid eating or drinking anything acidic at least 30 to 60 minutes before sleep to lessen the odds of uncomfortable burning in the chest. Over time, drinking undiluted vinegar can also erode your tooth enamel.

People who still want to consume apple cider vinegar can do it more safely and comfortably if they mix a small amount into a large glass of water or combine it with other ingredients in salad dressings.

Curcumin supplements might ease meal-related discomfort

Y ou might know turmeric as the golden-yellow spice used in curry powder and yellow mustard. Turmeric contains the naturally occurring chemical curcumin, which might have anti-inflammatory and antioxidant properties. And now a small randomized trial has found that taking curcumin supplements (derived from turmeric) helps reduce symptoms of functional dyspepsia—recurring, unexplained stomach pain, bloating, or early feelings of fullness. Scientists randomly assigned 206 people (ages 18 to 70) with functional dyspepsia to one of three treatments: taking 500 milligrams (mg) of curcumin (two 250-mg capsules) four times a day, taking 20 mg of the medication omeprazole (Prilosec, Zegerid) once a day, or taking both treatments each day. After about a month of treatment, people in all three groups said their dyspepsia symptoms had improved.

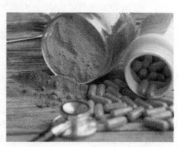

© Elis Cora | Getty Images

The results were even better after two months. The findings suggest that curcumin supplements are as effective at relieving dyspepsia symptoms as omeprazole (which curbs stomach acid), and that curcumin is safe and well tolerated. The 2023 study was published by *BMJ Evidence-Based Medicine.*

How to shop for healthier foods

Focus on sodium, fiber, and added sugars.

When it comes to dietary choices, many people keep coming back to old favorites. They find a few foods they enjoy and rotate them through their daily meals.

"There is nothing necessarily wrong with that as long as their diet includes plenty of whole foods like fruits, vegetables, legumes, and whole grains, and avoids high amounts of processed foods," says Eric Rimm, professor of epidemiology and nutrition at Harvard's T.H. Chan School of Public Health. "But everyone also should be more mindful about reading food labels when selecting their favorite foods to ensure they get more of the healthiest nutrients and much less of certain substances."

For those who stick their favorites, Rimm suggests they be especially mindful of adding more fiber and minimizing their intake of sodium and added sugars.

Sodium

FDA guidelines suggest people consume no more than 2,300 milligrams (mg) of sodium daily. (People with prehypertension and hypertension should limit their intake to 1,500 mg.) But the average person consumes about 50% more—3,500 mg per day.

Excess sodium in your bloodstream signals your kidneys to hold on to more water. The extra fluid can cause high blood pressure and lead to cardiovascular disease.

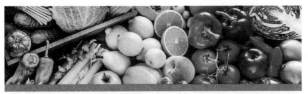

© fcafotodigital I Getty Images

Eat the rainbow

An easy way to increase the variety of produce you consume is to aim to eat a colorful variety of fruits and vegetables. Eating a broad range of fruits and vegetables—especially dark green, red, and orange ones—will ensure you take in a broad range of nutrients. So allow your eyes to guide you in the produce section and aim to eat as many colors as you can.

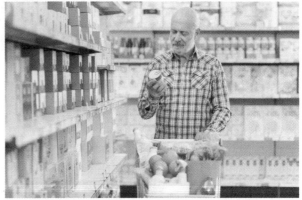

© demaerre I Getty Images

Reading food labels helps you get more fiber and avoid excess sodium and added sugars.

Shopping tip: Choose low-salt versions of packaged foods. Many products, including soups, crackers, and canned vegetables and beans, come in low-salt, reduced-salt, or no-added-salt versions. "Even bread can contain high amounts of sodium in a single slice," says Rimm. Select items with 150 mg or less of sodium per serving. For nuts, choose unsalted.

Fiber

A high-fiber diet helps keep body weight under control and lowers LDL (bad) cholesterol levels. Research has also linked eating enough dietary fiber with a reduced risk of heart disease and diabetes. Adequate fiber improves digestion, supports the immune system, and reduces symptoms in many people with irritable bowel syndrome. Men and women older than age 50 should consume 30 grams and 21 grams of fiber per day, respectively. However, most people consume, on average, only about half that amount.

Shopping tip: There are two types of fiber: insoluble and soluble. Rimm suggests focusing on getting both kinds. "This means loading up on whole plant foods like fruits, vegetables, legumes, nuts, seeds, and whole grains." Most men can meet their daily fiber requirement from two to four servings of fruit; two to five servings of vegetables, whole grains, and legumes; and one to two servings of nuts and seeds.

Added sugars

"Added sugars" refers to sugars and syrups in food products and beverages that increase sweetness and ▸▸

texture and extend shelf life. (This differs from the natural sugars found in fruit, vegetables, and dairy.) Research suggests that increased intake of added sugars is linked with obesity and cardiovascular disease.

Shopping tip: It's easy to predict high amounts of added sugars in products like sodas, cookies, and cakes. But many other seemingly innocent items, such as tomato sauce, yogurt, granola bars, and breakfast cereals, also have a lot of added sugars.

Labels now list added sugars under total sugar, so it's easier to know how much is included. "One teaspoon of sugar is equal to 4 grams, so that is something to keep in mind when looking at the amount of added sugar," says Rimm.

Also, note the number of grams of added sugar per serving and how much constitutes one serving. "The label might say 5 grams per serving, which is low, but you might typically eat three or four servings, so you will end up consuming 15 to 20 grams of added sugar," says Rimm.

You can also check the ingredients list of a food product to find added sugars. (See "Look closer at food labels.") "Especially avoid foods that list multiple forms of sugar or include a sugar among the first three ingredients," says Rimm.

Look closer at food labels

Added sugars are identified on a product's ingredient label. They often are called by names other than "sugar." Here are the ones you should look for, according to The Nutrition Source, a resource from the Harvard T.H. Chan School of Public Health:

- agave nectar
- brown sugar
- cane crystals
- cane sugar
- coconut sugar
- corn sweetener
- corn syrup
- crystalline fructose
- dextrose
- evaporated cane juice
- fructose
- fruit juice concentrates
- glucose
- high-fructose corn syrup
- honey
- invert sugar
- malt sugar
- malt syrup
- maltose
- maple syrup
- molasses
- raw sugar
- sucrose

Chapter 6

Coping with Chronic Conditions

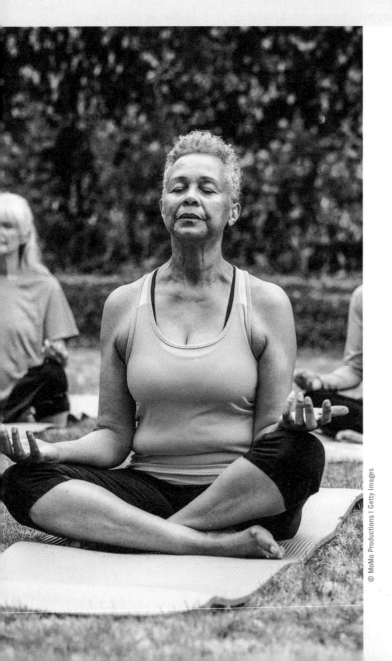

© MoMo Productions | Getty Images

Healthy Habits! 5 Things You Can Do Now

1 **Avoid COVID.** In addition to vaccination, a plant-based diet reduces risk of severe symptoms, while other healthy choices help head off long COVID. (pages 130 and 132)

2 **Fight fatigue.** If you're often tired, it's important to learn why. (page 136)

3 **Get a grip on Lyme.** Try a technique called pacing to manage your energy. (page 141)

4 **Treat persistent pain.** Free and reasonably priced treatments can be effective. (page 142)

5 **Reduce your allergy symptoms.** A saline rinse offers relief. (page 159)

by **ANTHONY L. KOMAROFF, M.D.,** Editor in Chief, *Harvard Health Letter*

How can I avoid long COVID?

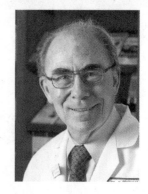

Q *I was pretty sick with COVID-19 but have improved somewhat. Now I'm worried about getting long COVID. How serious is long COVID, and what can I do to avoid it?*

A Some people who "recover" from COVID-19 unfortunately suffer persisting symptoms—such as fatigue, difficulty concentrating, and disrupted sleep—that seriously impair their ability to function at work and at home. This illness is called long COVID. While it is more likely to develop in people who were most severely ill when they first caught the virus, it also can occur in people who were only mildly affected. Initially, some people (including some doctors) suspected that such persisting illness was due purely to psychological problems or even that the patients might be faking their illness.

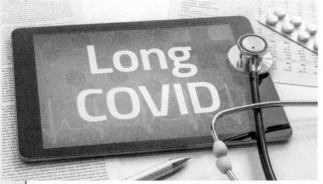

© Zerbor | Getty Imagess

Three years later, it is clear that tens of millions of people are affected by long COVID. Senior Harvard economists have estimated that the cost to the United States of caring for post-COVID illnesses may be as much as $3.7 trillion over the coming years. If the millions of people currently affected by long COVID remain sick for years—that is, if long COVID becomes a chronic illness—then the cost is likely to be considerably greater.

It also has become clear that the illness is due to physical problems caused by the virus. Two 2023 scientific reviews published in the journals *Nature Reviews Microbiology* and *Frontiers in Medicine* summarize the many underlying biological abnormalities that are found in people with long COVID, involving primarily the brain, the immune system, energy metabolism, and the heart and lungs.

How can you protect yourself from getting long COVID? Vaccines protect you against getting COVID-19, and you can't get long COVID without first getting COVID-19. But vaccines are not perfect: some people get "breakthrough" infections with the COVID virus despite having been vaccinated. Fortunately, a 2022 study published in the journal *Nature Communications* finds the risk of long COVID is reduced by vaccination.

Two 2023 observational studies in the *The BMJ* and in *JAMA Internal Medicine* found that people with COVID-19 who were prescribed the antiviral medicines nirmatrelvir/ritonavir (Paxlovid) and molnupiravir (Lagevrio) were 25% to 50% less likely to develop long COVID than people of similar age and state of health who did not get an antiviral. Randomized trials are needed to make sure antivirals truly protect against long COVID, and such trials are under way.

Long COVID is a real and serious problem, but fortunately vaccines and antiviral drugs appear to offer some protection against getting it. The National Institutes of Health has committed over $1 billion to discover how to better diagnose, effectively treat, and ultimately prevent long COVID—answers that we sorely need.

COVID-19's cardiac legacy

The virus may leave people more vulnerable to a host of heart-related issues. But vaccination can lower these risks.

Most Americans have been infected at least once with SARS-CoV-2, the coronavirus that causes COVID-19. It's clear that these infections can have lingering effects on the cardiovascular system, including among people with no previous evidence of heart disease. Even a mild infection with SARS-CoV-2 may increase your risk of a heart attack, stroke, or heart failure up to a year after you recover from the infection.

In addition, a recent study reveals a higher risk of additional heart complications in people with post-COVID conditions (PCC), commonly known as long COVID (see "Long COVID: Lingering effects throughout the body"). Published in 2023 in *JAMA Health Forum*, the study relied on health insurance claims data from more than 40,000 people throughout the United States during the first year of the pandemic.

Compared with people without a diagnosis of PCC, those with PCC were more than 3.5 times as likely to later have a pulmonary embolism (blood clot in the lung) and more than twice as likely to develop a heart rhythm problem such as atrial fibrillation. In addition, the risk of stroke, coronary artery disease, and heart failure were approximately twice as common in people with PCC.

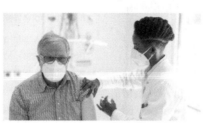

© Luis Alvarez | Getty Images

A COVID-19 infection raises your risk of serious heart problems for up to one year. But being vaccinated against the virus can lower those risks if you do contract the disease.

Vaccine victory

However, this evidence was gathered before COVID vaccines were widely available, starting in early 2021. "New research shows that being vaccinated against COVID can significantly lower the risk of serious heart problems, including heart attack, stroke, and death from heart disease, in people who get COVID," says cardiologist Dr. C. Michael Gibson, professor of medicine at Harvard Medical School. The benefits of vaccination are most pronounced in older people, who face the highest risk of heart problems, he notes.

Dr. Gibson is referring to another 2023 study of more than 1.9 million people in the United States ages ▸▸

Could this diet ward off COVID?

A study published in 2024 by *BMJ Nutrition, Prevention & Health* suggests that following a vegetarian or plant-based diet—higher in vegetables, legumes, and nuts, and lower in dairy foods and meat—is tied to lower risks of getting COVID-19. Researchers evaluated the self-reported information of more than 700 people in Brazil who were surveyed in 2022 about their health, medical history (including COVID vaccines), and diet. About 400 people said they regularly consumed meat. About 300 people said they ate a plant-based diet (either a "flexitarian" diet that included some meat or a strict diet that excluded some or all animal products). Almost half of the study participants reported having had COVID. But plant-based eaters were 39% less likely to have had a COVID infection, compared with meat eaters. Researchers speculate that plant-based diets might offer some protection against the virus due to beneficial plant chemicals. While the evidence that plant-based diets protect against getting COVID-19 is not yet solid, it is clear that plant-based diets help stave off many chronic diseases.

▶▶ 18 to 90 who had a COVID-19 infection between March 2020 and February 2022. Even partial vaccination was linked to a lower risk of heart problems, report the study's authors, whose results appeared in the *Journal of the American College of Cardiology*.

What about myocarditis?

Myocarditis—inflammation of the heart muscle—is a rare condition that can arise after a viral infection, including stomach "flu," the common cold, or COVID-19. Although mild myocarditis may go unnoticed, more serious cases can cause severe heart failure and rhythm disturbances.

Starting in 2021, reports from around the world, including the CDC, noted a possible increased risk of myocarditis after receiving an mRNA COVID-19 vaccine (made by either Pfizer or Moderna). However, the risk of developing myocarditis is substantially higher immediately following a COVID infection than during the weeks after getting a COVID vaccine. That's according to an analysis of nearly 43 million people in England published in 2022 in *Circulation*.

"Getting just one dose of a COVID vaccine cut the risk of myocarditis in half," says Dr. Gibson. But it's worth noting that severe myocarditis is very rare. In this yearlong study, just one in 15,000 people was hospitalized for or died of myocarditis.

Long COVID: Lingering effects throughout the body

An estimated 10% to 13% of people infected with COVID-19 have lingering, debilitating symptoms, known as post-COVID conditions (PCC). Also called long COVID, PCC is defined as new, returning, or ongoing health problems that occur or persist for four or more weeks after a COVID infection.

Symptoms might include fatigue, cough, pain (joint, throat, chest), loss of taste or smell, shortness of breath, brain fog, and depression. The CDC has a more detailed list; see health.harvard.edu/loncov.

The COVID Recovery Center at Harvard-affiliated Brigham and Women's Hospital treats people with long COVID, many of whom are young, previously healthy athletic women who now have many of the classic symptoms of postural orthostatic tachycardia syndrome, or POTS.

Because COVID vaccines also reduce the risk of other serious heart complications, the risk-benefit calculation is vastly in favor of getting vaccinated, says Dr. Gibson. Vaccines also appear to lower the risk of developing long COVID, so be sure to stay up to date with current CDC vaccination recommendations. 🛡

IN THE JOURNALS

Healthy habits might ward off long COVID

Women who practice many aspects of a healthy lifestyle are about half as likely as peers who don't to experience persistent symptoms after a COVID-19 infection ("long COVID"), a new study suggests.

The Harvard-led study, published in 2023 by *JAMA Internal Medicine*, analyzed data from more than 32,000 women in the Nurses' Health Study II. They reported information about their lifestyle in 2015 and 2017 as well as their COVID-19 status from April 2020 through November 2021. More than 1,900 participants were infected with the virus during that time, and 44% of those developed long COVID, with symptoms persisting beyond four weeks after the initial infection.

Women who practiced five or six of a list of healthy lifestyle habits—including weight control, not smoking, regular exercise, adequate sleep, high-quality diet, and moderate alcohol consumption—were 49% less likely to develop long COVID compared with women who practiced none. Of the six lifestyle factors, healthy body weight and adequate sleep (defined as seven to nine hours nightly) were most strongly linked with lower risk.

COPING WITH CHRONIC CONDITIONS

Ways to regain your sense of smell

Sniffing peanut butter, peppermint, and other strong scents may help you retrain your brain and restore your sense of smell.

Your smell sense gives you a superpower. Without moving a muscle or opening your eyes, it helps you detect danger, store or trigger memories, discern flavors, or get a rush of feel-good chemicals during a meal. So you can imagine that losing your sense of smell (a problem doctors call anosmia) can be devastating. Many millions of people have been experiencing it as a common side effect of COVID-19. Other conditions also can lead to anosmia.

When it occurs, you need to try to regain the sense as soon as possible. "The longer you go without it, the less likely you are to recover it," says Dr. Neil Bhattacharyya, an ear, nose, and throat specialist (otolaryngologist) at Harvard-affiliated Massachusetts Eye and Ear.

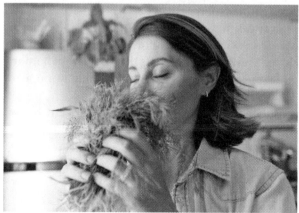

© Westend61 | Getty Images

You can use materials you have at home, such as fresh herbs, to stimulate your smell sense.

Why did you lose it?

Your sense of smell is made possible by your olfactory system. This includes thousands of sensory cells in the nasal cavity that detect odors (entering through the nose or mouth) and send information to the brain via olfactory nerves. If the olfactory nerves become inflamed or damaged, they may not function properly, and you may lose your sense of smell.

Causes of anosmia include nasal polyps, sinus problems, head trauma, chemotherapy side effects, brain tumors, neurological conditions such as Parkinson's disease, or viral infections such as COVID-19.

Why might a viral infection affect smell sense? "Some viruses infect the olfactory nerves or the cells near them, attack them, and damage them," Dr. Bhattacharyya says. "It could also be that inflammation surrounding the nerves causes damage."

Consequences of smell loss

Anosmia has serious consequences. It shuts down your ability to sniff out hazardous odors, and it also steals much of your ability to taste and appreciate food. Loss of taste occurs because your olfactory sensory cells are responsible for most of your perception of flavor. (By comparison, the taste buds in your tongue detect whether a food is sweet, salty, sour, bitter, or savory.)

When everything tastes like cardboard, you lose the pleasure of eating. "It hurts your quality of life,"

Dr. Bhattacharyya says. "I have a patient whose wife is an exceptionally good cook. When he first lost his smell and taste senses, he ate less, lost 50 pounds, and became depressed. Now he's underweight."

Will you get it back?

If you have anosmia from a chronic neurological problem, such as Parkinson's disease, Dr. Bhattacharyya says the chances of recovering your smell sense aren't great. If the anosmia is due to a temporary condition, such as COVID-19, the chances are better that your smell sense will return within a few months, though it's not guaranteed.

For example, a study conducted by Dr. Bhattacharyya and his colleagues, published in 2023 by *Laryngoscope*, found that about 21 million Americans reported losing smell and taste from COVID in 2021. Almost 30% said they still hadn't fully regained the senses approximately 12-to-18 months later.

But there's hope: Dr. Bhattacharyya says the sense of smell is neuroplastic, meaning it sometimes regenerates.

Smell retraining

If you've lost your sense of smell, don't wait around for it to come back. "We used to tell people to wait six months before they came to see us about it," ▶▶

▸▸ Dr. Bhattacharyya says. "But now we want you to begin smell retraining therapy as soon as possible to activate the body's recovery process."

Smell retraining therapy is simply a matter of sniffing a wide variety of odor-generating elements. About six to 10 different types of scents will do, such as lemons or oranges, flowery perfumes, peanut butter, eucalyptus, rosemary, cinnamon, pine, peppermint, or cloves. You can use materials that you have at home or buy a smell retraining kit online (commonly found on Amazon.com) for about $15 to $35.

"Once or twice a day, smell each scent for 30 seconds to two minutes. As you do, think about what you're smelling, and try to recall moments when you've smelled this before. For example, cut open an orange, inhale its aroma, and think about another time when you savored a fresh, delicious orange," Dr. Bhattacharyya says. "That triggers odor-particle recognition. It's deeply seated in the brain, but you have to stimulate it to re-establish function. You're retraining the brain."

Try this therapy every day for at least four weeks, Dr. Bhattacharyya suggests. If your sense of smell doesn't return, see an otolaryngologist to rule out underlying conditions that may be causing anosmia. Treating an underlying condition may restore it. ⬤

IN THE JOURNALS

Uncontrolled high blood pressure or diabetes tied to severe COVID-19 outcomes

Here's another incentive for people with high blood pressure or diabetes to lower their numbers: a study of almost 1.5 million people in the United States suggests that having uncontrolled high blood pressure or diabetes prior to getting COVID-19 sharply increases the risk for COVID complications. Researchers evaluated participants' health both before and during the time they developed COVID (from March 2020 to February 2022). Compared with people whose blood pressure was the best controlled before getting infected, those with the worst-controlled blood pressure had about 30% greater odds of needing hospitalization or critical care and 32% greater odds of being on a ventilator. Among participants with diabetes, those whose blood sugar was most poorly controlled before getting COVID had about 61% greater odds of being hospitalized, 42% greater odds of needing critical care, 12% greater odds of being on a ventilator, and 18% greater odds of dying, compared

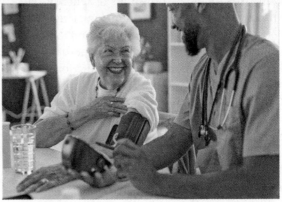
© Halfpoint Images | Getty Images

Treating high blood pressure and high blood sugar levels may reduce risk of hospitalization for COVID.

with those whose blood sugar was the best controlled. The study, published in 2023 by the *Journal of the American Heart Association*, was observational and doesn't prove that controlling diabetes and high blood pressure protects against COVID complications. But we know for sure that controlling these conditions also reduces the risks of heart or kidney disease and premature death—and that's reason enough.

COPING WITH CHRONIC CONDITIONS

Autoimmune diseases pose a threat to the heart

The growing field of cardio-rheumatology aims to improve cardiac care for people with autoimmune diseases.

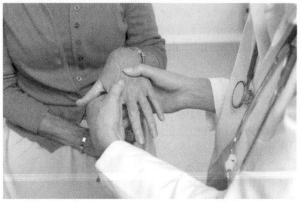
© Adam Gault/Spl | Getty Images

Autoimmune diseases such as rheumatoid arthritis raise your heart disease risk.

Your immune system, a network of specialized cells and organs, defends your body against viruses, bacteria, and other invaders. But sometimes, for reasons that remain largely mysterious, immune cells launch an inappropriate attack against the body's own tissues. The resulting outpouring of white blood cells and other substances causes inflammation, triggering the pain, redness, and swelling that characterizes many autoimmune diseases (see "Autoimmune diseases: From common to rare").

But inflammation also damages the linings of blood vessels, encouraging the buildup of fatty plaque that can narrow arteries (atherosclerosis), boost blood pressure, and raise the risk for a heart attack or stroke. This connection likely explains why people with autoimmune conditions, such as rheumatoid arthritis, have higher rates of heart disease. Until recently, the scope and severity of this problem have been unclear.

A heightened risk

However, in 2022, *The Lancet* published a study that looked at cardiovascular disease rates in combination with 19 of the most common autoimmune diseases. Depending on the specific condition, people with these diseases were up to three times more likely to develop cardiovascular disease than people without an autoimmune disease.

"My patients have said to me, 'I had no idea that my autoimmune disease could affect my heart,'" says Dr. Brittany Weber, a cardio-rheumatology specialist at Harvard-affiliated Brigham and Women's Hospital. Many of the people she treats have rheumatoid arthritis, psoriatic arthritis, or lupus—three common conditions linked to cardiovascular problems. ▶▶

Autoimmune diseases: From common to rare

In the United States, up to 8% of people have an autoimmune disease, which occurs when the immune system mistakenly attacks healthy organs or tissues. For unknown reasons, women are twice as likely as men to develop these conditions. Out of the more than 100 known autoimmune diseases, the three described below are among the most common and best studied. But the majority are rare and therefore less well understood.

Psoriasis. The inflammation in psoriasis affects the skin, causing a pink or dull-red, scaly skin rash that occurs in patches, usually on the back of the elbow, in skin folds, and on the scalp. About one in three people with psoriasis also has psoriatic arthritis, which causes joint inflammation (especially in the fingers, toes, or knees) and morning stiffness.

Rheumatoid arthritis. The immune system attack targets tissue lining the joints, creating inflammation marked by swelling, pain, and stiffness. It typically strikes multiple joints at once, especially in the hands and feet. Other symptoms include fatigue and lingering morning stiffness.

Lupus. The inflammatory process in lupus can affect almost any organ in the body, triggering a wide array of symptoms. Common early symptoms include fever and joint pain similar to rheumatoid arthritis. One distinct symptom is a "butterfly rash" across the bridge of the nose and cheeks. Damage to the heart, lungs, kidneys, and blood vessels can also occur.

▶▶ Awareness of this elevated risk is especially important because autoimmune disease typically strikes when people are in their 20s or 30s. In turn, heart problems may develop up to a decade earlier than in people without an autoimmune disease. A calcium scan, which detects early signs of atherosclerosis, can help assess a person's risk and guide treatment advice, says Dr. Weber. Sometimes, people blame rheumatoid arthritis for symptoms (for example, shortness of breath when climbing stairs) that are actually caused by heart disease, she adds.

Treatment advice

In addition to prescribing statins and other medications that lower heart attack risk, cardio-rheumatologists also work with rheumatologists to manage the appropriate use of disease-modifying biologic drugs, some of which carry a higher risk of cardiovascular side effects than others.

The same diets recommended for preventing heart disease (see page 105) are also beneficial for people with autoimmune diseases. Maintaining a healthy weight helps, too. Exercise is often particularly challenging for people with autoimmune diseases, especially those with severe cases of rheumatoid arthritis, who may have limited mobility. "Many of my patients like swimming, which is easy on the joints," says Dr. Weber. Others find yoga to be helpful, especially because of the added stress relief and relaxation yoga provides. Using an elliptical machine is another exercise that can raise the heart rate without putting too much pressure on the joints. ▮

When fatigue leaves you drained, depleted, and dumbfounded

When fatigue is persistent, it's essential to learn why.

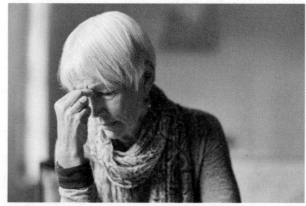
© Cecilie_Arcurs | Getty Images

Marked by everyday exhaustion, fatigue feels different from being merely tired or sleepy.

If you feel as though you're dragging through your days feeling weary, weak, and listless, fatigue has arrived at your doorstep.

But what's the line between feeling fatigued and merely tired? Fatigue means no amount of sleep helps you feel refreshed. Forget about mustering *joie de vivre*—you can barely get through the day without becoming exhausted.

"Being tired or sleepy is different from fatigue," says Dr. Daniel Sands, a primary care doctor at Harvard-affiliated Beth Israel Deaconess Medical Center. "It's true they can overlap, because if you're not getting enough sleep, you'll feel fatigued. But fatigue is different—everyday things like walking to the bathroom or doing the dishes wear you out."

You might chalk it up to getting older, since fatigue is commonly viewed as a normal part of aging instead of a symptom of an underlying ailment. But often, something is indeed amiss. Between 40% and 74% of older adults with a chronic condition deal with fatigue, according to a 2021 research review in *Rehabilitation Nursing*.

When it lingers for weeks or months, fatigue is a problem that needs to be solved. A long list of both obvious and more opaque conditions can lead to it, some of them serious.

"I get worried when people have stopped doing the things they love—like going for walks, babysitting their grandchildren, or cooking," says Dr. Soheyla Gharib, an internist at the Phyllis Jen Center for Primary Care

COPING WITH CHRONIC CONDITIONS

at Harvard-affiliated Brigham and Women's Hospital. "If they say they're not doing those things, that's a huge red flag, and we definitely want to find out why."

Gamut of causes

Some contributors to fatigue are abundantly clear. If you're not sleeping well, for instance, or have allergies, a cold, the flu, or COVID, you're likely to feel drained. Chronic illnesses such as heart disease, cancer, diabetes, kidney disease, multiple sclerosis, or rheumatoid arthritis are also widely known to sap energy.

But the list of less-recognized causes is just as long. You might not suspect

- sleep disorders
- depression or anxiety
- thyroid problems
- infections
- iron-deficiency anemia
- poor diet
- medication use.

Chronic fatigue syndrome—characterized by prolonged tiredness, fever, and aches—might be on your radar if you have unshakable fatigue, but it's rarely the case, Dr. Sands says, and only considered after other reasons are ruled out.

Pathway to answers

How do you know it's time to see a doctor about your fatigue? Not only when it's unexplained, prolonged, and debilitating, but also if it's joined by other symptoms such as

- weight loss or gain
- frequent headaches
- chronic pain
- muscle weakness
- thinking or memory problems
- mood changes
- sleep problems such as insomnia, severe daytime sleepiness, or restless sleep.

"If you have actual weakness, like you can't climb stairs; shortness of breath; or trouble getting dressed or making meals—or if you're nodding off in the middle of the day when you never used to—those are all big warning signs," Dr. Gharib says.

© Kathrin Ziegler | Getty Images

Fatigue can be caused by a wide variety of conditions.

In addition to performing a thorough physical exam, your doctor will likely ask about your sleep habits and use of alcohol and other substances as she carefully reviews your medical history. Additionally, comprehensive blood testing can unearth a variety of fatigue culprits, including anemia, thyroid issues, certain infections, and liver or kidney problems, as well as guide further testing.

Typically, doctors follow a well-worn credo when investigating fatigue and other such nebulous symptoms: "When you hear hoofbeats, think horses, not zebras." That means they first consider the obvious causes before looking to less likely possibilities.

"If someone gets almost no physical activity and tells me she's worn out all the time now, most likely she is deconditioned. I get more concerned when I see a patient who runs a 5K three times a week and suddenly can't run a mile," Dr. Sands says. "What goes along with fatigue often tells us whether something is serious or not. But in someone with no obvious clues, it's rare there's something serious going on," he adds.

Vitality-enhancing tactics

If your check-up didn't unearth anything worrisome—or you're now being treated after a new diagnosis—the next step is to proactively boost your oomph. Try these strategies:

Move more. Staying active helps maintain muscle mass and strength, which helps stave off fatigue. (See "To combat fatigue, rise up and exercise," page 138.) "It's paradoxical—you can't get good sleep if you're not exercising," Dr. Gharib says. "You'll feel even more tired, ironically. If you're starting from zero, even 15 minutes a day of exercise will get you going, with the goal of getting to 30 minutes of physical activity a day, five days a week."

Optimize your diet. You can't drink from an empty cup, as the adage goes. Fuel your body appropriately by filling your plate with high-protein options such as lean meat or fish, along with complex carbohydrates ▸▸

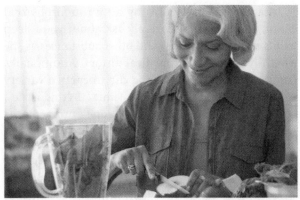
Eating healthy foods can help you avoid plummeting energy levels.

© Jose Luis Pelaez Inc | Getty Images

such as whole grains, fruits, and vegetables. These choices will help you avoid the plummeting energy levels common after eating processed, high-sugar foods. "Healthy eating and good hydration will do wonders for making you feel better," Dr. Gharib says.

Use caffeine strategically. There's no question it can help you feel powered up, but caffeine can also disrupt sleep patterns, especially when consumed in midafternoon or later.

Limit alcohol use. Alcohol has a sedative effect, ultimately causing an energy slump. Additionally, while it may help you doze off, the effect often wears off in the wee hours, leaving you awake when you should be sound asleep.

To combat fatigue, rise up and exercise

When you're tired, the last thing you may feel like doing is exercising. Yet that's exactly what can help break the cycle of persistent fatigue and reboot your energy levels, a recent study suggests.

The 2022 analysis, published in *Frontiers in Psychology*, reviewed 81 earlier studies that involved a total of more than 7,000 adults. Researchers found that regular exercise leads to small-to-moderate improvements in fatigue as well as feelings of energy and vitality. Regular exercise was defined as exercising at least once a week and included resistance training (such as weight lifting) and aerobic exercise (such as brisk walking, cycling, or swimming).

How can exercise beat back fatigue and boost energy levels? By increasing blood flow to muscles and organs, releasing feel-good chemicals called endorphins, and improving sleep quality, says Dr. Daniel Sands, a primary care doctor at Beth Israel Deaconess Medical Center.

"It increases your cardiovascular reserve—the ability of your heart and lungs to pump blood and extract oxygen from it," Dr. Sands says. "You're toning up your system."

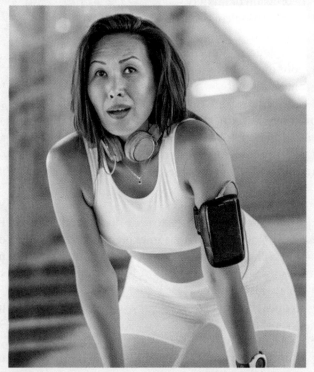

© RealPeopleGroup | Getty Images

Exercise perks us up by increasing blood flow to muscles and organs, among other benefits.

If you feel you can't begin exercising on your own, ask your doctor for help devising a plan to incorporate more physical activity into your days, Dr. Sands says. And start small by taking the stairs instead of an elevator, parking farther from the front door of a store, or getting off a train a stop earlier than planned and walking the rest of the way.

COPING WITH CHRONIC CONDITIONS

Living with Lyme: Post–Lyme disease syndrome

A variety of treatments can help alleviate persistent symptoms of this tickborne disease.

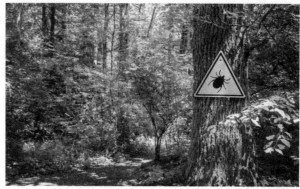

© 24K-Production I Getty Images

When Lyme symptoms persist after a course of antibiotics, options are available for managing pain and daily function.

Characterized by a distinctive "bull's eye" red rash during its initial stages—but sometimes by no symptoms at all—Lyme disease is becoming increasingly common in the Northeast, Mid-Atlantic, and Midwestern United States and has even expanded into parts of Canada, Europe, Asia, and Africa.

Lyme is usually successfully treated if it's caught early on. (For more on the symptoms, diagnosis, and treatment of Lyme, see Harvard Health Publishing's *Lyme and Other Tick-borne Diseases* and https://lyme.health.harvard.edu). However, for reasons that are still unclear to researchers, about 5% to 15% of those who are diagnosed and treated for any stage of Lyme disease may continue to have a range of symptoms. For most people, these symptoms go away within six to 12 months. But for others, they may continue for a year or longer. Doctors often refer to this as post-treatment Lyme disease syndrome or post–Lyme disease syndrome (PLDS).

Symptoms of PLDS are not specific and overlap with other post-infection syndromes such as myalgic encephalomyelitis/chronic fatigue syndrome. Most recently, similarities have been noted between PLDS and symptoms of post-acute sequelae of COVID-19, commonly called long COVID. Symptoms that are common with both PLDS and long COVID include fatigue, muscle and joint pain, and cognitive problems. However, people with PLDS do not typically experience ongoing shortness of breath or trouble breathing, as do some people with long COVID.

PLDS is a term that covers a very wide spectrum of disease. Some people have mild symptoms that steadily improve. Other people have more severe symptoms that disrupt their normal lives and can leave them unable to work, exercise, or concentrate on daily tasks.

In general, people who had more severe symptoms when first treated for Lyme disease or who were diagnosed at a later stage are those most likely to have severe symptoms after treatment. Recovery can be slow, although most people steadily improve. Some people, however, may never recover to their pre-infection state.

Treatment options

People who are very sick for a long time often seek out new doctors and new treatments in hopes of finding relief. Frustrated patients or caregivers may insist on continuing antibiotic treatment.

A small minority of doctors do advocate longer-term antibiotic treatment. Based on the results of some animal studies, they believe that Lyme can persist even after a standard course of antibiotics. These doctors and some patient advocacy groups prefer the term "chronic Lyme disease" rather than PLDS.

However, no study in humans has ever shown persistence of active Lyme disease after antibiotic treatment. In addition, multiple large, high-quality clinical trials have shown no benefit to additional antibiotic therapy beyond the established courses of 14 to 28 days. Based on available data, both the Infectious Diseases Society of America and U.S. Centers for Disease Control and Prevention strongly discourage additional antibiotic therapy beyond standard treatment. Both say symptoms that linger after recommended treatment with antibiotics should be treated individually, not with more antibiotics. This means that treatment choices will vary depending on the symptoms a particular person is having.

This is because long-term antibiotic treatment carries significant risks, including allergic reactions, rash, diarrhea, disruption of the body's natural collection of microorganisms (microbiome), and a higher risk of *Clostridium difficile*, a type of antibiotic-resistant bacteria that can grow rapidly in the intestines ▸▸

▶▶ after antibiotic treatment and cause life-threatening illness. Taking antibiotics that are not needed also increases the risk of antibiotic resistance among various types of bacteria, which can undermine the management of future infections.

As a result, treatment generally focuses on symptom management and improving daily function. It is important to note that most people do continue to improve over time, though the sluggish pace of recovery can be frustrating. Patients with severe disease may benefit from a multidisciplinary approach that includes some or all of the following strategies.

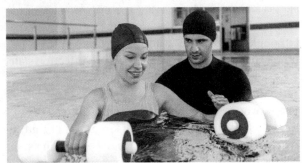
© andresr | Getty Images
Physical therapy for post–Lyme disease syndrome may include exercises done in a pool to make them easier for people whose strength is much diminished.

Physical therapy

This type of therapy can include a variety of techniques to help people manage pain and improve strength, mobility, and flexibility. A physical therapist performs a thorough evaluation and develops an individualized program for each person.

Physical therapy for PLDS may include the following activities:
- ▶ aquatic therapy (therapy in a pool) for people with profound weakness
- ▶ graded exercise programs that help people regain strength without suffering setbacks from overexertion
- ▶ restorative yoga, which uses props such as blankets, blocks, and straps to make yoga practice supportive, gentle, and stress-free.

Pain management

Pain that occurs in joints (arthritic pain) may require different treatments than pain that is nerve-related (neuropathic). Treatment may include a combination of medication and nondrug approaches.

NSAIDs. Treatments for joint pain may include nonsteroidal anti-inflammatory drugs (NSAIDs). These drugs reduce pain and swelling by blocking production of chemicals involved in the body's inflammatory response. Some NSAIDs, such as ibuprofen (Advil, Motrin) and naproxen (Aleve), are available without a prescription. Prescription NSAIDs include prescription-strength naproxen (Naprosyn), ibuprofen (Motrin), and indomethacin (Indocin).

NSAIDs may carry an increased risk of bleeding in the stomach or intestines. Long-term use may increase the risk of heart attack or stroke, especially in people with heart disease. Ask your doctor if NSAIDs are safe for you.

Pregabalin (Lyrica) and gabapentin (Neurontin). These drugs may be helpful if you have persistent neuropathic pain, which is caused by damaged nerves. This type of pain is often described as shooting, burning, or tingling. Side effects of these drugs may include dizziness, drowsiness, loss of balance, problems with memory or concentration, tremors, and blurred or double vision.

Acupuncture. The ancient Chinese practice of acupuncture involves insertion of thin needles into specific locations, depending on the condition being treated. The needles are left in place for 20 to 30 minutes and then removed. There's little scientific evidence that acupuncture is effective for PLDS. However, acupuncture has been used to treat many pain syndromes, and some people have found that it helps alleviate their PLDS symptoms. Complications are rare.

Chiropractic treatment. Chiropractic is best known for spinal manipulation, which involves quick but strong pressure on a joint between two vertebrae of the spine. The intent is to correct the body's alignment. Although chiropractic has been little studied as a treatment for PLDS symptoms, some people with Lyme disease say that it has helped them to relieve pain and improve function. Serious complications are rare.

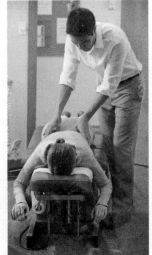
© AJ_Watt | Getty Images
Some people with post–Lyme disease syndrome say that chiropractic treatment has helped them.

COPING WITH CHRONIC CONDITIONS

Cognitive therapy

Several different therapies can be useful in addressing the cognitive or mental health manifestations of PLDS.

Cognitive rehabilitation. This form of therapy is used for people who have trouble with concentration and focus. It includes a broad array of structured cognitive exercises that address specific deficits in thinking, memory, or other brain-related functions. They can help train the brain to focus for longer periods of time. These exercises are also used as part of the recovery process for someone with traumatic brain injury.

Meditation or mindfulness practice. Meditation and mindfulness encompass a variety of spiritual and relaxation practices that involve focusing attention on a particular object or sensation, such as a repeated word or your own breathing. This discipline has not been studied extensively for relief of PLDS symptoms. However, mindfulness-based stress reduction programs have been shown to provide sustained benefit for people with chronic pain. Meditation may also help to modify thinking patterns and improve concentration.

Behavioral health treatments. Talk therapy may be particularly helpful for people who are struggling to adjust to new limitations. Some people with PLDS also have depression or anxiety. Treatment of these conditions may help to improve quality of life and coping skills for people with PLDS. Treatments that have been effective for anxiety and depression include medications and cognitive behavioral therapy, which teaches people to change negative thought patterns that can make pain and other symptoms worse.

Stimulants. Some people may benefit from a trial of medication to help with focus, such as amphetamine and dextroamphetamine (Adderall) or methylphenidate (Ritalin). While these medications can be very helpful in the short term, some people become dependent on them. If stimulants are part of your recovery plan, work closely with your doctor to find the right dose and duration of treatment.

Nutrition consultation

Appropriate nutrition is important for recovery from PLDS and overall well-being. But some people with severe symptoms also experience loss of appetite. In these cases, consultation with a nutritionist may help you to plan meals to ensure you are getting enough calories and all of the nutrients you need to help restore your health.

Occupational therapy

An occupational therapist can recommend ways to modify your day-to-day activities and environment to help conserve energy and reduce excess sensory stimulation at home and at work. These adjustments can help you cope with pain and other issues such as fatigue, sensitivity to sound and light, brain fog, and memory problems.

Pacing

Pacing is a strategy of planning when and how to use your limited energy so as not to overexert yourself and worsen symptoms.

Some suggestions for pacing:

▶ Prioritize tasks and spread them out over the day or week.
▶ Take advantage of times when your energy is good, and don't push your body when you are fatigued.
▶ At work, try dividing up a longer task into smaller segments and take breaks in between them.
▶ Give yourself more time to finish everyday tasks and projects.
▶ Ask for and accept help when you can.
▶ Look for opportunities to outsource strenuous chores such as cleaning your home or doing yardwork.
▶ Try to find ways to modify your work or school schedule to avoid long stretches of mental or physical exertion.

Note when it takes you a long time to recover from some activities, and try to avoid or reduce them in the future.

Rest

In addition to getting good-quality nightly sleep, taking mental or physical rest breaks during the day may help with brain fog and fatigue. Respond to what your body is telling you and allow yourself to rest when needed.

Sensory quiet time

If environmental stimuli such as light or sound are uncomfortable, it may help to incorporate sensory quiet time into your day, for example:

▶ Take short rest breaks throughout the day with an eye mask and noise-canceling headphones or earplugs.
▶ Turn off sound notifications on your phone or your work computer.
▶ Request a desk or floor lamp at work if the overhead fluorescent lighting is too bright. ▮

Pill-free pain treatments that won't break the bank

Many alternative therapies to relieve pain are free or low-cost.

One of the most effective elixirs for chronic pain is a total freebie. You can administer it at home, at any time, in any manner you choose. This bargain treatment? It's exercise. Physical activity has many pain-relieving benefits, yet not everyone takes advantage of them.

A recent CDC study found that one in four adults relies exclusively on over-the-counter or prescription painkillers to treat chronic pain, despite recommendations to use pill-free alternatives.

"Some people feel there's no care given unless they end up with a prescription. Or they have barriers to drug-free therapies, including cost, a lack of knowledge, and poor access to care. But many treatments are free or low-cost and easily accessible," says Dr. Jennifer Kurz, a physiatrist who specializes in alternative pain management strategies at Harvard-affiliated Spaulding Rehabilitation Hospital.

First, the free stuff

Many strategies that reduce pain are activities that support a healthy lifestyle. Take exercise, for example. While it is sometimes difficult to exercise if you are in pain, it also can bring relief. "It strengthens and loosens your muscles, reduces stress, promotes weight control, and helps improve mood and sleep. All of those work together to relieve pain," Dr. Kurz says.

Other activities that help relieve pain include yoga, stretching, tai chi, deep breathing, mindfulness meditation, stress management, sleeping seven to nine hours per night, and staying socially connected. Here are free (or very low-cost) ways to help you practice them.

Online videos. YouTube has thousands of free videos that relate to these methods of pain reduction. For example, you can find videos of exercise routines for chronic pain, ways to improve sleep, and meditation for beginners. Make sure the instructor in the video is certified in his or her field. Or search for videos on the websites of large hospitals and nonprofit groups you trust.

Apps. Health apps for chronic pain can guide you to meditate, exercise, and more. Look for apps that are

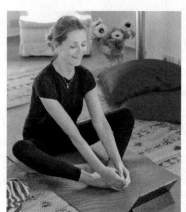

© Kathrin Ziegler | Getty Images

Many free apps can guide you through exercises that help reduce pain.

free (or have a small fee per month), have good reviews, don't collect too much information from you, and have hundreds of thousands or millions of downloads. Examples include Curable, Manage My Pain, Migraine Buddy, and Better Sleep. For meditation, try Insight Timer, Calm, or Headspace.

Health club memberships. Some health insurance plans, including some Medicare Advantage and Medigap plans, include a free fitness membership called Silver Sneakers. It gives you access to 14,000 fitness and recreation clubs across the country. You might even strike up conversations with other exercisers, which is great for staying socially connected.

Online lectures or classes. Large hospitals, academic research centers, and nonprofit organizations frequently offer free or low-cost lectures or classes related to chronic pain treatment. For example, Dr. Kurz founded a pain management program called FINER (www.finerprogram.org), which features free lectures from Harvard-affiliated physiatrists, physical therapists, and pain psychologists. It also has videos and links to helpful apps, books, podcasts, and more on its website.

And Spaulding Rehabilitation Hospital (https://www.health.harvard.edu/sascpaulding) offers numerous online exercise classes—most are designed for people with limited mobility—for a low fee (such as $5). Slots fill up quickly, so sign up early if you're interested.

Support groups. Support groups for chronic pain promote social connection and feelings of hope and control. Look for online groups on Facebook (search "chronic pain support") or through large nonprofit chronic pain associations, such as the U.S. Pain Foundation's Pain Connection (https://painconnection.org). Or join a local in-person support group (a local hospital can often connect you to one).

Reasonably priced treatments

If you can afford to spend money on drug-free strategies to treat pain, be careful: many are bogus. But the

COPING WITH CHRONIC CONDITIONS

following are safe, effective, and reasonably priced.

Physical therapy. The No. 1 treatment for pain reduction, physical therapy involves working with a therapist who assesses your physical strengths and weaknesses and designs a customized program that includes exercise and other therapies. It's covered under most insurance plans, though you'll have to make co-pays. Otherwise, physical therapy costs $100 to $200 per session.

Dietitian services. A dietitian can design a balanced eating plan to help you lose weight (if you need to) and eliminate many inflammatory foods in your diet. "That might help you reduce fat and chronic inflammation, which will have an effect on your mood, your sensitivity to pain, and your overall health," Dr. Kurz says. The average cost for a dietitian is $100 to $200 per session, and you may only need a few visits. Insurance might cover a portion of the costs.

Acupuncture. This ancient Chinese practice involves inserting hair-thin needles into nerve junctions. It doesn't work for everyone, but it's safe if administered by a certified acupuncturist. Acupuncture is covered by Medicare and many other insurance plans for common chronic pain diagnoses, like back pain, if

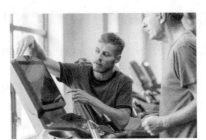

© Iza Habur I Getty Images

Though you may have co-pays, most insurance plans cover physical therapy.

the practitioner is a medical doctor. Otherwise, an average session costs about $100.

Massage. Therapeutic massage helps muscles, tendons, and joints; relieves stress and anxiety; and might interrupt pain messages to and from the brain. The average cost for a therapeutic massage is about $60 per hour. It's not covered by Medicare, but might be covered by other insurance plans.

In-person exercise classes. You might want to join a particular health club or perhaps a yoga, dance, or martial arts studio. Membership typically costs about $100 or more per month.

Talk therapy. There are many approaches to cope with the emotional and psychological side of pain, such as cognitive behavioral therapy, which redirects negative thoughts about pain; mindfulness-based psychologies, which help you focus on the present; and pain reprocessing therapy, which helps the brain "unlearn" the response to chronic pain. You can find free lectures for these online, but if you'd like to work with a therapist, it will cost $100 to $200 per hour. Insurance doesn't always cover visits. "Each therapy works in a different way," Dr. Kurz says, "but they all help you change your relationship with pain, which is essential for feeling better." ◗

Try mind-body techniques for head pain

A number of techniques can relax your muscles and ease tension, which should help reduce headache pain. But if you're prone to headaches, treating the stress, anxiety, and other psychological distress that can contribute to attacks is important. Mind-body therapies—such as mindfulness and other types of meditation, relaxation techniques, yoga, hypnosis, stress management, and biofeedback—seek to harness the power of the mind to relax the body and aid in health and pain relief. Mind-body techniques also lower stress and promote healthier lifestyle habits, such as getting adequate sleep, which can help keep headaches at bay. You can find many free yoga classes online, as well as information on how to try mindfulness

meditation. In addition, try these three relaxation techniques to help ease headache pain:

▶ **Deep diaphragmatic breathing.** Slow, controlled breathing in which your abdomen (rather than your chest) expands with each breath. This technique is most relaxing if you make the exhalation longer than the inhalation.

▶ **Meditation.** A process of sitting quietly and directing your attention to a single point of focus, such as the breath, a phrase, or bodily sensations.

▶ **Visualization.** A practice in which you imagine a peaceful scene that relaxes you. Some people find this easier to do with a recording, video, or in-person counselor who guides you through the practice.

Electricity as chronic pain medicine

Several types of "electroceuticals" might ease longstanding pain.

You might be willing to try anything to relieve chronic pain, even getting zapped with tiny shocks of electricity. The concept began evolving long before Ben Franklin conducted his famous experiments with a kite and a key; for example, the ancient Greeks used the natural electrical discharges of torpedo fish to relieve headache and gout. Eventually, as scientists figured out what electricity was and how to use it safely, they applied it to medicine. Today, there are several types of "electroceutical" therapies available to treat pain. Three have our attention.

TENS therapy

In transcutaneous electrical nerve stimulation (TENS) therapy, a machine sends pulses of non-painful, low-intensity electricity to electrodes placed on the skin. The strength of the current and the frequency of the pulses (the number per second) remain consistent throughout a 20-minute session.

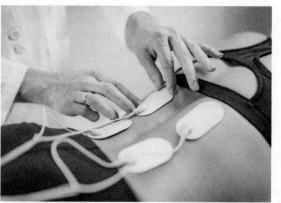
© microgen | Getty Images
Tiny zaps of electricity may bring temporary pain relief.

How does TENS work to quiet pain? "The electrical stimulation closes the 'gate' that allows pain signals to get to the brain. It's just like when you were a kid and got an 'ouch.' Your mom might have told you to rub it to make it feel better. That was enough to close the gate," explains Vitaly Napadow, director of the Scott Schoen and Nancy Adams Discovery Center for Recovery from Chronic Pain at Harvard-affiliated Spaulding Rehabilitation Hospital.

You can go to a practitioner (such as a physical therapist) for TENS therapy or purchase a home TENS unit (about $25 and up). Medicare sometimes covers the costs.

Electroacupuncture

Like TENS therapy, electroacupuncture interrupts pain signals by delivering a consistent frequency of jolts at a certain strength. Instead of being delivered via electrode patches on the skin, it's delivered with acupuncture—hair-thin needles inserted at specific locations in the body. Electrodes are clipped onto the needles and then charged with electricity. "The needles allow the current to penetrate deep underneath the skin, to muscles, tendons, and deeper nerves," Napadow says. "The treatment has the added benefit of acupuncture, which—in traditional Chinese medicine—is believed to affect energy channels. Modern medicine has found that acupuncture can adjust signaling molecules in the nervous system."

Electroacupuncture is available only from a private practitioner or clinic. Sessions cost about $100 per hour, which is often covered in part by Medicare or private insurance.

Scrambler therapy

Scrambler therapy is a newer treatment that sends low-intensity electrical currents to electrodes on the skin. But the frequency of the pulses isn't steady; it changes constantly, with a goal of scrambling—not inhibiting—pain signals and replacing them with non-pain messages. The information is then perceived as a pleasant sensation, tingling, or itching.

Scrambler therapy is found in hospitals or clinics, but it's not widely available. Most insurance companies don't cover the costs, which can be hundreds of dollars per session.

Are they effective?

Experts debate whether electroceutical therapies can zap away chronic pain. TENS therapy and electroacupuncture are well established, and some people swear by them for relief. But they don't work for everyone, and research has produced mixed findings.

"TENS therapy has lost some favor because it's thought that the effect isn't long-lasting. But I think a lot of that has to do with the parameters used in stimulation. At lower frequencies, you might be able to get longer-lasting results," Napadow says. "And some

COPING WITH CHRONIC CONDITIONS

evidence has shown that electroacupuncture can last for months after therapy. But you can't do it by yourself at home, like you can with TENS."

What about scrambler therapy? A review of small preliminary studies published in 2023 in *The New England Journal of Medicine* found that scrambler therapy reduced chronic pain in 80% to 90% of study participants, that it might have long-lasting effects (months or years), and that it might be more effective than TENS therapy. But we'll need more research to confirm the findings.

Is it right for you?

Stay away from electroceuticals if you have any kind of implanted stimulation device, such as a pacemaker or bladder stimulator.

Good candidates for electroceutical therapies are people who have chronic pain, such as arthritis, neuropathy (chronic tingling or pain in the limbs), neck or back pain, or pain from cancer treatment. Potential side effects include skin irritation from electrode patches, burns (which are rare) from electrodes, bleeding from acupuncture needles, dizziness, headaches, nausea, or worsened pain. "Yes, there are risks, but in general they are lower than the potential for side effects from many pain medications," Napadow says.

Get your doctor's okay before seeking treatment, especially if you have a heart condition such as an abnormal heartbeat. And make sure your electroceutical therapy clinician is a licensed health professional who's trained to provide treatment. ▮

Opioid use disorder in older adults: More common than you might think

Overuse and deaths from opioids among older adults have skyrocketed. Could you have a problem and not know it?

You've had a stressful few months: major surgery led to lingering pain worsened by anxiety and the unsettled sense you aren't quite back to normal. Your pain has subsided, but you've decided to ask your doctor for another refill of the opioid painkillers she prescribed after your operation. *Just a little longer ... just until the nerves shake out,* you think.

Seems harmless enough, right? But staying on opioids to allay anxiety, rather than pain, is a slippery slope, Harvard experts say. It's also one of the most common ways well-meaning people slide into opioid addiction (formally called opioid use disorder), a problem responsible for about three-quarters of the nation's overdose deaths.

In contrast to drug addiction stereotypes, astounding numbers of people with opioid use disorder are older adults. Indeed, people over 60 are the largest users of prescription opioids in the United States—with women outpacing men, according to the CDC. And the toll is stunning: opioid use disorder in adults

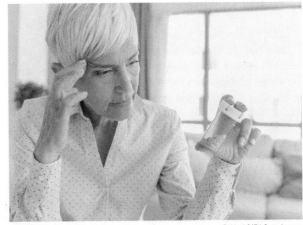
© blackCAT | Getty Images

It's vital to work with your doctor to prevent opioid use from sliding into misuse.

65 and older more than tripled between 2013 and 2018, while opioid-related deaths among Americans 55 and older increased nearly 19-fold between 1999 and 2019, according to a 2022 study published in *JAMA Network Open.*

"One question to ask yourself is, 'If I didn't have pain, would I still have the desire to take these medications?' If the answer is yes, that raises some serious concern," says Dr. Christopher Gilligan, associate chief medical officer at Harvard-affiliated Brigham and ▸▸

Women's Hospital. "You may not realize you have an opioid problem."

Someone who continually seeks opioid refills, asks for higher doses, or tries to obtain prescriptions from multiple doctors is probably also in trouble. "If she comes up with excuses such as 'I lost it' or 'someone took it,' or asks me if I can help her get more, those are not good indicators," says Dr. Robert Jamison, a clinical psychologist and professor of anesthesia at Brigham and Women's Hospital Pain Management Center.

Who's more vulnerable?

A class of pain relievers also called narcotics or opiates, opioids include some familiar names. In addition to the illicit street drug heroin (often laced with fentanyl), prescription versions include morphine, hydrocodone, short-acting or long-acting oxycodone (OxyContin), tramadol, and hydromorphone (Dilaudid). They're typically prescribed to treat pain after surgery or injury, or extreme chronic pain from diabetic neuropathy, arthritis, or cancer.

While opioids carry indisputable dangers, "they're not necessarily a bad thing," Dr. Jamison says. "They're some of the best medications we have to manage postoperative pain," he says. "Quieting pain after surgery is really important, and opioids can do that."

However, certain factors can make someone susceptible to misusing opioids or becoming addicted. You're more at risk if you smoke cigarettes; have anxiety, depression, or another mood disorder; or have a family or personal history of abusing substances, including alcohol.

These scenarios can also make someone more vulnerable to opioid abuse:

Earlier drug use. Baby boomers who overdose on opioids often used drugs recreationally when they were younger and kept it up, according to the 2022 study in *JAMA Network Open*.

Quick discharge after surgery. Pandemic pressures and limitations imposed by health insurance companies have shortened hospital stays for many joint replacement patients, who may return home in significant pain and, in turn, may take more opioids than they would under close medical monitoring, Dr. Jamison says. (See "After joint surgery, less really is more.")

Longstanding use. People who take opioids for chronic pain conditions can develop tolerance, meaning the same dosage provides less relief. Then they might start taking more, Dr. Jamison says.

Prevention strategies

Seeking treatment for opioid use disorder doesn't carry the stigma it once did. Treatment is common and reflects the understanding that opioid use disorder

---

After joint surgery, less really is more

Joint replacement patients prescribed fewer doses of opioids after surgery don't require more refills than those whose prescriptions include a greater number of pills, a new study suggests.

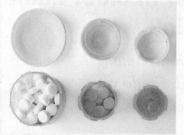

© SeanR1 | Getty Images
Opioid prescriptions with fewer doses may be safer.

Researchers evaluated national insurance data that included nearly 121,000 total joint replacements among adults up to age 75 whose surgeries took place from January 2015 to November 2019. None had previously used opioids. People who had knee replacement were far more likely (nearly 60%) than those who had hip replacement (26%) to refill their opioid prescription within 30 days. But patients whose initial prescriptions included fewer tablets weren't more likely to refill them than those whose prescriptions included more of the medication. The analysis was published in 2022 by *The Journal of Arthroplasty*.

The study bolsters evidence indicating doctors can prescribe smaller amounts of opioids without sacrificing pain control or creating a need for urgent refills, says Dr. Christopher Gilligan, associate chief medical officer at Brigham and Women's Hospital. Smaller prescriptions lower the chances that patients will have leftover opioids in their homes after recovery—potentially tempting them or others to abuse the medication. "We're recognizing that prescribing excessive opioids after surgery inadvertently increases the problem of other people obtaining the medications, leading to misuse," says Dr. Gilligan.

COPING WITH CHRONIC CONDITIONS

is just as much a disease as, say, diabetes or high blood pressure. Often, treatment blends behavioral therapies with medications such as buprenorphine (Butrans), naltrexone (Vivitrol), or a combination of buprenorphine and naloxone (Suboxone), which work by binding to the same pain receptors as opioids, easing cravings.

It's ideal, of course, to prevent opioid use from ever slipping into misuse. To do so, Dr. Gilligan and Dr. Jamison suggest these strategies:

Take opioids for the shortest possible time. Use them for only a few days or less—and at the lowest possible dose—before switching to non-opioid, over-the-counter pain relievers such as such as ibuprofen (Advil), acetaminophen (Tylenol), or naproxen (Aleve).

Tap a non-opioid option. You can turn down opioids if offered after a minor procedure, such as dental work, Dr. Gilligan says. For longer-lasting pain, certain medications used for other conditions can provide notable relief. These include the antidepressant duloxetine (Cymbalta) as well as the antiseizure drugs pregabalin (Lyrica) and gabapentin (Gralise, Horizant). "If you can achieve pain control with zero opioids, your risks are typically much lower," he says.

Try alternative approaches for pain relief. Comfort measures such as heat, ice, and massage "all make a difference," Dr. Jamison says. So too can complementary therapies, such as deep breathing, mindfulness meditation, and acupuncture. Cognitive behavioral therapy can also be "very helpful in coming off medications," he says.

Wean off opioids slowly and with a doctor's guidance. Abruptly stopping opioids can trigger a temporary pain flare-up and bring on other withdrawal symptoms, such as nausea and sweating. "Continual monitoring and gradual tapering is helpful," Dr. Jamison says.

Discuss pain relief before you need it. If you're scheduled for surgery, ask your care team what types of pain measures are appropriate, including regional anesthesia that can block pain to a specific body area for hours to days. "Many different pathways can reduce opioid use after surgery while still delivering pain control," Dr. Gilligan says.

Try yoga to relieve stress and ease symptoms of PTSD

Practicing yoga on a regular basis can help modulate the stress response and reduce anxiety symptoms, calming your heart rate and breathing and lowering your blood pressure. The practice might also have some application in the treatment of generalized anxiety disorder, and some studies have examined yoga as a treatment for post-traumatic stress disorder. Participants have reported reductions in insomnia, depression, anxiety, and fear; improvements in interpersonal relations; and an increased sense of control over their lives. The results are impressive enough that many Department of Veterans Affairs facilities offer yoga-based programs.

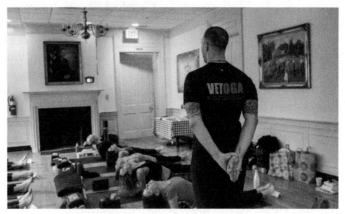

© The Washington Post I Getty Images

Yoga helps reduce a variety of symptoms of PTSD, improving quality of life for those who practice it.

Surprising symptoms of chronic heartburn

Your dentist, cardiologist, or another doctor might spot the signs of heartburn before you do.

With a name like heartburn, it's easy to assume that the condition always shows up as a fiery feeling in your chest or stomach. While that's certainly the classic symptom, chronic heartburn can also make its presence known in other ways, such as a tingling feeling in the nose, chest pressure, a bitter or metallic taste, a hoarse voice, tooth damage, or a dry cough.

What's the link between these symptoms and that spicy spaghetti you had for dinner? Stomach acid. It can leak up into the esophagus, the tube that carries food from the mouth to the stomach. Chronic leakage is a condition called gastroesophageal reflux disease (GERD) and is responsible for symptoms that you might mistake for other conditions.

© ljubaphoto | Getty Images

A chronic dry cough could be a sign of previously unsuspected heartburn.

Heart symptoms

Sometimes acid reflux irritates the upper part of the stomach or the esophagus, which can cause chest pain or pressure, mimicking pain from a partial blockage in a heart artery or even a heart attack.

What you should do: If you're worried about sudden pain in your chest, don't try to figure out if it's heartburn. "This is especially true for people with heart disease risk factors," says Dr. Christopher Cannon, a cardiologist and editor in chief of the *Harvard Heart Letter*.

But discerning the difference between heartburn and heart problems is complicated, and it's best to talk to a doctor about it.

"Chest pain can come from many causes, like acid reflux, but also stress, lung irritation, or muscle aches," Dr. Cannon says. "We have to consider your heart disease risk factors. For example, do you have high blood pressure or diabetes? Does the pain come with exercise? Those could all point to heart trouble, and we might order tests. If the pain comes when you lie down after eating a heavy meal, and taking an antacid makes it better, then it's likely heartburn."

Nose or throat symptoms

In GERD, stomach acid can get up high in the throat and even the area behind the nose, triggering a number of potential symptoms.

"The upper airway isn't built to have the same protections as the stomach or esophagus, so when reflux comes up, it causes injury, almost like a low-level chemical burn. It can cause a dry cough, a sore throat, a hoarse voice, a feeling like there's a lump or mucus plug in the back of the throat, or a tingling feeling in the nose," says Dr. Neil Bhattacharyya, an ear, nose, and throat specialist (ENT) at Harvard-affiliated Massachusetts Eye and Ear.

Because these symptoms overlap with many other conditions, such as a cold or allergies, it can be a long time before you recognize that you have GERD.

What you should do: If you suspect GERD might be causing your symptoms, talk to your primary care provider or an ENT. "We usually recommend that someone go on a four-week trial of heartburn medications, such as over-the-counter omeprazole, and make temporary lifestyle changes to avoid heartburn triggers," Dr. Bhattacharyya says. (See "Lifestyle strategies to combat heartburn," page 149.)

"If symptoms improve after four weeks, it's a good indicator that you probably have reflux disease," Dr. Bhattacharyya says.

Mouth or dental symptoms

For some people, GERD symptoms might seem more like mouth or dental problems. "If the acid reaches your mouth, you might develop mouth sores or ulcers, erosion or wear on your teeth, or cavities. The cavities could be due to the acid, sugary heartburn medications, your diet, poor oral hygiene, or a combination of those factors," says Dr. Tien Jiang, a prosthodontist in the Department of Oral Health Policy and Epidemiology at the Harvard School of Dental Medicine. Acid reflux can also create a bitter or metallic taste in the mouth.

What you should do: If you suspect that acid reflux is reaching your mouth, rinse frequently with water to neutralize it and protect your gums, soft tissues, and teeth. "Wait 30 minutes after meals or after detecting reflux to brush your teeth. This allows your saliva—and water that you rinse with or drink—to neutralize the mouth's acidity," Dr. Jiang says. "Just before brushing, rinse with water to eliminate the acid first, so you don't accidentally brush the acid against your teeth and cause more extensive wear. And get your teeth cleaned at least twice a year." ▼

Lifestyle strategies to combat heartburn

Lifestyle habits are an important part of thwarting heartburn. Try as many of the following as possible:

Avoid foods and drinks that seem to trigger heartburn symptoms, such as anything spicy, fatty, fried, greasy, or acidic (like tomato sauces or citrus); foods with onions or garlic; alcohol; soda; and anything with caffeine, such as coffee, tea, or chocolate.

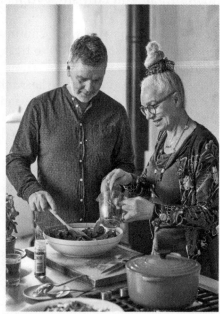

- ▶ Eat smaller meals.
- ▶ Stay upright for at least two hours after meals.
- ▶ Avoid late-night eating or drinking (especially alcohol).
- ▶ Sleep on a wedge pillow.
- ▶ Quit smoking.
- ▶ Lose weight if you need to.

© Gary Burchell | Getty Images

Aim to keep your heartburn under control

Acid reflux (heartburn) can keep you up at night. Steer clear of foods that contribute to heartburn, as lying down can provoke or worsen the problem. Common culprits include coffee, chocolate, alcohol, peppermint, and fatty foods. If you're prone to acid reflux, elevate your upper body with an under-mattress wedge or blocks placed under the bed's legs. Over-the-counter and prescription drugs that suppress stomach acid secretion can also help. Finally, if you sleep on your right side, try to sleep on your left side instead, as several studies suggest that sleeping on your right side aggravates heartburn.

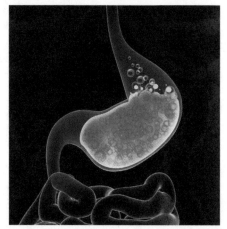

© decade3d | Getty Images

CPAP machines and masks: Which ones are right for you?

We've boiled it down to several tips to help you make decisions and begin treatment, so you can start to feel better.

Your doctor says you need continuous positive airway pressure (CPAP) to treat your sleep apnea, and you're eager to begin treatment. You're also a little worried, since you've heard that using a CPAP system can be uncomfortable and challenging. How do you choose a system that will give you the best odds of success? Here are some tips to help.

Understand the treatment

CPAP is the first-line treatment for people with obstructive sleep apnea, a sleep disorder marked by repeated pauses in breathing caused by a blocked airway.

The CPAP system's job is to keep your airway open. It does that by pushing a forceful stream of air through a tube and into a mask you wear while you sleep. The air comes from a small bedside pump (an air compressor).

Other forms of positive airway pressure (PAP) may be helpful for people with central sleep apnea,

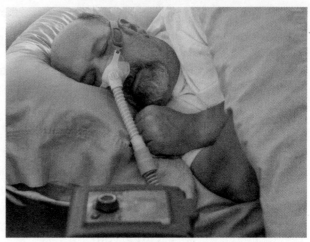

© grandriver | Getty Images

Some CPAP masks are less intrusive than others, covering the nose but not the mouth.

although pauses in breathing in this type of sleep apnea are related to garbled messages from the brain, not blockages (see "What is sleep apnea?").

Trust your doctor

Your physician will determine what kind of CPAP device you need. "The device and its settings are by prescription, just like a medication," says Dr. Noah Siegel, director of Sleep Medicine and Sleep Surgery at Harvard-affiliated Massachusetts Eye and Ear.

With CPAP, a single fixed air pressure is used throughout the night. Other types of PAP therapies include

- **auto-adjusting positive airway pressure, or APAP,** which provides a range of preset pressures throughout the night
- **bilevel positive airway pressure, or BiPAP,** which provides two different preset pressures—a more powerful one when you inhale and a less powerful one when you exhale
- **adaptive servo ventilation, or ASV,** an advanced device that provides pressure based on breathing patterns throughout the night.

"Generally speaking, people with obstructive sleep apnea respond better to CPAP or APAP. People with central sleep apnea may respond better to BiPAP or ASV," Dr. Siegel says.

Investigate face mask options

You get to choose the face mask for your PAP system, and it's an important decision.

What is sleep apnea?

Sleep apnea is a potentially life-threatening condition characterized by pauses in breathing during sleep. The pauses last at least 10 seconds, lead to poor-quality sleep, and put a strain on your body. Untreated sleep apnea may increase your risk for high blood pressure or stroke.

In obstructive sleep apnea, pauses in breathing occur when the airway briefly becomes blocked. This can be caused by too much tissue in the airway (often due to excess weight), large tonsils, or a large tongue.

In central sleep apnea, pauses in breathing occur when the brain fails to deliver electrical impulses to the muscles that help you breathe.

COPING WITH CHRONIC CONDITIONS

Face masks often feel bulky, making people reluctant to wear them. Dr. Siegel recommends looking at mask options online and trying on a few before making a selection. That might happen at a medical supply store or during a home visit from your medical equipment supplier.

The masks fall into two categories.

Full-face masks. These cover the nose and mouth and deliver air to them both. They are ideal for someone who breathes through the mouth or has nasal or sinus problems.

Nasal masks. These masks deliver air through the nose only. They are less bulky than full-face masks and come in styles that fit over, under, or in the nose.

An important consideration for both mask types, Dr. Siegel says, is the site where the tube from the pump enters the mask. "Traditional-style masks connect the tubing in the front of the mask, near the nose. That's not great for people who roll over a lot in bed or people who are claustrophobic," he says. "Newer styles attach at the top of the mask. It's much less intrusive."

Give it time

Adjusting to any PAP system takes time. You may need to try a few masks to find the right fit and comfort. "And if allergies or frequent sinus congestion keep you from using a nasal mask, we have interventions—such as nasal sprays or surgery—that might make a nasal mask more tolerable," Dr. Siegel says. Also, your doctor may need to make adjustments to your machine, such as changes to settings for pressure and humidification.

Just stick with it, and remember that using a PAP system, like taking a medication, is an ongoing therapy that needs regular evaluation. ♦

New thinking about tinnitus

Harvard Medical School scientists close in on a mysterious cause of ringing in the ears.

Experts have long debated the most common cause of tinnitus—a ringing, whooshing, roaring, or hissing in the ears without an external sound source. Some have maintained that tinnitus is triggered by hearing loss: with less sound coming in, the brain compensates by becoming hyperactive and generating a phantom noise.

But that theory hasn't explained the problem for people with normal hearing tests who still have tinnitus. What causes tinnitus in those cases?

Mounting evidence

Increasingly, Harvard Medical School scientists are finding evidence that some people have "hidden" hearing loss: damage to the auditory nerve—which carries sound signals from the ear to the brain—that isn't picked up by conventional tests.

Researchers first discovered the phenomenon in lab mice in 2009. "From there, it wasn't difficult to add two and two by suggesting that the loss of these

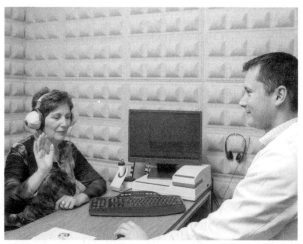
© Maica | Getty Images

Sometimes people with normal hearing tests can have "hidden" hearing loss and tinnitus.

nerve fibers in people with normal hearing tests could be associated with tinnitus," says Stéphane Maison, a tinnitus researcher and associate professor of Otolaryngology–Head and Neck Surgery at Harvard Medical School.

Subsequent studies began making the connection. The latest—believed to be the largest and most nuanced to date—was published in 2023 ▸▸

▸▸ in *Scientific Reports*. Maison and his colleagues at Harvard-affiliated Massachusetts Eye and Ear recruited almost 300 people (ages 18 to 72) with normal hearing tests who had chronic tinnitus, no tinnitus, or intermittent tinnitus.

Scientists measured participants' auditory nerve responses and brainstem activity. Compared with not having tinnitus, having chronic tinnitus was associated with a loss of auditory nerve fibers as well as increased brain activity. "That fits with the idea that as a result of hearing loss, the brain increases its activity, which is possibly why you perceive a tone or a sound that isn't there," Maison says.

What this means for treatment

For people with measurable hearing loss, getting hearing aids sometimes reduces the perception of tinnitus. But hearing aids aren't recommended for people with normal hearing test results—even if your doctor suspects hidden hearing loss—since we don't have tests outside of research labs to measure it.

Still, the new evidence linking hidden hearing loss and tinnitus offers hope for people with tinnitus. "When you have hidden hearing loss, only a portion of the auditory nerve has degenerated. Another portion remains alive for years or decades. And a number of experiments by others have found that it's possible to regenerate nerve fibers in animal models," Maison says. "If we can one day regenerate those fibers in humans, perhaps it might bring back missing information to the brain, reducing its hyperactivity and the perception of tinnitus."

Until that day comes—and it's unclear when or if it will—we have only limited ways to cope with the problem.

What you can do

If you have tinnitus despite a normal hearing test, report it to your primary care doctor or ear, nose, and throat specialist. In rare cases, the noise can be caused by a tumor or cyst pinching the auditory nerve, a buildup of earwax, or blood vessel damage. Sometimes treating underlying conditions like these can reduce or even eliminate the noise.

More often, we can only learn to how to live with or reduce tinnitus. The following strategies may help.

Distract your brain. Listening to white noise or nature sounds might make tinnitus seem quieter. Use a white noise machine, sleep headphones, earbuds, or a wearable sound-masking device.

Use mind-body therapies. Cognitive behavioral therapy, mindfulness-based tinnitus treatment, and biofeedback can help you redirect negative thoughts and emotions linked to tinnitus.

Join an online support group. Look for tinnitus groups on Facebook or through the American Tinnitus Association (www.ata.org; click on "Support"). You may pick up tips that work for other people, or at least feel empowered by camaraderie.

Reduce stress. Stress may increase both your perception of tinnitus and your reaction to it. Try yoga or tai chi to help manage stress; since you'll be concentrating on movement and breathing, you might not focus on the tinnitus as much.

Live a healthier lifestyle. Practice good sleep hygiene, exercise daily, and limit alcohol intake. Each one of those healthy habits can help reduce the frequency and intensity of tinnitus, while also reducing stress.

Consider trying bimodal stimulation. These new devices for home use provide two types of stimulation—for instance, sound along with gentle taps to the wrist delivered by a bracelet. "They aren't yet widely recommended as there's not enough evidence that they work, but preliminary results are encouraging," Maison says. "Ask your physician about your options." ▰

What should you do when sciatica flares?

These options can help calm the searing pain of an irritated sciatic nerve.

People with diagnosed sciatica have no trouble recognizing a flare-up. It strikes as numbness, tingling, or pain in the buttock and down the leg, caused by irritation to the sciatic nerve, which begins in the spine and travels downward into the leg.

While it's easy to identify a flare-up, it's trickier to tamp it down. It may take a combination of approaches to ease discomfort.

Pill-free approaches

Coping with sciatica discomfort starts with pill-free strategies that you can try immediately.

Stay active. One of the most important things you can do when sciatica flares is to avoid bed rest. "Part of low back pain is muscle-related, possibly because muscles surrounding the irritated nerve roots tighten and try to protect the area. Movement keeps the muscles loose and working correctly. If you don't move, they can get tight and increase pain," says Dr. Max Epstein, a physiatrist at Harvard-affiliated Spaulding Rehabilitation Hospital.

Modify activities. If activity is painful, do only what you can tolerate. "Think of a green, yellow, or red zone of pain. The green zone is a mild amount of pain while doing an activity. That's okay. But if you get into the yellow zone, it's time to pull back and modify an activity," Dr. Epstein says. "For example, if it hurts to carry a full laundry basket, take out a few things. Or if it's painful to stand at the sink and do dishes, open the cabinet below the sink and rest your foot on the bottom of the cabinet. That will take tension off the nerve."

Stretch. Keep the muscles loose and limber with gentle stretching, but only within the green zone of pain. For example, you might stand and try to touch your toes to stretch your back and leg muscles. Or try some yoga poses. Dr. Epstein recommends the cat-cow: Rest on "all fours," with your hands directly beneath your shoulders and your knees beneath your hips. Next, inhale and lift your head and tailbone toward the ceiling, while curving your lower spine toward the floor. As you exhale, round your back, bringing your chin toward your chest and tucking your tailbone under. Repeat the exercise 10 times.

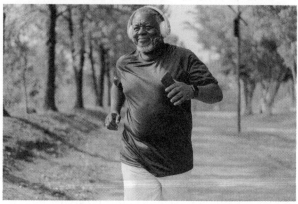

© andreswd | Getty Images

Stay active when sciatica flares. Inactivity only tightens muscles and increases back and leg pain.

Use hot or cold therapy. Hot or cold therapy for sciatica can take many forms. For example, you might soak in a warm bath or apply a hot pack or a cold pack to your leg or back. "What works for one person might not work for another, so you may have to experiment to see what's best for you," Dr. Epstein says. How does it help sciatica? "Heat may loosen muscles, and cold may tamp down inflammation, but we don't know for sure," Dr. Epstein explains.

Relaxation. Staying relaxed is an important part of controlling both acute pain (the kind that's sudden and temporary) or chronic (ongoing) pain.

"All pain is processed in the mind. If you're able to calm the processing centers, the perception of pain may decrease," Dr. Epstein says. He recommends trying breathing exercises, meditation, yoga, or tai chi. Practicing mindfulness—focusing attention on the present moment—might also help ease discomfort by helping you to accept it.

Drugstore remedies

Several over-the-counter remedies can also play a part in relieving sciatica.

Oral painkillers. Oral nonsteroidal anti-inflammatory drugs (NSAIDs) such as ibuprofen (Advil, Motrin) help reduce inflammation, which reduces pain. But they may cause stomach ulcers and bleeding, liver or kidney damage, or an increased risk of heart attacks. So get your doctor's okay before using them, and find out the dose and frequency that's safe for you.

▶▶

▶▶ Acetaminophen (Tylenol) is often less effective at relieving sciatica pain than NSAIDs, but it's also less risky—unless you take it in very high doses, which can cause liver damage. The usual limit is no more than 3,000 milligrams (mg) per day, but your doctor might set a lower limit depending on your health.

Topical painkillers. Applying painkillers to your skin as creams, gels, or patches can also bring sciatica relief. Topical NSAIDs such as diclofenac gel (Voltaren) may have fewer risks than NSAID pills, since topicals stay close to the site of application and aren't well absorbed by the rest of the body. But it's still wise to check with your doctor before using them. Other types of topicals with fewer risks than NSAIDs include creams, sprays, and patches that contain anesthetics such as lidocaine; pain signal interrupters such as menthol or capsaicin; or arnica gel, an herbal remedy thought to have anti-inflammatory properties.

Turmeric supplements. Turmeric (a golden-yellow spice) contains curcumin, which appears to have anti-inflammatory and antioxidant properties. "Although there have not yet been studies that prove

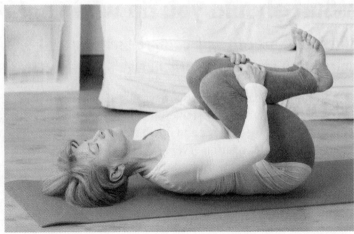

© KatarzynaBialasiewicz | Getty Images

Yoga poses, such as bringing your knees to your chest while lying down, may help ease sciatica.

its benefit, it's the one supplement that I would support for pain relief. There's no clear recommendation for dosage, but 1,000 mg per day might help. You can take it all at once or break it up into morning and evening doses," Dr. Epstein says.

Call your doctor

A typical flare-up lasts for a few days to a week or two. If it's not improving or responding to home remedies, it's time to make an appointment with your doctor.

Your doctor might order imaging tests and prescribe a prescription anti-inflammatory drug, such as oral or injected prednisone. "That will buy you a window of time to strengthen muscles without pain and keep them flexible," Dr. Epstein says. "That will help keep your body strong and protected, so you'll be in a better place than where you started."

What if you don't reach out for help? "At times the nerve stays irritated for years," Dr. Epstein says. "So try not to delay treatment. Usually our interventions are able to put out the fire or at least calm the severity of the symptoms in a meaningful way."

If you'd like more information, check out the Harvard Special Health Report *Finding Relief for Sciatica* (www.health.harvard.edu/frfsc). ♥

What is sciatica?

Sciatica is the term for discomfort caused by irritation of the sciatic nerve. This nerve starts at each side of the low back and extends down through the buttocks, back of the thigh, and lower leg.

Irritation usually occurs in the spine, with one of the nerve roots that eventually form the sciatic nerve. Anything pressing against a nerve root—such as a bony growth from arthritis in the spine or a bulging disc in between the spinal bones—can inflame the nerve root and send pain, numbness, or tingling all the way down one of the sciatic nerves.

"If you've never had it before, it's common to worry that you may have damaged your sciatic nerve. It's usually more of an irritation, however, as opposed to an outright injury," says Dr. Max Epstein, a physiatrist at Spaulding Rehabilitation Hospital. "But if you also experience muscle weakness or significant changes to your bowel or bladder habits, that could be a sign of nerve damage. In either case, you should speak to a health care provider as soon as possible."

A look at dry eye

Everyone's eyes occasionally get irritated. But for people with dry eye syndrome, it's an almost daily frustration.

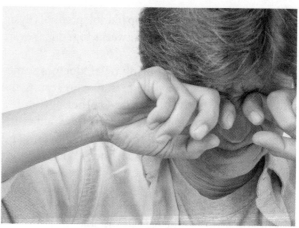
© makotomo | Getty Images

Burning and itching that provoke the urge to rub your eyes are common symptoms of dry eye.

Who hasn't grappled with the occasional itchy or bothersome eyes? It may be caused by allergies, dust, pollutants, or over-rubbing tired peepers. But suppose your eyes constantly have a gritty feeling, or they're sensitive to light, or your vision fluctuates? In that case, you may be one of the millions of people with dry eye syndrome.

"Dry eye syndrome is one of the most common eye problems among older adults," explains Dr. Nandini Venkateswaran, an ophthalmologist with Harvard-affiliated Massachusetts Eye and Ear. "People with the condition can have good and bad periods, but by following prevention methods and seeking treatment when the disease flares, they can keep dry eye from interfering with their lives."

The eyes have it

Every time you blink, a film consisting of tears, oil, and other lubricants coats your eyes. The tears are produced by the lacrimal gland in each of your upper lids. The oil, from tiny meibomian glands that line the upper and lower lids, prevents the tears from evaporating too quickly. A layer of protein called mucin that covers the eye's surface acts as a lubricant.

As we age, tear and oil production decline, making the tear film less abundant and leaving the eyes feeling dry. Eye issues like glaucoma or cataract surgery also can lead to dry eye. "People who are longtime contact wearers or who had laser eye surgery when they were younger also may be more prone to dry eye as they age," says Dr. Venkateswaran.

Dry eye syndrome can be a side effect of certain medications, such as antidepressants, antihistamines, decongestants, anti-anxiety agents, and diuretics and other drugs for blood pressure. Dry eye syndrome can cause any of the following symptoms:
- burning or itchy eyes
- painful eyes when you wake up
- a feeling of something gritty, like sand, in the eyes
- sensitivity to light
- difficulty wearing contact lenses
- excessive tearing
- a sticky sensation caused by mucus
- trouble focusing or needing to repeatedly blink to see clearly.

Don't ignore symptoms of dry eye syndrome. "Dry eye syndrome shouldn't cause permanent eye damage, although severe cases can result in corneal scarring. But left untreated, it can affect your quality of life," says Dr. Venkateswaran.

Treatment options

Dry eye syndrome is diagnosed by adding a special stain to the eye that highlights dry spots. The doctor can then evaluate the quality and quantity of the tear film and how quickly it evaporates. A Schirmer's test can also be used to measure tear production. Here, a thin strip of filter paper is placed inside the lower lid, and after five minutes, the amount of moisture in the paper is measured.

Treatment for dry eye takes a stepladder approach, where you begin with conservative options and progress to more intensive treatments if needed, says Dr. Venkateswaran.

The most common treatment is over-the-counter preservative-free artificial tears, which are eye drops that mimic natural tears. These can be used multiple times a day and for the long term. Over-the-counter ointments and gels applied before bedtime also may be helpful. For more severe cases, your doctor may recommend prescription eye drops, such as lifitegrast (Xiidra) or cyclosporine (Cequa, Restasis), which reduce eye inflammation and increase tear production. Short ▸▸

▶▶ courses of a steroid eye drop like loteprednol (Eysuvis) can be used for two to four weeks to reduce severe dry eye flares.

If artificial tears don't bring relief, doctors sometimes prescribe eye drops made from your serum, the clear liquid part of your blood. Another option is a nasal spray with varenicline (Tyrvaya), which stimulates the nerve connected to the lacrimal gland and meibomian glands. The spray can be used alone or with other dry eye therapies.

Your doctor also may try to make the most of your natural tears by placing tiny plugs made of collagen or silicone into the tear drain holes at the inner corners of the eyes. "These help maintain longer periods of lubrication on the eye's surface," says Dr. Venkateswaran. ▼

Protect your eyes

To lower your risk of developing dry eye syndrome, or to reduce eye sensitivity if you have dry eye, try the following:

▶ Reduce exposure to elements that can cause or aggravate the condition, such as wind, smoke, chemical vapors, dry heat, and fans.

▶ Wear protective glasses or sunglasses when outdoors.

▶ Use an indoor humidifier.

▶ Take regular breaks if you spend long hours at a computer screen.

IN THE JOURNALS

Antidepressant may help manage irritable bowel syndrome symptoms

Amitriptyline, a tricyclic antidepressant also used to treat nerve pain, may be one of the best pharmacologic choices to help improve symptoms of irritable bowel syndrome (IBS).

IBS causes abdominal pain and changes to bowel movements, with symptoms fluctuating in severity over time. IBS has no cure, and standard treatments like dietary and lifestyle changes and taking antispasmodic or antidiarrheal medications yield varying benefits.

In a 2023 study published in *The Lancet,* 463 people with IBS took either amitriptyline (10 to 30 milligrams based on the severity of each person's symptoms) or a placebo every day for six months. Afterward, people who took amitriptyline were almost twice as likely as those taking a placebo to report an overall improvement in their symptoms

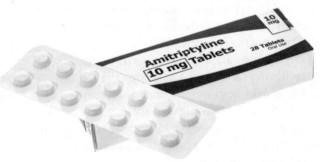

© clubfoto | Getty Images

New evidence for the antidepressant amitriptyline.

and had significantly lower IBS severity. It's believed amitriptyline helps by increasing people's threshold for IBS pain and discomfort.

The researchers suggested that doctors should consider low-dose amitriptyline for managing IBS when dietary and other lifestyle changes are not sufficient.

COPING WITH CHRONIC CONDITIONS

Get moving to manage osteoarthritis

Exercise may be the best medicine for healthy joints.

The estimated 32 million Americans with osteoarthritis face a dilemma: exercise is often difficult and painful, but it is precisely what they should do to help manage their pain.

"Regular exercise and movement can help people with osteoarthritis in many ways," says Dr. Jeffrey Katz, professor of medicine and orthopedic surgery at Harvard Medical School. "Besides helping with pain management, it can improve patients' level of function and may delay the need for a joint replacement."

Casing the joints

Osteoarthritis, the most common type of arthritis, is a chronic and progressive disease characterized by loss of the cartilage that covers and protects the ends of the bones where they meet at a joint.

"The condition slowly wears away joint cartilage so that forces usually absorbed by the cartilage are transferred to bone, which has pain sensitive nerve fibers," says Dr. Katz. "Cartilage breakdown can also lead to pain, swelling, inflammation and activity limitation."

Osteoarthritis most often occurs in the knees, hips, and lower back. The condition becomes more common with age, but other factors can increase a person's risk, such as a family history of the disease, previous injury, and excess weight.

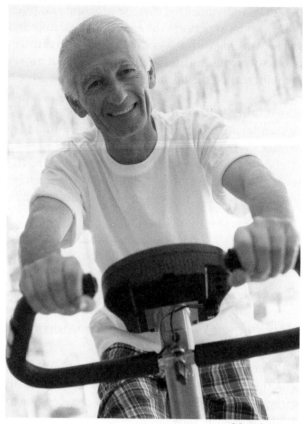

© Fuse | Getty Images

Low-impact activities like riding a stationary bike help improve your joints' range of motion.

Preventing the pain of osteoarthritis

Not only can exercise keep osteoarthritis from possibly becoming worse, but it may reduce the risk of developing the condition. One study that looked for a connection between running and osteoarthritis risk in the hip or knee found that only 3.5% of people who ran for exercise eventually got knee or hip osteoarthritis, compared with 10% of inactive people. Another study found that among people who had mild knee osteoarthritis or were at higher-than-average risk for the disease, those who walked an average of almost 7,000 steps per day (more than three miles) did not experience additional cartilage loss over two years.

There is no cure for osteoarthritis. Nonsteroidal anti-inflammatory drugs, such as ibuprofen (Advil, Motrin), naproxen (Aleve), or aspirin, can temporarily soothe pain and inflammation. Steroid injections also may offer short-term relief.

Another way to manage symptoms is to get moving. "Exercise can't help replace lost cartilage or necessarily slow its natural decline," says Dr. Katz. "It has a supporting role—strengthening the bones and surrounding muscles to protect the affected joints from excess stress so they can work better."

Get evaluated

If you have osteoarthritis, and are having difficulty initiating an exercise program, Dr. Katz recommends seeing a physical therapist.

▶▶

▶▶ "An expert evaluation can help identify alignment issues, weakness, and limitations in joint motion that can make joint pain worse and make movements more difficult," he says. "Physical therapists can also design an individualized exercise program and teach patients how to perform the exercises accurately and safely. Working with a physical therapist also can help people overcome any fear or hesitation about movement increasing their pain."

Exercising your options

A standard exercise program typically includes aerobic exercises and resistance training to increase strength in the major muscle groups supporting the joints, like the buttocks, thighs, and the muscles in the lower back. You might use weights, exercise bands, body weight, or another means of providing resistance.

"Your program will depend on various factors, including which joints are involved, how severe the pain is, your fitness level, and whether you have other medical conditions," says Dr. Katz.

Low-impact aerobic activities are also part of an overall exercise strategy, as they help strengthen muscles, improve endurance, and increase your joints' range of motion. Examples include power walking, swimming, using an elliptical trainer, cycling, or riding a stationary bike.

"Your physical therapist can recommend the best low-impact activities to complement your exercise program and how long and often to do them," says Dr. Katz. ▍

Get ready for allergy season

Here's how to manage the symptoms of pollen allergies.

Allergy season typically runs from around March through October. Tree pollen dominates in spring, grass pollen in summer, and ragweed pollen in late summer to early fall.

If you have an allergy, when you inhale pollen, your immune system generates antibodies called immunoglobulin E that trigger the release of chemicals like histamine, leukotrienes, and prostaglandins. These chemicals eventually spread to tissues in the eyes, nose, throat, and lungs. Too much pollen exposure can cause the immune system to go haywire and trigger the hallmark allergy symptoms, such as sneezing, watery eyes, stuffiness, scratchy throat, wheezing, and coughing.

Allergies may also cause "brain fog." "Allergy symptoms often disrupt sleep and make people feel tired and groggy," says Dr. Mariana Castells, an allergist and immunologist in the division of Allergy and Clinical Immunology at Harvard-affiliated Brigham and Women's Hospital. "Plus, your body can become weaker as it fights the inflammation triggered by allergies, contributing to fatigue and making it harder to concentrate and focus."

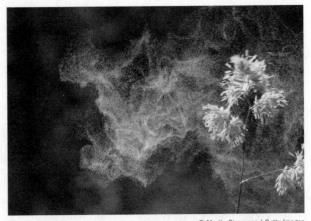

© Martin Siepmann I Getty Images

Pollen from trees, grass, and ragweed are the main sources of spring and summer allergies.

Managing symptoms

Allergy symptoms vary in severity and length, depending on your specific sensitivity to particular pollen, the amount of exposure, and your major symptoms. "This is why some people may experience allergy symptoms only during a certain time of allergy season or only for a few days or weeks," says Dr. Castells.

COPING WITH CHRONIC CONDITIONS

Reaction to pollen also can vary from year to year because of weather changes. "Pollen levels increase when it's drier and go down when there is more rain," says Dr. Castells.

There are many ways to manage allergy symptoms. Dr. Castells advises treating symptoms at the first sign of a sniffle, scratchy throat, or itchy eyes. "This way, you can help manage inflammation before it rages out of control." (Note that symptoms that affect only one side, like one nostril, ear, or eye, should be checked by your doctor, as this could be something unrelated to allergies such as an infection.)

Here are the most effective methods for treating seasonal allergies.

Over-the-counter medication
Over-the-counter drugs fall into three main categories.

Non-drowsy antihistamines. These come as pills and nasal sprays and work to block the effects of the excess histamine that causes itchy and watery eyes, sneezing, and a runny nose. Sprays also help with congestion and postnasal drip. The less sedating oral antihistamines include loratadine (Claritin), cetirizine (Zyrtec), fexofenadine (Allegra), levocetirizine (Xyzal), and desloratadine (Clarinex).

Decongestants. These are available as pills, liquids, and nasal sprays. They shrink tiny blood vessels, which decreases fluid secretion in the nasal passages, helping to unclog a stuffy nose. Oral decongestants like pseudoephedrine (Sudafed) can increase heart rate and blood pressure, so check with your doctor before taking them if you have heart or blood pressure problems.

Nasal steroid sprays. These reduce inflammation that causes congestion, runny or itchy nose, and sneezing. People with glaucoma should take these with caution, as they can raise pressure inside the eye and lead to vision loss. "Antihistamines and decongestants are sometimes enough to relieve allergy symptoms," says Dr. Castells. "If that is insufficient, then a combination of antihistamines and nasal steroids is the next step."

Allergy shots and oral immunotherapy
If your allergy symptoms are severe or not sufficiently relieved by over-the-counter remedies, one option is a preventive regimen of immunotherapy, given in the form of injections ("allergy shots") or sublingual tablets (which are placed under the tongue to ▸▸

Rinse and repeat

One drug-free way to get relief from allergies is by rinsing your nasal cavity twice daily using a saline solution. You can do a nasal rinse using a small bulb syringe or a neti pot, which resembles a small teapot with a long spout. Both are found at most drugstores and online. Here's how a nasal rinse is done:

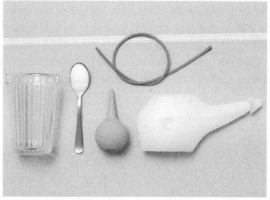
© Koldunova_Anna | Getty Images
A saline nasal rinse can be surprisingly effective for reducing allergy symptoms.

1. Stir two to three teaspoons of non-iodized salt (not table salt, which has too many additives) and ¼ to ½ teaspoon of baking soda into 2 cups of lukewarm distilled water. (You can use tap water, but always boil it and let it cool to a lukewarm temperature first.) Another option is an over-the-counter sinus mix; add one packet to the neti pot with the water.

2. Pour the solution into a neti pot or pull it into a bulb syringe.

3. To rinse your nose, stand over a sink, bend forward, and tilt your head to one side. Insert the tip of the pot or syringe inside one nostril, and gently pour or squeeze the bulb to release about ½ cup of the solution. The water will run back out the nostril or the opposite nostril and into the sink. Repeat the procedure in the other nostril. Then gently blow your nose. Perform twice a day until your sinuses are clear.

4. Thoroughly rinse (with distilled or cooled boiled water) and dry the neti pot or bulb syringe after each use.

dissolve). "These do not eliminate your allergy, but they change your immune response to better tolerate it," says Dr. Castells.

An allergist does skin and blood testing to identify your specific pollen allergy and then develops a personalized vaccine. Allergy shots are done in two phases: buildup and maintenance. The buildup phase involves increasing exposure to the pollen once or twice weekly for three to six months. For the maintenance phase, you get monthly injections for three to five years.

When you've finished this regimen, the protective effect can last several years, says Dr. Castells. Sublingual tablets offer similar protection. There is no buildup period. Instead, you take the tablets daily for a few weeks before and during pollen season.

Reduce pollen exposure

Another way to manage symptoms is to lower your exposure to pollen. For example, keep your windows closed, and occasionally run the air conditioner to help remove pollen from the indoor air. Restrict outside time to the afternoon or evening when the pollen count is lower. (Pollen is usually highest from about 4 a.m. to noon). Check daily pollen counts in your area and sign up for high pollen alerts at www.pollen.com.

If you are outside when pollen is high, wear a mask, which can block 70% to 80% of pollen, according to Dr. Castells. When you come inside, immediately shower and wash your clothes to keep any pollen out of the indoor air.

Exercising outside in the cold and have asthma? Cover your mouth and nose

Exercising in cold weather can bring on asthma symptoms. Experts suspect that the cold, dry air narrows bronchial tubes and causes cells lining your airway to release chemicals that trigger inflammation, further constricting airways. If you have asthma and are exercising in cold weather, try to breathe through your nose, and wear a scarf, bandanna, or other covering over your mouth and nose. The cloth will retain some of the moisture from your breath as you exhale, humidifying the air drawn in as you inhale. Dress properly for cold-weather workouts. Depending on the temperature, wear layers you can peel off as you warm up, and don't forget gloves.

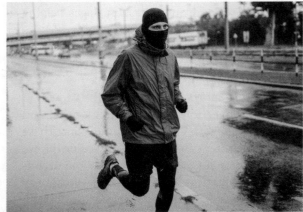

© bojanstory | Getty Images

COPING WITH CHRONIC CONDITIONS

Chapter 7

Cancer Prevention and Early Detection

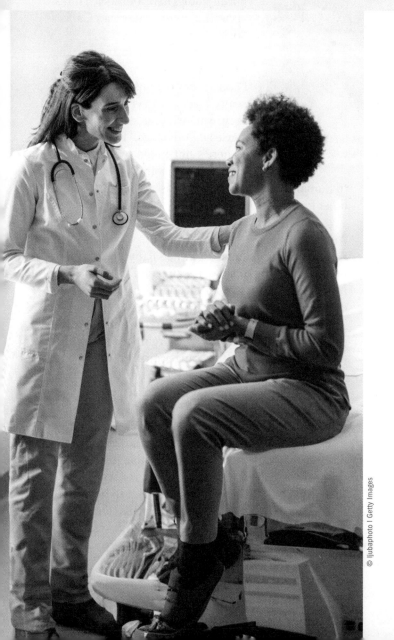

© ljubaphoto I Getty Images

Healthy Habits! 5 Things You Can Do Now

1 **Perform a skin self-exam.** Learn how to spot skin cancer early. (page 164)

2 **Learn to let go of survivor's guilt.** Taking time to grieve can help you move on after successful cancer treatment. (page 174)

3 **Shed fat.** Extra pounds are associated with a higher risk of prostate cancer. (page 178)

4 **Add a vegetable or two to your daily meals.** Making healthy dietary changes gradually makes them more likely to stick—and reduces cancer risk. (page 179)

5 **Rethink frequent PSA testing.** Overtesting may lead to unnecessary, invasive treatment. (page 181)

Cancer concerns from everyday products

Some items are linked with increased risk. But how much should you worry?

In the span of a few days in the summer of 2023, the simple act of sipping a diet soda became a bit more fraught.

Why? International health authorities issued a statement classifying aspartame—an artificial sweetener widely found in diet drinks and foods like gum, yogurt, and ice cream—as possibly carcinogenic in humans. But limited evidence supports any cancer-causing effects of aspartame, especially at the amounts most people consume, the International Agency for Research on Cancer noted.

Nevertheless, the announcement spurred much confusion and consternation—most of it needless, says Timothy Rebbeck, a professor of cancer prevention at Harvard-affiliated Dana-Farber Cancer Institute. "A lot of people thought that statement meant they'd better not use aspartame, that it causes cancer. But that's not what it said, or how to interpret it," Rebbeck says. "There's not much meaningful evidence that aspartame confers cancer risk at all."

The muddle also reignited simmering concern that products we use every day—what we eat or drink, apply to our skin, or live with in our homes—might raise our risks for cancer, which causes one in every six deaths globally each year. But Rebbeck says fear may trump knowledge when it comes to knowing which products we routinely use pose a meaningful cancer risk.

"Most consumer products people are exposed to confer very low cancer risks, if any," says Rebbeck, who is also director of the Zhu Family Center for Global Cancer Prevention at the Harvard T.H. Chan School of Public Health. "People's estimate of the risk is probably higher than it actually is."

What other household goods might prompt cancer concerns? Rebbeck offers context around the evidence gathered for an array of products.

Nonstick cookware

Some pots, pans, and other cookware are coated with a synthetic chemical called polytetrafluoroethylene,

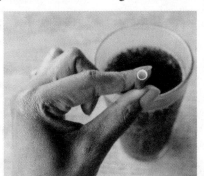
© Grace Cary | Getty Images
Evidence linking aspartame in diet drinks to cancer is very limited.

commonly known as Teflon and one of a group of related chemicals known as perfluoroalkyl and polyfluoroalkyl substances, or PFAS.

The evidence: PFAS can be found at very low levels in just about everyone's blood worldwide. Research examining cancer rates in people living near or working in PFAS-related chemical plants, as well as in the general population, suggest—but don't prove—a link between PFAS exposure and certain cancers. And not all studies have found such links, according to the American Cancer Society (ACS).

Expert take: "The interesting thing about nonstick compounds is, because they're nonstick, they don't really react with very much when they're in their solid state. They don't cause DNA damage," Rebbeck says. "There's not much evidence that nonstick cookware is carcinogenic in humans, but some compounds related to Teflon in other forms have been associated with cancer."

Mattresses

Some mattress manufacturers add flame retardants to prevent burning or slow the spread of fire. This may mean the mattress you're sleeping on every night is coated in those chemicals.

The evidence: Certain flame retardants contain chemicals known as volatile organic compounds (VOCs), which means they can become airborne. Some research suggests these flame retardants can interfere with hormone levels and may be associated with cancer, according to the National Institute of Environmental Health Sciences.

Expert take: One pitfall of linking cancer risk with flame retardants is there aren't reliable measures of exposures to these chemicals in people and populations, Rebbeck says. "Epidemiological studies in people are limited, and these studies either offer mixed messages or say they have no effect on cancer risk," he adds. "But in any case, the effects are really small. I personally see no reason for people to change their behavior."

Cleaning products

Some household cleansers, dish soaps, and detergents contain chemicals known as endocrine disruptors. These are substances that interfere with human hormones and the reproductive or other biological processes they regulate.

The evidence: A 2022 study in the journal *Indoor Air* suggested that using household cleaning products can expose us to potentially hazardous VOCs. Some VOCs, such as benzene and formaldehyde, have been linked with cancer, according to the American Lung Association. And a study published in 2023 by the *Journal of Exposure Science and Environmental Epidemiology* suggested that exposure to certain endocrine-disrupting chemicals may contribute to cancers of the breast, ovaries, skin, and uterus.

Expert take: "Our ability to measure these relevant exposures is very limited," he says, "so the studies we do in humans cannot estimate risks accurately. We believe that if the effects were large enough, we'd have already seen them—like we did with cigarette smoking and lung cancer."

Personal care products

Some cosmetics, skin care, hair dyes, deodorants, hair relaxers, and other personal care products contain chemicals such as parabens, formaldehyde, coal tar dyes, and more.

The evidence: Research is scant that examines the long-term effects of most cosmetics on health, so there's little evidence to suggest using them increases cancer risk, according to the ACS.

But certain chemicals stand out. In October 2023, the FDA proposed a ban on formaldehyde in hair relaxers, products used to smooth or straighten hair. Repeated exposure has been linked to certain cancers, according to the National Cancer Institute. And a 2023 study of 33,000 women conducted by the National Institutes of Health suggested that those who used hair-straightening chemicals more than four times in the prior year

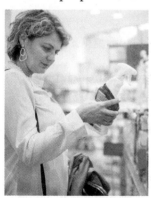
© credit | Getty Images
Cleaning products can be suspect.

were twice as likely to develop uterine cancer—the most common malignancy of the female reproductive system—compared to women who didn't use them.

Expert take: Most personal care products today contain lower amounts of potentially toxic chemicals

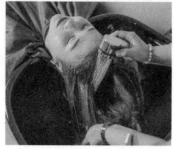
© credit | Getty Images
Cancer risks may climb for people who work with hair products that contain certain chemicals.

than in years past, Rebbeck says, "so your past exposure may still matter to your cancer risk, but those exposures have really changed."

For people who work around these chemicals, the risks may climb. Earlier studies suggested that hair stylists, for example—who work with hair dyes and related chemicals in large amounts—faced higher odds of cancer. "If you're exposed to gallons of hair dye a month, that's very different from the small amounts most women are exposed to," he says. "The amount and way you're exposed is very relevant. But even with occupational exposure, the risk is still quite low."

Cancer prevention basics

If you're worried about your exposure to any of these common substances, Rebbeck's advice is simple: find alternatives. A back-to-basics approach to cancer prevention is also paramount.

"There are so many things you can do to reduce your cancer risk that are really meaningful and measurable and large: stop smoking, don't drink alcohol, get exercise, and maintain a healthy weight," he says.

To stay updated on new evidence emerging on cancer risks associated with everyday products, Rebbeck also advises visiting reputable websites such as the Harvard T.H. Chan School of Public Health's Cancer FactFinder (https://cancerfactfinder.org), the ACS (www.cancer.org), and the National Cancer Institute (www.cancer.gov).

"There's a lot of misinformation out there," he says. "That's why it's so important to turn to the right sources of information—not social media or what your neighbor tells you. There's much you can do to lower your cancer risks and empower yourself to make better decisions." 🛡

Check out your skin

A routine full-body skin exam can catch early skin cancer and other potential problems.

You probably look at your face in the bathroom mirror a couple times each day. But do you ever take a close-up look at your entire skin? Devoting time to regular full-body check-ups can help you identify abnormalities that may signal skin cancer.

"Many skin spots and growths are related to normal aging and are not cause for concern," says Dr. Abigail H. Waldman, director of the Mohs and Dermatologic Surgery Center at Harvard-affiliated Brigham and Women's Hospital. "But you should note and monitor anything new or unusual."

Do a self-check

Dr. Waldman recommends doing a head-to-toe self-exam every three to six months. Use a full-length mirror, plus a handheld mirror for hard-to-see spots, and a magnifying glass to examine smaller areas. "If possible, have someone assist you so you don't miss anything," says Dr. Waldman. Here's how to do it.

- Look at your face, neck, ears (especially behind them), and scalp. Use a comb or a blow dryer to move your hair so that you can see better.
- Look at the front and back of your body in the mirror. Then, raise your arms and look at your left and right sides.
- Bend your elbows. Look carefully at your fingernails, palm and back of each hand, forearms (including the undersides), and upper arms.
- Check the back, front, and sides of your legs. Also, check the skin all over your buttocks and genital area.
- Sit and examine your feet, including the soles of your feet, the spaces between your toes, and your toenails.

Note any new or questionable moles, sores, painful or itchy spots, raised or firm bumps, dark flaky patches, and black or brown lines along fingernails and toenails. Make sure to feel any suspicious areas for firmness, too. "We often feel something troubling before we see it," says Dr. Waldman.

Write down the date of your self-exams and record what you find, including the exact locations.

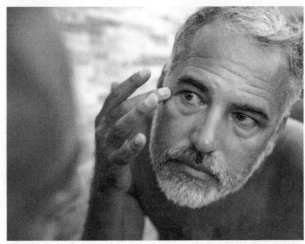

© CasarsaGuru | Getty Images

A close-up look at your skin may reveal spots and growths that need medical attention.

Take photos with your phone to share with your doctor or dermatologist. "After six to eight weeks, look at the trouble spots again, and get them checked out if they have not improved, or have changed color or size, have become painful, or easily bleed," says Dr. Waldman.

Looking for skin cancer

Melanoma is the most lethal type of skin cancer, and the earlier you can catch it, the better the outcome. The first sign of melanoma is usually a change in an existing mole. However, it also may appear as a new mole. Melanoma often appears on sun exposed areas, however, it also can occur in areas protected by the sun like nails. To recognize possible melanoma, follow the ABCDE guide:

Asymmetry: the shape of one half doesn't match the other half

Border: ragged or blurred edges

Color: red, brown, blue, black, or white, and the shades may be uneven

Diameter: about a quarter of an inch or larger, although some can be smaller

Evolution: any changes in size, shape, or color.

Here are some other skin issues to look out for during your self-exam:

Freckles. Monitor large, irregular ones. If they grow or change appearance, this can be a prelude to a specific form of melanoma called lentigo maligna melanoma. Problem freckles often appear on the face, upper shoulders, chest, and arms.

CANCER PREVENTION AND EARLY DETECTION

Basal cell carcinoma (BCC) and squamous cell carcinoma (SCC). "Both are types of skin cancer, but they are slow-growing, usually not life-threatening, and easy to treat if caught early," says Dr. Waldman. BCC may look like a bleeding pimple, an open sore, a red patch, a shiny pink growth, or a scar. SCC resembles a crusted, scaly red bump, patch, or wart. Both cancers appear in areas frequently exposed to the sun, such as the face, rim of the ear, lower lip, balding scalp, neck, hands, arms, shoulders, back, and legs.

Actinic keratoses (AKs). These growths are rough, gritty, and sometimes painful. They can be flat or slightly raised and appear in different colors, such as red, tan, pink, skin-colored, brown, or silver. AKs often appear on the face, tips of the ears, bald spots, and backs of the arms and hands. "While AKs are not initially dangerous, get them looked at, as they may lead to squamous cell carcinoma if left alone," says Dr. Waldman.

Cosmetic changes

Father Time brings us wrinkles, lines, bags under the eyes, age spots, raised rough lesions, and sagging skin. Many cosmetic treatments can treat these issues, such as botulinum toxin (Botox) injections, chemical peels, freezing liquid nitrogen sprays, laser treatments, prescription creams, and plastic surgery. Speak with your dermatologist about available options.

IN THE JOURNALS

Quick bursts of activity tied to reduced cancer risks in people who don't exercise

If you've been meaning to start an exercise regimen but you can't find the motivation to get going, consider this: a 2023 study published in *JAMA Oncology* found that just a few minutes of intense daily activity, like house cleaning or stair climbing, is linked to significantly lower cancer risks among people who don't exercise. Scientists evaluated the health data of more than 22,000 cancer-free "non-exercisers" (average age 62) who wore activity trackers for about a week and were then followed for about seven years. People who racked up three-and-a-half minutes of vigorous activity per day, accrued in one-minute bouts, had an 18% reduction in their risk of developing cancer during the study period, compared with people who didn't do any vigorous activity. Doing four-and-a-half minutes of vigorous activity per day

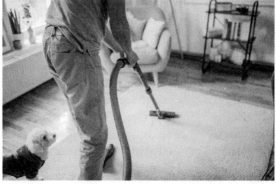
© South_agency | Getty Images
Even a few minutes of daily activity matters.

was associated with a 32% risk reduction. The findings are observational and don't prove definitively that short bursts of activity prevent cancer. But we already know that more substantial amounts of exercise are associated with lower risks of many types of cancer. So pour on the steam a few times a day—it may even inspire you to start exercising more regularly.

Screening advice that's not just skin deep

Despite perceptions, most people don't need an annual skin cancer exam. Here's who does.

After decades of public service campaigns, the message has clearly sunk in: melanoma kills. Awareness about the deadliest skin cancer—which claims 8,000 lives each year—has soared over the past two decades.

But now there's a new bulletin to absorb. Contrary to popular wisdom, the vast majority of people don't need to see a dermatologist each year to check for the malignancy. Skin checks every two to three years are sufficient for 80% of us, says Dr. Katherine Brag, a dermatologist at Harvard-affiliated Beth Israel Deaconess Medical Center.

Many dermatologists are flooded by calls from "worried well" patients who request annual skin exams they don't need, Dr. Brag says. They've paid attention to statistics indicating that melanoma is diagnosed in 200,000 Americans each year, with rates doubling between 1982 and 2011. An estimated one in 40 women will develop melanoma in her lifetime, according to the American Academy of Dermatology, while 1 in 27 men will develop it.

"Everyone is understandably afraid of melanoma. Even though it represents only a small fraction of diagnosed skin cancers, it accounts for more than 70% of deaths," Dr. Brag says. "It's hugely concerning—and deservedly so. But most people who get a skin check get a perfectly clean bill of health."

The case against hypervigilance

Much research reinforces Dr. Brag's approach. In 2023, the U.S. Preventive Services Task Force—which offers science-based recommendations about disease prevention—said there isn't enough evidence to support annual melanoma screenings for people with no symptoms who are at average risk for the disease. The benefits don't clearly outweigh the risks, which include unnecessary—and potentially disfiguring—biopsies, along with higher health care costs, the task force said.

Additionally, most cases of melanoma aren't found during skin cancer screenings. More than half are

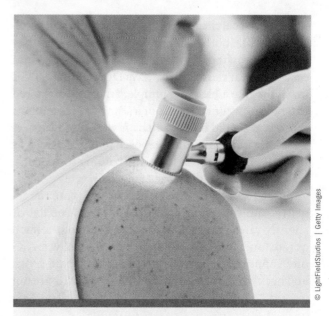

Watch for melanoma signs

Most melanoma lesions are found by the patient or a partner, not by a doctor. Staying vigilant is as easy as remembering the alphabet—look for the "ABCDE" features in body moles described on page 164 and see your dermatologist immediately if you notice any.

self-detected—usually because they're bleeding—and women spot these cancers more often than men, according to a 2016 study in the *Journal of the American Academy of Dermatology*.

Deaths from melanoma also don't drop when clinicians detect the malignancy during routine skin checks, according to a 2021 study in *JAMA Dermatology*. "Screenings don't necessarily improve outcomes from melanoma itself, and that's the point of a screening," Dr. Brag says.

Risk-increasing scenarios

So who *can* benefit from a yearly skin exam? The 20% of people who have any of the following risk factors:

Dozens of atypical moles. Most of us have between 10 and 40 common moles, which are small, round, and smooth. Atypical moles tend to be larger, with irregular or blurred borders. If you've got several dozen, a yearly skin check is warranted, since there's a slight chance they can develop into melanoma.

Family history of melanoma and atypical moles. If a first-degree relative—such as a parent, sibling, or child—has had melanoma or many atypical moles, your risk rises. "When someone tells me her grandfather had melanoma at 89, that's different from telling me her mother had it at 40," Dr. Brag says. "One is a function of age and many years of sun exposure, and the other may be more familial."

Previous skin cancer of any kind. Depending on how long ago you had a skin malignancy, this risk factor may warrant getting skin checks even more frequently, such as every three or six months. Ask your doctor.

Genetic mutations or predisposition. People with BRCA gene mutations, a family history of certain inherited cancers, or dysplastic nevus syndrome (an inherited skin condition marked by unusual moles and melanomas) all face higher melanoma odds.

Organ transplantation or inflammatory bowel disease. Both of these scenarios can involve taking immune-suppressing drugs that can increase patients' chances of developing skin cancer.

History of blistering sunburns. Three sunburns before age 15 substantially increase your melanoma risks.

Tanning bed use. Multiple tanning bed sessions—especially before age 20—dramatically increase melanoma risks.

ASK THE DOCTOR

by **TONI GOLEN, M.D.,** Editor in Chief, *Harvard Women's Health Watch*

What's the difference between age spots and sun spots?

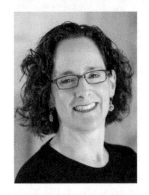

Q *I have a couple of brown skin patches that look like age spots. But my friend says they might be sun spots, which can develop into skin cancer. How can I tell the difference?*

A It's an important question, since distinguishing sun spots from age spots—or "liver" spots, as our grandmothers called them—can help us determine when to seek a doctor's evaluation. Both spots tend to appear on areas that get a lot of sun exposure, such as the face, hands, arms, and shoulders.

The color of age spots ranges from pink to tan to brown. They're bigger than freckles and usually oval-shaped. They're often found in clusters. Age spots can be unsightly, but they are harmless.

Sun spots, known medically as actinic keratoses, come in a

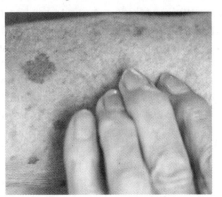

© Cristina Pedrazzini/Science Photo Library | Getty Images
Texture defines the difference between age spots and sun spots.

variety of colors. The biggest difference between harmless age spots and sun spots (actinic keratoses) is the texture. Age spots are smooth and flat, but potentially dangerous actinic keratoses usually feel rough and scaly. Actinic keratoses can develop into skin cancer, so it's vital that you show any such spots to your doctor. And if you're in doubt about any type of skin changes, it's also wise to point those out.

The best sun-protective clothing

Suit up in densely woven fabrics and a hat to stay safe from ultraviolet rays.

If you're spending time in the sun—no matter the season—in addition to using a strong sunscreen when you go outside, it's a good idea to wear sun-protective clothing. That's not just any hat or long-sleeved shirt in your closet; sun-protective clothes are made of materials that effectively shield your skin from harmful ultraviolet (UV) rays.

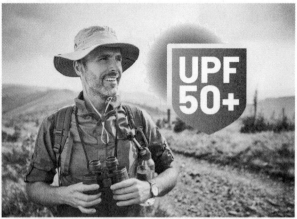

© Westend61, Calin Hanga | Getty Images

Look for sun-protective clothing with an ultra-violet protection factor rating of 50 or more.

Protective fabrics

Loosely woven fabrics of summer (such as gauze and linen) do very little to keep UV radiation from reaching your skin. The best defense comes from tightly woven fabrics with high thread counts, in dark or bright colors (which absorb light). Examples include polyester, nylon, lightweight wool, or canvas.

Many clothing manufacturers now use high-tech fabrics for sun-protective garments. High-tech fabrics offer at least as much protection as regular densely woven fabrics, and maybe more. Often these fabrics wick away moisture and dry quickly. Some are even embedded with chemicals used in sunscreens (such as zinc oxide and titanium dioxide). Note, however, that such chemical protection may last for only a limited amount of wash cycles, such as 20 to 40.

UPF protection

You'll know for sure if clothes are sun-protective if they have an Ultraviolet Protection Factor (UPF) rating on the label. That's a measure of how much UV radiation penetrates the fabric.

"Look for a UPF rating of 50, which should block about 98% of the sun's rays. It's comparable to sunscreen with a sun protection factor [SPF] of 30, so wearing the clothes is consistent with actually putting sunscreen on," says Dr. Abigail Waldman, director of the Mohs and Dermatologic Surgery Center at Harvard-affiliated Brigham and Women's Hospital.

Can you skip sunscreen if you're wearing UPF-rated clothes? "Yes, but only for areas covered by the clothes," Dr. Waldman says. "Any exposed skin still needs sunscreen, such as your neck, ears, hands, and feet."

And keep in mind that all clothes, UPF-rated or not, provide less UV protection when they get wet or if they're stretched and light can peek between the fibers. "So make sure clothing fits loosely. And it's not a bad idea to wear a waterproof sunscreen beneath sun-protective clothes if you know you'll be perspiring a lot or going into water," Dr. Waldman says.

Options and costs

If you're looking to buy UPF-rated clothing, you'll find a wide range of options to shield every inch of your skin, including hats, scarves, gloves, face masks, neck gaiters, shirts, hoodies, dresses, skirts, shorts, pants, leggings, shawls, swimwear, unitards, and more.

Which items do you really need? "The more skin you cover, the better, especially if you're doing yard work or going to the beach," Dr. Waldman says. "A hat, long-sleeved shirt, and pants are preferable. That can be a challenge on a really hot day, so make sure the fabric feels breathable and has moisture-wicking properties."

UPF-rated clothing can be pricey. A man's long-sleeved tee from some of the largest retailers (such as Coolibar Sun Protective Clothing, Columbia Sportswear Company, Lands' End, or L.L. Bean) goes for about $50. Brimmed hats for men and women also start at about $50.

To save some money, Dr. Waldman recommends using a laundry aid that adds sun-protective chemicals to densely woven clothes you already own (dry-fit nylon or polyester-blend tees are good candidates). The laundry aid is called Rit SunGuard, and it can give clothes a UPF of 30. "It's a powder. You just throw it in

    CANCER PREVENTION AND EARLY DETECTION

with normal washing, and it lasts for 20 washes. The clothes look the same," Dr. Waldman says.

A word about hats
You need a hat that protects more than just the crown of your head from UV rays, and that means you need a wide brim. "A lot of people fall short by using a baseball cap. But it doesn't cover the ears, the chin, or the back of the neck. So get as wide a brim as possible, at least three inches," Dr. Waldman says. "If you're not wearing a hat with a wide brim, apply sunscreen on exposed areas. And that goes for when you wear bike helmets, too. They have slits that allow for sunburns."

A hat's materials and construction are also important considerations. "You don't want a lot of mesh or large holes in the hat, because UV rays can reach your skin. The best material would be canvas, polyester, or nylon. They'll provide more protection than a straw hat," Dr. Waldman says.

Remember why you're doing this
Taking the time to wear protective clothes outside has a big payoff for your skin. "Even one sunburn can result in skin cancer in a few years," Dr. Waldman says. "If you can cover up and avoid burning now, you'll be better off later."

The bumpy truth

Most skin lumps and bumps aren't harmful, but here's what to watch.

Noticing a new lump or bump on your skin is never a happy discovery, especially if it's something unfamiliar—not your garden-variety wart, mole, or hives—and you're not sure whether to worry.

Even the term "lump" or "bump" can be confusing. Located on or just under the skin, these growths can be almost flat or "cause the skin to pooch out over them," says Dr. Rachel Reynolds, interim chair of dermatology at Harvard-affiliated Beth Israel Deaconess Medical Center. Beyond that, their characteristics run the gamut: soft and squishy or rock-hard, movable or fixed in place, round or irregularly shaped, or growing slowly or quickly.

Regardless, they seldom signal something serious. "People feel a lump and often immediately think it's cancer," Dr. Reynolds says. "But that's quite rare."

Most common types
Aside from highly common basal and squamous cell skin cancers—which can appear as shiny or wartlike domes—the vast majority of other skin bumps are either epidermal cysts or lipomas, Dr. Reynolds says. What are their qualities?

Epidermal cysts often appear on the face or back and "may feel like a marble under the skin," she says. They

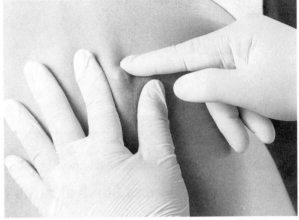

© jarabee123 | Getty Images

Doctors can typically diagnose most skin lesions on sight alone.

grow as benign "buds" off hair follicles, filling with a cheesy protein called keratin. (Pilar cysts are another version, but on the scalp.) As they grow, epidermal cysts can become inflamed or infected.

"Sometimes, even after being present for many years, they act like a boil, enlarging and becoming red and tender," Dr. Reynolds says. "If that happens, see a doctor, since some will require drainage or antibiotics."

Lipomas are benign fatty tumors that often appear on the trunk or shoulders. They usually grow slowly and can run in families. "You can't see most lipomas unless they get really big," she says. "But if you are able to feel them, they're really squishy, without any sharp edges."

▸▸

▶▶ A lipoma can become uncomfortable if it presses on surrounding nerves. In this case, your doctor can remove it surgically or with liposuction, or dissolve it by injecting it with a drug called deoxycholic acid (Kybella).

Diverse list

Other types of skin growths are defined by a variety of diverse features.

Cherry angiomas are smooth, red bumps representing an overgrowth of superficial blood vessels in the skin. They can range in size from a tiny dot to the diameter of a pencil eraser. Cherry angiomas tend to appear suddenly, especially on the torso, and are more common in people over 40.

Dermatofibromas are small, firm, brown or pink spots that contain scar tissue, sometimes appearing after a skin injury or insect bite. They might itch or pucker inward if you pinch them, but they aren't painful.

Keloids occur when scar tissue continues to grow beyond an injured area. These large bumps aren't harmful, although "they can become itchy and unsightly," she says.

Sarcomas are cancerous tumors that can appear deceptively similar to cysts or lipomas, but typically grow more quickly. "A sarcoma may feel firmer under the skin, but not like a marble, as an epidermal cyst does," Dr. Reynolds says. "It's a little more ill-defined, and sometimes it's painful." If the lump hurts even when it's left alone, that's a particularly concerning sign.

When to act

While sarcomas are one of the few types of skin lumps that are dangerous, Dr. Reynolds urges caution about any lump appearing near lymph nodes—immune system nodules located in the armpits, groin, and neck. While lymph nodes can enlarge from a cold or other

IN THE JOURNALS

Early breast cancer survival rates increasing

Encouraging news about breast cancer survival: most women treated for early breast cancer are likely to become long-term survivors, according to a 2023 study published in *The BMJ*. Researchers analyzed the health data of more than 512,000 British women who had been diagnosed with early breast cancer (confined to one breast and possibly the lymph nodes under an arm) between 1993 and 2015. The women in the study (most were age 50 or older) were treated initially with surgery and then followed for up to 20 years. Scientists determined that the five-year risk of death from breast cancer fell from about 14% for women diagnosed in the 1990s to about 5% for women diagnosed later in the study. For example, among women diagnosed between 2010 to 2015, more than six in 10 had a five-year death risk of 3% or less. The study was observational and merely suggests (but doesn't prove) that death risk has decreased in general. It also doesn't explain why the death risk dropped among women in the study. The scientists speculated that better treatments, improved imaging, and increased breast cancer awareness and screenings have contributed to better outcomes.

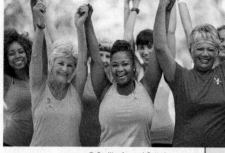

© Cecilie_Arcurs I Getty Images

Improvements in treatment have led to significant drops in mortality.

CANCER PREVENTION AND EARLY DETECTION

infection, swollen nodes sometimes signal cancer. Other symptoms might also be present, including weight loss, fever, and chills.

"Get checked," she says. "Some lymph nodes become temporarily inflamed, enlarge, and then go back down, but it's something that should be monitored."

A dermatologist can usually diagnose a skin bump or lump on sight alone. Occasionally, imaging tests or a biopsy may be needed to determine the culprit. You can be proactive by doing the following:

Pointing it out. At your next primary care appointment, ask your doctor to take a look. "Seek a more urgent visit if something is growing quickly, bleeding, feels painful, looks infected, or is red or tender," Dr. Reynolds says.

Speaking up. Your doctor might not focus on a benign bump unless you mention that it's painful, irritating, or cosmetically unappealing. 🛡

Not your grandmother's breast cancer treatment

Recent advances have transformed a one-size-fits-all approach into a personalized treatment arsenal.

Some things never change: a breast cancer diagnosis still evokes a storm of anxiety—just as it did decades ago—despite the fact that survival rates have soared. Indeed, while more than two million women worldwide receive a breast cancer diagnosis each year, the average risk of dying in the following five years has dropped from 14% to 5% since just the 1990s, according to a 2023 study involving more than a half-million women.

"For many women, a breast cancer diagnosis is particularly unsettling because we often don't know why a patient developed it," says Dr. Harold Burstein, a medical oncologist at Harvard-affiliated Dana-Farber Cancer Institute. "But the good news is, outcomes are getting better and better."

There's good reason for this survival swing. While breast cancer was once believed to be a single disease requiring a single treatment approach, scientists can now categorize breast tumors by cell type, opening the door for treatment combinations tailored toward each. (See "Types of breast cancer," page 172.)

Nowadays, surgery is still *de rigueur* for most types of breast cancer. But once-mainstay chemotherapy may be used in smaller amounts or skipped entirely. Meanwhile, newer drugs have enabled doctors to personalize each woman's arsenal of options. These include immunotherapy—which harnesses the power of the immune system to kill cancer cells—and targeted

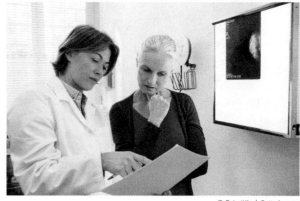

© Bsip/Uig | Getty Images

Doctors can now tailor each woman's breast cancer treatment to its specific cell type and stage.

therapies aimed at gene mutations or proteins active in cancer growth.

"As we recognize these important subsets of breast cancer, we're tailoring treatment to the individual and the special characteristics of each breast cancer," Dr. Burstein says. "There isn't an infinite number of treatments, but the toolbox keeps getting bigger."

Why treatments are improving

Even the past 10 years brought marked shifts in treatment approach, thanks to extensive research that clarifies how genes and cells behave in various cancer subtypes. This, in turn, fueled the development of ▸▸

groundbreaking tests. Some can identify women with BRCA gene mutations that drastically raise their risk of developing breast cancer, while other tests help predict the likelihood a tumor will grow or spread to better pinpoint treatment needs.

These efforts have revealed that some types of breast cancer may respond to less intensive chemotherapy, while one especially aggressive type needs more.

ER-positive, HER2-negative breast cancer, which accounts for up to three-quarters of all cases, has undergone a treatment overhaul, Dr. Burstein says. "By the year 2000, we were giving chemo to almost every woman with this type of cancer. We understood it was overkill, that most women received very little benefit, but we didn't have a robust tool to distinguish who did and didn't need chemo," he says. "Now we have powerful genomic tools that allow us to say a patient might not need chemo as part of her treatment plan."

Additionally, a class of medications called CDK4/6 inhibitors—which target proteins that can fuel growth of ER-positive breast cancers—is often added to a patient's blend of treatments if her cancer is considered at high risk for spread (metastasis).

HER2-positive breast cancer, a more aggressive subtype that constitutes about one in five cases, has become more curable thanks to targeted therapies that disrupt the HER2 proteins that fuel its growth. The monoclonal antibody trastuzumab (Herceptin) revolutionized treatment over the past two decades, making chemotherapy less necessary, though doctors may combine the two to maximize effectiveness.

In the wake of this development, a newer approach known as an antibody drug conjugate pairs chemotherapy with manufactured proteins to deliver potent results with fewer side effects. "It acts like a smart bomb, delivering chemo directly to tumor cells," Dr. Burstein says. "This has emerged as a very powerful tool for the treatment of metastatic breast cancer. Hopefully, we'll see this approach used soon in early-stage breast cancer because it looks more effective than any chemotherapy option."

Triple-negative breast cancer is a rapidly growing type that remains a holdout in attempts to reduce chemotherapy. "We're actually using more and more treatment because we've found more drugs that are effective," Dr. Burstein says. "We've amped up chemo, started adding immunotherapy, and have some specific therapies for women with hereditary breast cancers as well."

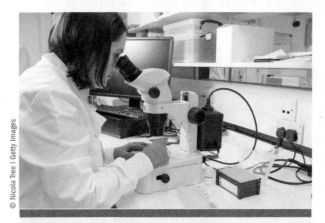

© Nicola Tree | Getty Images

Types of breast cancer

Breast cancer types are typically named for the kinds of hormone receptors present in tumor cells. Knowing the type enables doctors to choose the most appropriate treatments.

ER-positive. The cancer cells contain hormone receptors for estrogen.

HER2-positive. The cancer cells have high numbers of receptors for HER2, a protein that fuels cancer growth.

ER-negative, HER2-negative. Cancer cells don't contain receptors for estrogen or HER2, respectively.

Triple negative. Cells don't have receptors for estrogen, progesterone, or HER2.

Reasons for optimism

In coming years, nascent technologies not yet in widespread use are likely to hit the mainstream, Dr. Burstein says. These include so-called liquid biopsies: blood tests that look for the presence or absence of DNA from tumor cells in the bloodstream. "The test results will help us decide who needs more or less treatment based on circulating cell tumor DNA," he says.

Many women with metastatic breast cancer, which isn't yet curable, now thrive for many years as a parade of new treatments extend their lives while bolstering energy levels and the ability to live more normally.

"Patients are living longer and doing better with metastatic breast cancer," Dr. Burstein says. "It's fair to

CANCER PREVENTION AND EARLY DETECTION

say that most women will live for many years after that diagnosis, and many are likely to be treated with drugs that don't exist today because progress is happening so quickly."

Tips for better care

Women who've been diagnosed with breast cancer can help maximize treatment results with these strategies.

Seek a multidisciplinary care team. Blending clinicians in medical oncology, radiology, surgery, genetics, and other specialties, this care model promotes collaboration that can lead to better outcomes for women with early-stage breast cancer. Patient navigation and social work services can also be valuable parts of a multidisciplinary team. "Go to a center where everyone is familiar with each other," Dr. Burstein says. "Women with early-stage disease almost always need surgery, medications, and radiation, so it's important the team works together effectively."

Speak up. Don't take a passive role in your treatment. While your care team may possess great expertise, clinicians may not understand your personal priorities or concerns. "Make sure your questions are being answered by the team, so you understand where things are and where they're going," he says. 🛡

Without a telltale lump, inflammatory breast cancer can be deceiving—and deadly

If your breast seems red or swollen, feels unusually warm, or the skin has thickened or dimpled, don't pass it off as a bug bite or heat rash. Even without a discernible lump, breast cancer could be the culprit.

A form of the disease called inflammatory breast cancer (IBC), which is responsible for just 1% to 5% of all cases of breast cancer, shows up very differently from most breast cancers. Because it's so rare and initial signs are easy to miss, many women aren't on the lookout for IBC—but they should be, says Dr. Filipa Lynce, director of the Inflammatory Breast Center at Harvard-affiliated Dana-Farber Cancer Institute.

IBC is especially dangerous because symptoms often develop rapidly, over a few weeks or months. By then, the disease is already at an advanced stage because cancer cells have grown into the skin.

"Someone wakes up and notices her breasts feel heavier. A couple of weeks later, she may notice redness," Dr. Lynce says. "Then the skin around her nipples looks like the skin of an orange. It's all relatively quick."

Many women with such symptoms are treated with antibiotics, since their symptoms can resemble a breast infection. A doctor may also attribute symptoms to an allergic reaction or other minor problem. "A diagnosis that's missed or delayed is one of the challenges associated with this disease," Dr. Lynce says.

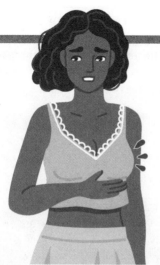

© Anastasia Boyko | Getty Images
Unusual symptoms characterize IBC.

Don't wait to see a doctor, especially if these signs don't quickly resolve. Diagnosing IBC involves breast imaging such as a mammogram, which is often followed by an ultrasound of the breast and nearby lymph nodes, a breast MRI, or both. A biopsy is required to confirm the diagnosis.

"Any woman who develops inflammatory changes in the breast, even without a lump, should understand it can be cancer," she says. "If your symptoms don't resolve right away with a short course of antibiotics, don't sit on it. Further workup is needed."

Silent suffering

Conquering cancer can be a double-edged sword when survivor's guilt creeps in. Here's how to move forward.

After your cancer diagnosis, you put your chin down and plowed through the task at hand—beating it. But you didn't necessarily expect to be smacked with another huge challenge soon after: survivor's guilt.

This psychological phenomenon, which includes strong, persistent feelings of sadness and remorse, is an unwelcome intrusion at the end of cancer treatment—a time that should, by all accounts, be joyful. And it doesn't just include guilt itself, but also an overwhelming sense of distress, helplessness, and injustice. But the tension between trauma and relief is exactly what poses difficulty to scores of survivors who'd hoped to be free of cancer's consequences, Harvard experts say.

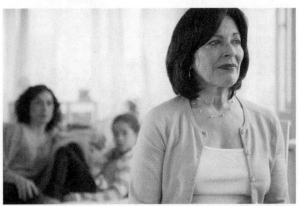
© JGI/Jamie Grill | Getty Images

Far more people are surviving cancer now than in decades past, making survivor's guilt more prevalent.

"Survivor's guilt is a lot more common than we think," says Cristina Pozo-Kaderman, a clinical psychologist in the Department of Psychosocial Oncology and Palliative Care at Harvard-affiliated Dana-Farber Cancer Institute. "Patients who express it are often met with others who minimize their feelings and tell them to just feel happy that they're okay."

"But admitting survivor's guilt doesn't mean you don't feel grateful," she adds. "Those emotions coexist."

Rising ranks

Recent innovations in cancer treatment have led to unprecedented numbers of survivors. Thanks to a 32% drop in the cancer death rate between 1991 and 2019, more than 18 million people in the United States now count themselves as cancer survivors, according to a 2022 report by the American Association for Cancer Research. Their ranks increased by more than one million over the past three years alone and are expected to rise to 22.5 million by 2032, according to the National Cancer Institute (NCI).

Cancer survivors comprise everyone who's living after a cancer diagnosis, including those still getting treatment. (See "Worried about cancer coming back?" on page 175.) Nearly 70% of survivors have lived five or more years since their diagnosis, and 47% have lived 10 or more years, according to the NCI. About 67% of survivors are 65 and older.

But this advance presents a double-edged sword. More survivors means more battle-scarred folks who've bonded with others facing cancer—and feel bereft when some of their compatriots die and they live.

Survivor's guilt isn't exclusive to cancer, of course. It can also strike people who've lived through other types of traumatic experiences that claimed others, including natural disasters, mass shootings, or military conflict.

Pozo-Kaderman points out that survivors may also face guilt that they
- can go on to have children when others can't
- had access to good medical care when others didn't
- burdened their family and friends during the rigors of treatment
- tested positive for a cancer-causing genetic mutation that may jeopardize family members.

"It's not just feeling bad you survived, it's many thoughts and feelings that go along with it," Pozo-Kaderman says.

Who's more at risk?

Predicting who will be affected by survivor's guilt is challenging, since many factors may contribute, Harvard experts say. But you could be more prone because of unusual circumstances: perhaps your family has been shaken by the deaths of multiple members from hereditary forms of cancer. Or maybe you beat a type of cancer with historically low survival rates.

According to a 2019 study in the *Journal of Psychosocial Oncology* that polled 108 lung cancer survivors, 55% reported feeling guilty. (The five-year survival rate for lung cancer is less than 19%, according to the American Lung Association.) "Guilt scores" among participants with the highest levels of guilt revealed five recurring themes, including frequently wondering, "Why not me?"

"I've witnessed wonderful friendships develop through cancer treatment, and when patients have friends with a similar diagnosis who don't survive, they're likely at higher risk of survivor's guilt," says Dr. Katharine Esselen, a gynecologic oncologist at Harvard-affiliated Beth Israel Deaconess Medical Center.

Feeling pressure to do something that confers "meaning" to an otherwise terrible experience can also pile on to survivor's guilt. But Pozo-Kaderman says it's perfectly okay if you're not inclined. "If you want to, that's great, but it doesn't mean you have to," she says. "You survived, and that's enough. You don't now have to do something to validate that you survived. It's a really heavy burden."

Ways to move forward

It's important not to let survivor's guilt fester. Downstream effects can include mood problems, trouble concentrating or sleeping, anger and irritability, loss of motivation, and a sense of detachment. Harvard experts offer these coping strategies: ▶▶

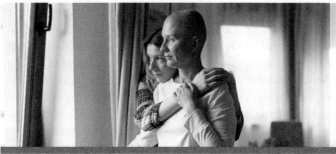

It's normal to worry that cancer will recur, but you can take charge of how you respond to your fears.

© NoSystem images | Getty Images

Worried about cancer coming back?

It's a feeling like no other: after months or even years of grueling therapy such as surgery, chemotherapy, radiation, or immunotherapy, you've been told there's no evidence of cancer left in your body. But will it come back?

The fear of recurrence is front and center for most cancer survivors, says Dr. Katharine Esselen, a gynecologic oncologist at Beth Israel Deaconess Medical Center. Not only can it steal your joy, but about 7% of cancer patients develop severe, disabling fear marked by dark thoughts and distorted worries.

"Fear of recurrence is perhaps the biggest emotional hurdle a cancer patient deals with after treatment ends," Dr. Esselen says. "Once you've been diagnosed with a disease that's completely out of your control, you realize that that anything is possible—and it can happen again."

Worrying your cancer will return is normal, especially during the first year after treatment. Certain events can trigger fears, such as scheduling follow-up medical visits and scans (also known as "scanxiety"); feeling symptoms similar to those you had when you were first diagnosed; and learning that someone you know with cancer has died.

"This is very normal and expected," says Cristina Pozo-Kaderman, a clinical psychologist at Dana-Farber Cancer Institute. "But if that fear of recurrence becomes immobilizing—not just a couple of days before follow-ups or scans, but weeks before—then you should get help."

Harvard experts also offer these tips:

Be open about your worries. Expressing strong feelings can release their power over you. "It's important not to bury your fears," Dr. Esselen says.

Control what you can. Ask your doctor what you can do to reduce the chances your cancer will return, and keep up with follow-up appointments. "Taking care of yourself, in many cases, reduces your risk of recurrence and developing other health conditions," Dr. Esselen says. "Doctors do the necessary tests and look out for you so that if it does come back, there are other options for treatment."

Stay active. Get back to doing things you enjoyed before cancer, whether that's working, pursuing hobbies, or spending time with family and friends. "You've worked hard to get to this point, so make choices that make you feel happy and fulfilled," Dr. Esselen says. "Surrounding yourself with people and things you love doing reminds you how to adjust to a new normal."

▶▶ Realize your feelings are normal. "It's important to not beat yourself up about them, to accept that this is the normal course of what you're going through," Dr. Esselen says.

Take time to grieve. Time may not heal all wounds, as the adage goes, but it can help you accept you couldn't have done anything to alter other cancer patients' outcomes.

Find ways to work through grief. Some people plant a tree for a friend who died or participate in charity events. Others channel their feelings through art, music, or photography. "There's no one strategy that works for everyone," Pozo-Kaderman says.

Seek support. In-person or online support groups can help you connect with others who know only too well the path you're on. Some groups are geared toward survivors of certain ages or diagnoses. "Programs with other survivors can often help you acknowledge feelings of guilt, just by having a name for the feeling," Pozo-Kaderman says. "It's very validating, and often you'll problem-solve together to tackle the issues you're dealing with."

Get help. Pervasive sadness, anxiety, or depression signals a need for counseling, Dr. Esselen says. A therapist can also help you explore any underlying contributors to your feelings of guilt. ▌

IN THE JOURNALS

National task force updates breast cancer screening recommendations

Women at average risk for breast cancer should get screened every other year starting at age 40, according to new guidelines from an independent national panel of experts.

The U.S. Preventive Services Task Force (USPSTF) has updated the group's earlier advice, lowering the starting age to 40 from 50. The new USPSTF recommendations also largely align with 2022 guidelines by the National Comprehensive Cancer Network, an alliance of leading cancer centers, which recommends annual mammograms for women at average risk of breast cancer.

The update resulted from new scientific evidence that indicate biennial mammograms starting at 40 may prevent at least one additional breast cancer death for every 1,000 women. Each year, about 264,000 American women are diagnosed with breast cancer and 42,000 die from the disease, according to the CDC.

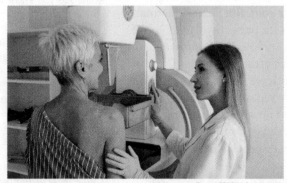

© peakSTOCK I Getty Images

Most women are now advised to start screening at 40.

Some women need earlier or more frequent screening, the task force said. These include women who had breast cancer before age 40; abnormal findings on a breast biopsy; chest radiation at a young age; or a test showing a genetic marker for breast cancer, such as a BRCA gene mutation.

CANCER PREVENTION AND EARLY DETECTION

by **HOWARD LeWINE, M.D.,** Editor in Chief, *Harvard Men's Health Watch*

What lifestyle changes can help me avoid prostate cancer?

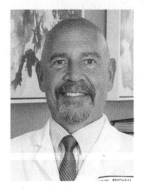

Q *I don't have a family history of prostate cancer, but I still want to lower my risk. Are there daily lifestyle changes I should adopt to help?*

A If men live long enough, most will develop cancer cells in their prostate gland. About 80% of men ages 80 and older live with some prostate cancer.

However, only a small percentage will develop an aggressive form of cancer that affects their quality of life and longevity. Therefore, the more important questions are what lifestyle changes might delay the onset of prostate cancer and decrease the risk of developing advanced prostate cancer. Here are three areas that observational studies have found may help.

Diet. Research has shown that the same types of diets associated with better heart and brain health are linked to a reduced risk of aggressive prostate cancer. In a 2022 study published in *The American Journal of Clinical Nutrition*, researchers who followed 47,239 men over 28 years found that men who reported eating primarily a plant-based diet, like the Mediterranean or DASH diets, had a significantly lower risk of developing aggressive prostate cancer. Other studies have shown following these healthier diets also may lower the odds of dying from prostate cancer. While this benefit might be related to the high amounts of omega-3 fatty acids in fish (a staple of the Mediterranean and DASH diets), taking a fish oil supplement has not been shown to reduce prostate cancer risk.

What you don't eat also matters. Maintaining a healthy weight and avoiding obesity is linked to a lower chance of developing advanced prostate cancer. Also, limiting meat and added sugars may be good for prostate health.

Exercise. Some evidence suggests that regular exercise can lower a man's likelihood of getting prostate cancer. In 2019, Harvard researchers published findings that showed men who engaged most frequently in vigorous activity had a 30% lower risk of developing advanced prostate cancer and a 25% lower risk of dying from prostate cancer compared with men who exercised the least.

Ejaculation frequency. Men who ejaculate frequently appear to have a lower risk of prostate cancer. According to one long-running large study, men who ejaculated more than 21 times per month had a 20% lower prostate cancer risk than those who ejaculated four to seven times monthly. It's not clear why frequent ejaculation is protective. Some experts believe the release of semen flushes harmful substances from the prostate. However, this study did not address the risk of advanced prostate cancer.

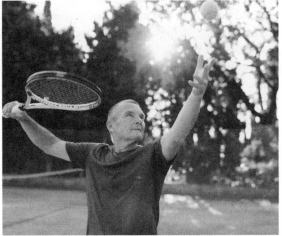
Oleg Breslavtsev | Getty Images

Regular vigorous exercise is linked with a lower risk for prostate cancer.

Can weight loss slow prostate cancer?

For men following active surveillance, maintaining a healthy weight may improve their prognosis.

You've had a biopsy and have been diagnosed with low-grade prostate cancer, defined as a tumor that is confined to the prostate gland and unlikely to grow or spread. You decide to follow active surveillance, a protocol in which you regularly follow up with your doctor for routine PSA tests, prostate biopsies, and possibly MRI scans. If at some point it looks like the cancer has progressed, then you can consider treatment (radiation or surgery).

For some men, this wait-and-see period lasts for years. But can you do anything to help slow your cancer's growth and delay treatment for as long as possible? Your bathroom scale might give you the answer.

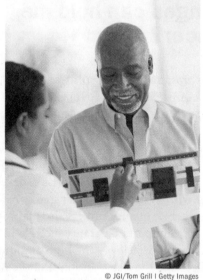
© JGI/Tom Grill | Getty Images

Maintain a healthy weight to help prevent aggressive prostate cancer.

How monitoring works

The reality is that most low-grade prostate cancer does not transform over time and become more aggressive, according to Dr. Mark Pomerantz, a medical oncologist with Harvard-affiliated Dana-Farber Cancer Institute.

"Being on active surveillance is more about looking out for cancer that the original biopsy missed," he says. "It's not necessarily that the original low-grade cancer becomes more aggressive—although that is possible in some cases—but rather, high- or medium-grade cancer is hiding, and we're looking for changes in PSA levels that might suggest it's there and become aggressive."

About 45% to 60% of men on active surveillance will not need cancer treatment over the 10 to 15 years following their initial diagnosis, according to Dr. Pomerantz. While those are encouraging figures, they still leave the chance you may need treatment sooner.

Controlling factors

You can't control two factors that can increase the risk of undetected high- or medium-grade cancer from becoming aggressive: genetics and family history. But one aspect you may be able to change is your weight.

"While excess weight doesn't appear to increase the likelihood of low-grade prostate cancer, there appears to be a strong association between being overweight or obese and the risk of developing aggressive prostate cancer," says Dr. Pomerantz. People with a body mass index (BMI) of 25 to 29.9 are considered overweight, while those with a BMI of 30 or higher are classified as obese.

Scientists reported in 2019 in the journal *Cancer* that, over a 10-year period, men diagnosed with prostate cancer whose waist size and BMI increased the most had greater risks of advanced and fatal prostate cancer compared with men who maintained a healthy weight.

Specifically, a five-point increase in BMI was associated with a 50% higher risk for advanced or fatal prostate cancer, and a 4.1-inch increase in waist size was associated with a 40% higher risk. Where that extra fat lies also is a driving factor. The same study discovered that extra visceral fat (the hidden kind that lies deep in the abdomen and surrounds the major organs) was linked with a 31% higher risk of developing advanced prostate cancer.

Your past weight gain also may play a role in future cancer growth, suggests research presented at the European Congress on Obesity in 2023. Researchers found that men who gained an average of 2.2 pounds each year from ages 17 to 29 increased their risk of developing aggressive prostate cancer later in life by 13%.

"So losing excess weight may be one way to possibly keep prostate cancer from growing more rapidly," says Dr. Pomerantz.

The weight connection

Experts don't fully understand the relationship between excess fat and prostate cancer growth. Some theories suggest that extra weight leads to higher levels

CANCER PREVENTION AND EARLY DETECTION

of inflammation, which in turn acts like fuel to prostate cancer cells. Overweight and obese men also are more likely to have higher levels of blood sugar, which stimulates the pancreas to release more insulin. Some studies have shown a link between higher insulin levels and an increased risk of prostate cancer. "This could be another factor raising the chance of more aggressive cancer," says Dr. Pomerantz.

While weight loss and weight management are never easy, Dr. Pomerantz says many men on active surveillance often embrace the situation as an opportunity to make overall health changes.

"Increasing exercise and adopting a healthy, plant-based diet, both of which can help men lose extra pounds, not only can help with their prostate cancer, but can reduce their risk of heart disease and other cancers," he says. "Most men on active surveillance will die of something other than prostate cancer, so this can be a wake-up call for men to get serious about their health." 🛡

Diet and prostate cancer

Can following a plant-based diet offer extra protection?

A plant-based diet can help people lower their risk for heart disease and diabetes. But what about prostate cancer? Can this medically touted eating pattern protect you from the most common cancer among men?

"Unfortunately, there is no miracle prostate cancer diet," says Dr. Bradley McGregor, an oncologist with Harvard-affiliated Dana-Farber Cancer Institute. "But as we learn more about the role diet plays in disease prevention, there is growing evidence that plant-based diets may lower your risk of prostate cancer and even help slow its spread."

What the science says

With some minor variations, the most studied plant-based diets—Mediterranean, MIND, and DASH—are similar. They emphasize eating plenty of fruits and vegetables (especially cruciferous vegetables), beans and legumes, whole grains, fatty fish, nuts and seeds, and olive oil while reducing the intake of red meat and processed foods. Plant-based diets also can include similar eating patterns, like vegetarian, vegan, and pescatarian (which adds seafood to an otherwise vegetarian diet). So what does current science say about plant-based diets and prostate cancer? Let's begin with the overall risk.

Much research supports the conclusion that following a plant-based diet is linked with a lower risk of

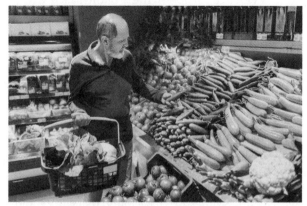

© Oleg Breslavtsev | Getty Images

The staples of a plant-based diet include healthy amounts of vegetables and fruits.

cancer in general. Studies that have looked at only prostate cancer have been promising, too. For instance, a 2022 study published in *BMC Medicine* that involved more than 409,000 people found that, compared with meat eaters, vegetarians and pescatarians had a 43% lower risk of prostate cancer over 10 years.

If you have prostate cancer, can a plant-based diet help slow its growth? In a 2021 study published in the journal *Cancer*, 410 men on active surveillance for localized prostate cancer recorded their daily diets for three years. In those who ate more fruits, vegetables, legumes, grains, and fish, the cancer was less likely to grow to the point of needing treatment.

Another analysis of this connection—part of the ongoing CaPSURE Diet and Lifestyle Study—was presented in 2023. Approximately 2,000 men (average age 72) with early- to mid-grade prostate cancer periodically completed questionnaires about how much and ▸▸

how often they consumed 140 different foods. After about 7.5 years, those who reported diets with the highest amount of plant foods had a 52% lower risk of prostate cancer progression and a 53% lower risk of recurrence than those who ate the lowest amount of plant foods.

However, other research has not been as supportive. For instance, a 2020 study in *JAMA* found that increasing vegetable intake did not lower the risk of prostate cancer progression in men on active surveillance.

Foods that fight cancer

These contradictions arise because most diet-related research only shows an association rather than cause and effect, says Dr. McGregor. "While the observational evidence for following a plant-based diet is strong, we can't be sure if certain foods or combinations are better than others, or even what specific amounts are ideal for managing prostate cancer."

Still, when researchers have looked at individual foods common in plant-based diets and their effect on prostate cancer, the results have been promising.

For instance, large studies have found that men with moderate to high fish intake are less likely to develop prostate cancer or die from it than men who do not eat fish. The fish's high levels of omega-3 fatty acids, known to fight inflammation, are often cited as protective benefits. Studies also have found that carotenoids

Planting the seeds for a better diet

Many men find following a plant-based too strict. One way to overcome this barrier is to begin making small changes in your diet and build from there. For instance, focus only on replacing red meat with fish, add more vegetables to meals, and choose fruits and nuts for snacks instead of processed foods. To learn more about how to adopt a plant-based diet, visit www.health.harvard.edu/meddiet.

(compounds that occur naturally in certain plants) have antioxidant properties that may protect the body against unstable molecules that damage DNA and cause cancer cells to form.

What you don't eat

Another part of diet and prostate cancer is what you don't eat. "Following a plant-based diet means you eat fewer processed foods, red meat, and foods high in cholesterol and saturated fat, all of which are linked to a higher risk of aggressive prostate cancers," says Dr. McGregor. "You also probably consume fewer calories over all, which can help manage excess weight, another risk factor linked with prostate cancer." ◗

IN THE JOURNALS

Cardiorespiratory fitness may protect men from some cancers

Better cardiorespiratory fitness (also known as cardio fitness or aerobic fitness) may help men lower their risk of death from cancer of the colon, lung, or prostate, suggests a study published in 2023 by *JAMA Network Open*. Researchers collected health data on more than 170,000 men that included measurements of their VO_2 max while they pedaled a stationary bike. VO_2 max is the maximum amount of oxygen the body can use during exercise. The higher the VO_2 max, the greater a person's cardio fitness.

After a mean follow-up time of 9.6 years, the men with greater cardio fitness were less likely to die from these cancers. These findings highlight that improving cardio fitness through moderate- to high-intensity aerobic exercises is not only important for heart health, but could lead to a better prognosis in men with these common cancers.

Rethinking PSA testing

Doctors are exploring better ways to use this test for detecting and managing prostate cancer.

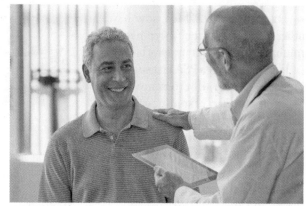
© Jose Luis Pelaez Inc/Blend Images LLC I Getty Images
Men should discuss the pros and cons of regular PSA testing with their doctor.

Prostate-specific antigen (PSA) testing has a complex role in prostate cancer diagnosis. On the one hand, it can help identify early prostate cancer. On the other, routine PSA screening can lead men to have biopsies or invasive treatments they may not need.

This has caused the medical community to re-evaluate how best to use the PSA test.

"While men in their 40s should begin a dialogue with their doctor about the pros and cons of PSA screening through middle age, work is ongoing to achieve the ultimate goal: developing a screening regimen that identifies only the prostate cancers that need to be cured," says Dr. Mark Pomerantz, an oncologist with Harvard-affiliated Dana-Farber Cancer Institute. "And there is a way for PSA testing to help achieve this."

The ABCs of PSA

PSA is a chemical made by the prostate. A PSA test measures the amount in a man's blood. A PSA level of less than 4 nanograms per milliliter (ng/mL) is considered normal.

"Though there is no level below 4 that guarantees freedom from prostate cancer, a level higher than 4 is the conventional threshold for considering a biopsy to look for cancer," says Dr. Pomerantz.

The PSA test initially was developed for use in men already diagnosed with prostate cancer and undergoing treatment, and it's highly reliable in this regard. PSA levels can reveal whether cancer has returned after surgery or whether the tumors have grown or shrunk after treatment with hormones or radiation.

But decades ago, research showed that in men not known to have prostate cancer, PSA levels higher than 10 ng/mL often indicated the presence of the disease. Soon after, it became the go-to prostate cancer screening test. However, PSA screening is far from perfect, especially when a man's level is between 4 ng/mL and 10 ng/mL.

These somewhat higher PSA levels frequently happen for reasons other than cancer, such as a benign enlarged prostate, an inflamed prostate (prostatitis), bike riding, or recent ejaculation. A man with this screening result often ends up proceeding with a biopsy—an invasive procedure with its own potential complications—just in case cancer is present.

And even when a biopsy confirms that cancer is the source of a rising PSA level, many men end up undergoing treatment for low-risk, slow-growing cancer that might never affect their longevity or quality of life.

"Treatments like surgery and radiation, beyond the stress and invasiveness associated with the procedures, also involve possible side effects like incontinence and erectile dysfunction," says Dr. Pomerantz.

In addition, research has produced mixed results on whether regular PSA screening helps men in the long run. "Even after 30-plus years of using the PSA test for screening, it still isn't clear how well it prevents prostate cancer deaths," says Dr. Pomerantz. "And the reality is that, even among men with prostate cancer, most will die from something else."

The main problem with using PSA tests to find prostate cancer? Most older men already have some traces of the cancer.

"You could take 100 random middle age or older men off the street, examine their prostates, and more than half would probably have some low-risk cancer, even though they may be healthy and unaffected by it for life," says Dr. Pomerantz. "If you go snooping around for prostate cancer, you will find it."

Better ways to use testing

So the question has become this: what role does PSA testing now play in prostate cancer screening?

"The result of a PSA test no longer needs to be the final word in who does or doesn't get a biopsy," says ▶▶

Dr. Pomerantz. "Men now have other ways to check for cancer that can minimize the need for invasive biopsy."

For example, if a PSA test suggests possible cancer, doctors now can order magnetic resonance imaging (MRI) of the prostate. The technology produces a high-resolution image of the entire prostate gland. Cancerous tissue has different magnetic properties than normal tissue, and an MRI scan can capture these differences.

If MRI reveals no cancer, your doctor may recommend you continue to monitor your prostate with PSA testing. If the scan does show the possibility of cancer, the detailed image can help the doctor determine the tumor's size and which part of the prostate should be sampled with a biopsy.

"This targeted approach can help with a more accurate diagnosis and avoid the need for repeated biopsies," says Dr. Pomerantz. "It brings us closer to our goal in prostate cancer screening—reliably finding the

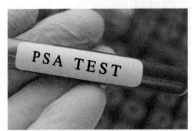

© Wladimir Bulgar/Science Photo Library | Getty Images
PSA blood testing has uses beyond cancer screening.

aggressive prostate cancers and avoiding overdiagnosis."

Another role for PSA testing

Periodic PSA testing is regularly used during active surveillance, a wait-and-see approach to prostate cancer management in which men monitor their cancer for changes and explore treatment options only if it becomes more active.

"The monitoring approach of active surveillance is ideal for many men diagnosed with low-risk cancer," says Dr. Pomerantz.

After an initial biopsy, active surveillance involves more frequent PSA testing to look for any changes. If your PSA level increases, your doctor may order an MRI scan to determine whether a repeat biopsy is needed.

"In this way, PSA tests can help men better monitor their condition and avoid jumping into treatment," says Dr. Pomerantz. "It can help men feel proactive about managing their prostate cancer." ▮

IN THE JOURNALS

Older men continue to have excessive PSA testing

The U.S. Preventive Services Task Force (USPSTF) recommends against routine prostate-specific antigen (PSA) testing in men ages 70 and older. Even so, men in this age group still have too many PSA tests, according to two studies published in 2023.

In the first study, published in *Urology*, researchers identified 3 million men who had regular PSA tests between 2003 and 2019. Men ages 70 and older were more likely than younger men to have high-frequency PSA testing, defined as having tests more than once every nine months.

The results also showed that the older men with high-frequency testing were significantly more likely to have prostate biopsies and receive prostate cancer diagnoses compared to older men screened less frequently. However, there was no difference in rates of immediate cancer treatment. According to the researchers, this was an indication that having prostate biopsies, even ones that showed cancer, did not lead to significant differences in recommendations.

The second study, published by *JAMA Network Open*, surveyed more than 32,000 men ages 70 and older. Among this group, 55.3% of men ages 70 to 74 had recent PSA screenings. The rate dropped with age, to 52.1% for those ages 75 to 79 and to 39.4% in those 80 and older. Still, the survey found that many men who would not benefit from routine PSA testing were still receiving screening at ages greater than those recommended by the USPSTF. The results also suggested that older men tend to perceive PSA screening as having more advantages than disadvantages. No matter what a man's age, his decision to continue PSA testing should be based on a balanced discussion with his doctor.

New test may help some men with elevated PSA avoid biopsy

The results can help men avoid unnecessary procedures.

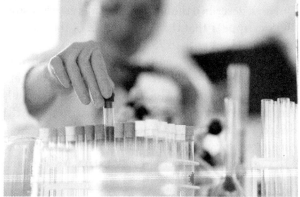
© Tsikhan Kuprevich | Getty Images

A noninvasive new urine test may offer a way to avoid biopsies and specialized imaging.

When a prostate-specific antigen (PSA) blood test produces an abnormal result, the next step is usually a prostate biopsy. A biopsy can confirm or rule out a cancer diagnosis, but it also has certain drawbacks. Prostate biopsies are invasive procedures with potential side effects, and they often detect low-grade, slow-growing tumors that may not need immediate treatment—or any treatment at all.

Researchers are exploring various strategies for avoiding unnecessary biopsies. Specialized magnetic resonance imaging (MRI) scans, for instance, can be useful for predicting if a man's tumor is likely to spread. A blood test called the Prostate Health Index (PHI) measures various forms of PSA, and can help doctors determine if a biopsy is needed.

In April 2024, researchers at the University of Michigan published results with a test that screens for prostate cancer in urine samples. Called the MyProstateScore 2.0 (MPS2) test, it looks for 18 different genes associated with high-grade tumors. "If you're negative on this test, it's almost certain that you don't have aggressive prostate cancer," said Dr. Arul Chinnaiyan, a professor of pathology and urology at the university, in a press release.

Gathering data and further testing

To create the test, Dr. Chinnaiyan and his colleagues first turned to publicly available databases containing over 58,000 prostate cancer-associated genes. From that initial pool, they narrowed down to 54 genes that are uniquely overexpressed in cancers classified as Grade Group 2 (GG2) or higher. The Grade Group system ranks prostate cancers from GG1 (the least dangerous) to GG5 (the most dangerous).

The team tested those 54 genes against archived urine samples from 761 men with elevated PSA who were scheduled for biopsy. This effort yielded 18 genes that consistently correlated with high-grade cancer in the biopsy specimens. These genes now make up MPS2.

Then the team validated the test by performing MPS2 testing on over 800 archived urine samples collected by a national prostate cancer research consortium. Other researchers affiliated with that consortium assessed the new urine test's results against patient records.

Interpreting the results

Study findings showed that MPS2 correctly identified 95% of the GG2 prostate cancers and 99% of cancers that were GG3 or higher. Test accuracy was further improved by incorporating estimates of the prostate's size (or volume, as it's also called).

According to the team's calculations, use of the MPS2 would have reduced unnecessary biopsies by 37%. If volume was included in the measure, then 41% of biopsies would have been avoided. By comparison, just 26% of biopsies would have been avoided with the PHI.

Dr. Chinnaiyan and his co-authors emphasize that ruling out high-grade cancer with a urine test offers some advantages over MRI. The specialized multi-parametric MRI scans needed to assess high-grade cancer in men with elevated PSA aren't always available in community settings, for instance. Moreover, the interpretation of mpMRI results can vary from one radiologist to another. Importantly, the MPS2 can be updated over time as new prostate cancer genes are identified.

What this means for you

Dr. Boris Gershman, a urologist at Harvard-affiliated Beth Israel Deaconess Medical Center in Boston, ▸▸

and a member of the advisory and editorial board for the *Harvard Medical School Guide to Prostate Diseases*, described the new study results as promising. "It does appear that the performance of the 18-gene urine test is better than PSA alone," he says.

But Dr. Gershman adds that it will be important to consider how such a test will fit into the current two-stage approach for PSA screening, which entails prostate MRI when the PSA is abnormal. Where MRI delivers a yes/no result (meaning lesions that look suspicious for cancer are either present or not), the MPS2 provides numerical risk estimates ranging between 0% and 100%. "The challenge with clinical implementation of a continuous risk score is where to draw the line for biopsy," Dr. Gershman says.

"This research is very encouraging, since many men in rural areas may not have access to prostate MRI machines or the added sophistication that is needed in interpreting these MRI scans," says Dr. Marc Garnick, the Gorman Brothers Professor of Medicine at Harvard Medical School and Beth Israel Deaconess Medical Center. "A widely available urine test may eventually help provide more precision in determining who should undergo a prostate biopsy, and may also help to assess the probability that a cancer is clinically significant and in need of treatment."

ASK THE DOCTOR

by **HOWARD LeWINE, M.D.,** Editor in Chief, *Harvard Men's Health Watch*

Does my prostate cancer increase my risk for other cancers?

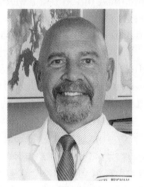

Q *I was recently diagnosed with prostate cancer. Does the occurrence of one type of cancer indicate a danger of developing other types of cancer?*

A It can, but it depends upon the type of cancer and the treatment. In general, prostate cancer that occurs after age 60 probably does not increase the risk of getting a second, different cancer.

Prostate cancer is the most common cancer among men. Almost every man develops prostate cancer if he lives long enough. So, an older man who has been diagnosed with prostate cancer is no more likely than any other man to develop a different type of cancer.

There are probably some exceptions. Some men inherit genes that increase the risk of developing a particularly aggressive type of prostate cancer, often at an early age (younger than 50). These same genes could increase the risk of other cancers, too.

Another possible reason for a higher risk of cancer may be related to lifestyle. For example, men who are obese are more likely to develop a more aggressive form of prostate cancer. And we also know that maintaining a healthy weight, eating a plant-based diet, and exercising regularly may lower the risk of other cancers, like colon cancer (the third most common cancer in men).

There may be a small increased lifetime risk of developing rectal or bladder cancer in men who have been treated with radiation therapy for prostate cancer. However, this is related to the treatment, not the prostate cancer itself.

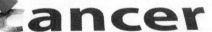

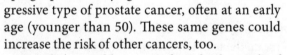

© maurusone | Getty Images

In general, having prostate cancer does not raise the risk of developing other cancers.

Chapter 8

Fit and Active

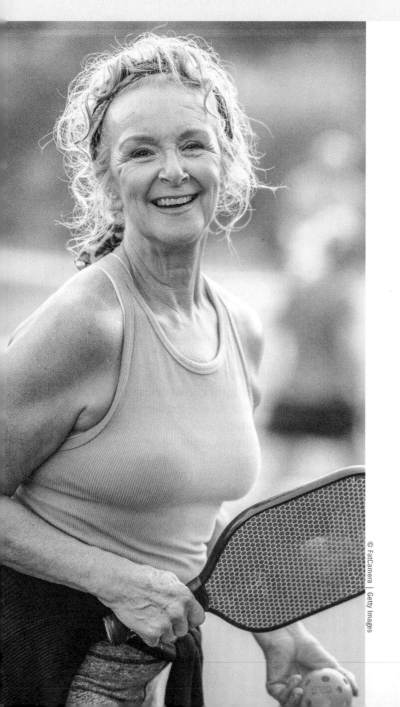

© FatCamera | Getty Images

Healthy Habits!
5 Things You Can Do Now

1 **Reboot your exercise routine.** If you've recently been inactive, learn tips to stay safe as you regain fitness. (page 186)

2 **Find your preferred time to exercise.** Evidence suggests no specific time or day of the week is best, so go ahead—choose what suits you. (page 190)

3 **Try a water workout.** This fun, gentle form of exercise offers multiple benefits. (page 202)

4 **Find the right shoes.** Caring for your feet is essential to maintaining activity levels. (page 210)

5 **Consider yoga.** Numerous varieties mean there's a style available for every body type and personality. (page 211)

Staying in shape: A case of "use it or lose it"

Fitness can quickly diminish if we stop exercising. Here's how to safely get back in the game.

Everybody needs a little time away—from jobs, people, and even exercise. But if you've stayed fit and strong from diligent, regular workouts, it's astonishing how quickly it can all slip away if you take weeks or months off, either voluntarily or because of illness or injury.

Beyond losing exercise's immediate benefits—including sounder sleep and stress relief—the disadvantages of stopping become rapidly apparent. The phenomenon is called deconditioning, and it happens to both recreational exercisers and elite athletes. Certain factors influence how quickly you'll lose strength and endurance—including age, prior fitness level, and any medical conditions—but it's universal, says Dr. Beth Frates, a clinical assistant professor in the Department of Physical Medicine and Rehabilitation at Harvard Medical School.

"It will happen no matter who you are," Dr. Frates says. "We say exercise is medicine, and it's true. When you take the medicine—or in this case, do the exercise—you reap the benefits. But it's 'use it or lose it.'"

Endurance and strength suffer

What does it mean to lose fitness, and how quickly does it erode? That depends on the category.

Cardiovascular fitness is the fastest to decline. Within just a few days of our last aerobic exercise session, our hearts pump less blood around the body, and the blood that's circulating to cells and muscles contains less oxygen. Only a few weeks later, you'll find yourself huffing and puffing to complete the same brisk walk, cycling route, or swim routine you'd once done with ease. Your heart might be pounding, too.

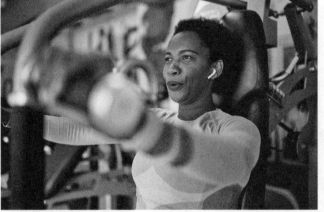

© Drazen Zigic | Getty Images

Muscle mass and strength you may have lost during an exercise break can come back quickly.

"Perhaps you'll notice that you can't talk while you're walking up that hill like you did four weeks ago," Dr. Frates says. "Something that was moderate-intensity exercise for you before is now vigorous, and you might feel like stopping earlier."

Muscle strength takes longer to lose after you've been inactive—about two months. You won't be able to lift as much or do as many repetitions as before your hiatus. The same weights or body-resistance exercises will prove far more fatiguing, and your muscles will likely feel extremely sore within a day of working out again.

The good news? "Muscle memory" is real, meaning shrunken muscle fibers can indeed rebound, Dr. Frates says. "You can get back to muscle strengthening a little more quickly than you can get back to the same level of cardiovascular conditioning," she says.

Staging your comeback

The first step in getting fit again is believing you can do it. There's no question it will get harder before it gets easier, Dr. Frates says.

"No one has a precise equation for how long it will take a particular person to regain fitness," she says. "The longer you were away from it, the longer it will take. It will not happen immediately—it will take at least several weeks."

Dr. Frates offers this guidance for safely rebooting your exercise routine:

Get your doctor's okay. This is crucial if you haven't exercised in a long time—many months or years—or have chronic conditions such as heart disease or diabetes. And if you experience any alarming symptoms when first exercising again, such as chest pain or pressure, stop immediately and seek medical attention.

Start small. Instead of reverting to your toughest workouts, try lighter activities or weight levels to get comfortably moving again. "Don't go off and do sprints at the track on your first day," she says. "Build up slowly. Even taking a walk can help."

Do what worked before. Perhaps you felt on top of your fitness when you took group classes or biked dozens of miles a week. So ease into doing it again. "Think back to when you were routine-consistent and successful and consider using a similar strategy this time around," Dr. Frates says.

Channel your inner kid. We learned as children that movement can be fun. If you loved hula-hooping or paddleboarding when you were younger, consider returning to it.

Set up a support system. Accountability partners aren't a new idea, but they work—which is why getting an exercise buddy should be top of mind when you're resuming a regimen. If you don't have a ready workout buddy, consider working with a health coach.

Track your progress. Wearable devices can fuel renewed exercise efforts by tracking step count, resting heart rate, and other metrics. But an old-school pen-and-paper log can also do the trick. "You can look at how you did and make adjustments," she says. "If Week 1 doesn't go the way you wanted, there's no shame or guilt. This is definitely a case where some exercise is better than none." 🛡

Hitting the activity mark

Guidelines recommend 150 minutes per week of moderate-intensity physical activity, but how can you consistently reach this number?

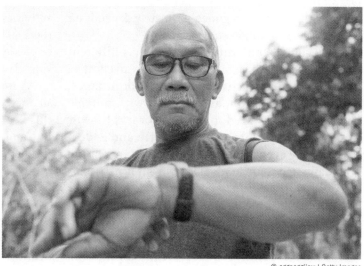

© eggeeggjiew | Getty Images

Breaking up your workout time into smaller segments is one way to reach your exercise goal.

When it comes to staying healthy, just how much exercise is enough? The Physical Activity Guidelines for Americans, issued by the U.S. Department of Health and Human Services, recommend a minimum of 150 minutes (2.5 hours) of moderate-intensity physical activity as well as two muscle-strengthening workouts per week. (Alternatively, you also can do half that amount—75 minutes per week of activity—but at a more vigorous intensity.)

Organizations like the American College of Sports Medicine and the American Heart Association also support these guidelines, which have been the standard for over a decade. "However, it is important to remember that these guidelines are meant for a broad population, and for many older adults, hitting just the 150 minutes per week poses a challenge," says Dr. George Ross Malik, a sports medicine physician with Harvard-affiliated Spaulding Rehabilitation Hospital.

What's in a number?

While both physical activity and muscle strengthening are important, experts tend to place more emphasis on the 150 minutes per week, since it helps keep people active and less sedentary. "Some research has suggested that people who regularly sit more than seven hours ▸▸

a day with limited activity have a higher mortality risk, similar to that posed by obesity and smoking," says Dr. Malik.

So where did the number 150 come from? "When scientific advisory committees and other experts combed the body of evidence linking exercise with chronic conditions like diabetes, cancer, and heart disease, a minimum of 150 minutes per week of moderate-intensity activity was repeatedly seen as the threshold for offering health benefits," says Dr. Malik. "People who regularly met this criterion often had a lower risk for disease and risk factors like weight gain, high cholesterol, and high blood pressure."

But the key word here is *minimum*. The guidelines set the low end at 150 minutes, and research has found that going beyond this number offers additional benefits.

Individual needs

Dr. Malik says that the 150-minute target is good to aim for, but your best regimen ultimately depends on your physical condition and goals.

"Everyone is built differently and has different health concerns, which can dictate what is an effective and safe amount of activity," he says. "For instance, people returning from an injury or with notable health issues may need to exercise for less time or less intensity until they build strength and endurance. It may even be as subtle as simply increasing your daily step count totals at first." Your fitness goals also play a role. Older people may need to focus more on strength training (doing more than the recommended two days per week) to help offset sarcopenia, the natural loss of muscle mass that occurs with age (see "Practical pointers about protein" on page 112). Or they may need to do more stretching, flexibility, and balance exercises to address range-of-motion and mobility issues.

"Consulting your doctor or a personal trainer can help you establish specific fitness goals and determine how much activity you require," says Dr. Malik.

Break it up

While the 150 weekly minutes is still a mark older adults should strive for, the number can feel daunting. Instead of focusing on the entire 150 minutes, break it down into manageable segments, suggests Dr. Malik. For example, 150 minutes equals 30 minutes done five days a week. Another option is to divide those 30 minutes into even smaller segments. "You don't have to do the entire 30 minutes at once to reap the benefits," says Dr. Malik. "Try doing 10 minutes of exercise three times a day, or two workouts of 15 minutes each."

You also need not do the same activity every time. "You can always squeeze in moderate-intensity activity throughout the day," says Dr. Malik. For instance, hold planks during TV commercials, go for a walk after lunch, and do counter push-ups or squats in the kitchen while waiting for the coffee to brew. Everyday activities like yard work and household chores also count toward your daily number, says Dr. Malik.

Another strategy is to focus on diversity. Find new activities of interest that can supplement your usual routine. For example, join a recreational sports league or pickleball group, or do a Peloton workout or take a yoga class.

As for doing shorter amounts of higher-intensity activity to meet your quota, Dr. Malik suggests this is a level that should be reached with preparation and adequate training. "It is important to reduce the risk of injuries by working gradually toward this more advanced type of exercise and incorporating cross-training to avoid overuse injuries," he says.

The bottom line is that while it is good to be mindful about reaching 150 weekly minutes, don't focus on the number itself, but rather on living a healthier lifestyle. "If necessary, begin with doing a smaller amount, like 50 minutes per week, and progress from there," says Dr. Malik. "Ultimately, it is about reducing sedentary time, staying active, and enjoying what you do. If you focus on that, you'll gradually reach the 150 minutes consistently—and likely even exceed it." ◗

Are you an everyday exerciser or a weekend warrior?

As long as you meet the recommended exercise goals, working out just one or two days a week may lower your heart disease risk as much as exercising throughout the week.

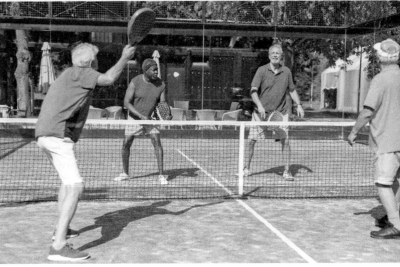

© RgStudio | Getty Images

Weekend warriors fare just as well as daily exercisers when it comes to heart health.

The standard advice about exercise is to do about 30 minutes a day, most days of the week. But in terms of heart-related benefits, does it matter if you rack up most of your exercise minutes over just one or two days instead of spreading them out over an entire week?

Earlier research has suggested that both patterns are equally beneficial. But those findings relied on people to self-report their exercise, which can be unreliable. Now, a study of nearly 90,000 adults who used wristband monitors to record their physical activity has reached a similar conclusion.

"The findings add to the body of literature showing that it doesn't matter when you get your exercise, as long as you get the recommended amount each week," says Dr. I-Min Lee, a professor of medicine at Harvard Medical School and an expert on the role of physical activity in preventing disease.

Volume matters more than pattern

The 2023 study, published in *JAMA*, doesn't define the term "weekend warrior" in quite the same way that most people do, says Dr. Lee. "Usually, weekend warriors are seen as people who don't exercise on weekdays but then take a long hike or play two hours of tennis on Saturday or Sunday," she says.

Instead, researchers used participants' physical activity data, which were recorded over seven consecutive days, to categorize them into different groups. About two-thirds of them met the federal physical activity guidelines (see "Hitting the activity mark," page 187). About 42% were deemed "weekend warriors," meaning they met the guidelines but got half or more of their total physical activity—not just exercise—on just one or two days. Another 24% were "regularly active," meeting the guidelines with activity spread out over the week. The remaining 34% didn't meet the guidelines.

After roughly six years, the researchers found that participants who followed either activity pattern had a similarly lower risk of heart attack, stroke, atrial fibrillation, and heart failure compared with people in the inactive group. Historically, experts have encouraged people to be regularly active, mainly because anecdotal reports suggest that weekend warriors may be more prone to injuries. But this study didn't find any difference in injury rates between the two active groups. That's likely because of the definition used in the study: the "warrior" group wasn't necessarily doing the types of high-intensity ▸▸

How much exercise?

The Physical Activity Guidelines for Americans advise adults to:

DO at least 150 minutes (two hours and 30 minutes) a week of moderate-intensity aerobic physical activity

OR 75 minutes (one hour and 15 minutes) a week of vigorous-intensity aerobic activity

OR an equivalent combination of moderate- and vigorous-intensity aerobic activity.

►► activities or sports often associated with muscle sprains and related injuries, Dr. Lee says.

Short bouts of activity count

Wristband devices enable researchers to capture all the short bouts of activity people do throughout the day that they may not remember. "If you do jumping jacks occasionally while watching television, you won't necessarily recall that activity the way you remember that you play tennis three times a week," says Dr. Lee. Similarly, people whose daily commutes include a few 10-minute bouts of walking may not consider that as counting toward their moderate-intensity activity minutes. But these small spurts of activity—sometimes referred to as exercise "snacks"—seem to be beneficial. If you're sitting for a long stretch, stand up and move around for a few minutes every hour. Activating your muscles even just briefly can help improve your body's ability to keep your blood sugar, blood pressure, and cholesterol in check. (For more on the benefits of short bursts of movement, see "Everyday activities count as exercise, but intensity matters," page 191.)

It's also worth noting that if you don't meet the physical activity guidelines, you'll still benefit from doing even small amounts of exercise—and every minute counts. ▮

Best time of day to exercise? Whatever works for you

Are there any pros or cons associated with exercising at certain times of the day? Research results tend to be all over the map, says Harvard Medical School professor Dr. I-Min Lee (though see "For weight loss, early morning exercise may be most effective," page 191). The best strategy is to exercise when it's most convenient and comfortable for you, whether that's the first thing in the morning, early evening, or anytime in between.

If you exercise early in the day, you can check it off your to-do list and can take advantage of the "feel-good" brain chemicals, serotonin and dopamine, that are released during exercise. But afternoon workouts also have some benefits. Your joints and muscles may be more limber later in the day, which may make exercise feel less taxing. If you experience a midafternoon lull, exercise can be a good way to reinvigorate yourself. If you can, find a buddy who likes to exercise at the same time, so you can go together and hold each other accountable.

Likewise, there's little evidence to suggest that coordinating your exercise with respect to mealtimes has any good or bad effects.

Some people find that vigorous exercise right before a meal curbs their appetite, while others find the opposite is true. A pre-breakfast workout works well for certain people. But having a small, carbohydrate-rich snack (like a banana or a slice of whole-grain toast) at least half an hour before exercising may provide a helpful energy boost, says Dr. Lee.

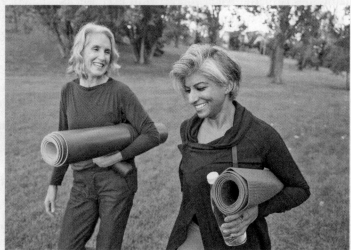

© Hero Images Inc | Getty Images

Scheduling time to do a workout with a friend can be a good way to help you meet exercise goals.

For weight loss, early morning exercise may be most effective

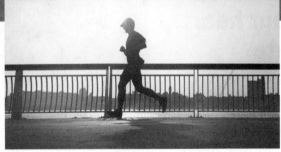
© Oli Kellett | Getty Images

Starting the day with exercise is linked with a lower obesity risk.

While there may be no "best" time to exercise, an observational study suggests that early morning may be ideal when it comes to weight management.

Researchers reviewed data from the CDC's National Health and Nutrition Examination Survey. The survey recorded the activity levels of 5,285 participants and what times of day they exercised: morning, midday, and evening.

Among people who met the recommended guidelines of 150 minutes per week of moderate-to-vigorous activity, those who consistently engaged in morning activity (usually between 7 a.m. and 9 a.m.) had a lower risk for obesity than those who were most active in the midday or evening.

Specifically, the morning group had a lower average body mass index and waist size than the other two groups. The findings were published in 2023 by *Obesity*.

Everyday activities count as exercise, but intensity matters

Can doing short bursts of everyday activities offer health benefits?

Researchers used wrist activity trackers to measure daily activities of more than 25,000 people ages 42 to 78 who did not exercise formally. Activities were defined as any continuous movement done at a faster-than-normal pace: for example, taking stairs, mopping

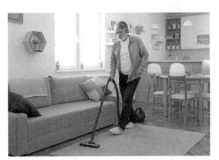
© milan2099 | Getty Images

Doing daily household tasks helps you stay active.

the floor, gardening, and playing energetically with children. Everyone's movements were tracked for one week, and the results were compared with their health status eight years later.

The researchers found that people who did multiple bouts of daily activities lasting from one to 10 minutes—for a total of about 28 minutes per day—had a lower risk for heart attacks and strokes compared with those who were active for less than a minute at a time. (There was no statistical advantage for being active longer than 10 minutes.)

Intensity was key, as the more vigorous the activity, the greater the benefit. However, the results suggested you don't need to maintain a high intensity all the time. The researchers found that doing at least 15% (about 10 seconds for every minute) at a vigorous level and the rest at a moderate level was enough.

The results were published in 2023 in *The Lancet Public Health*.

All about your heart rate

Here's what you should know about target and maximum heart rates during exercise—and other things that can speed up or slow down your heart.

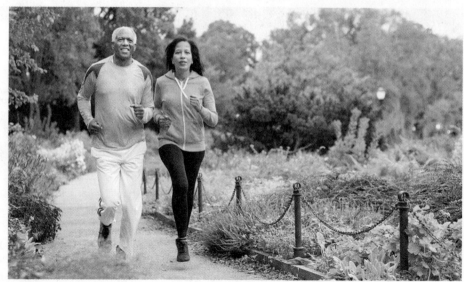

© Cultura RM Exclusive/yellowdog I Getty Images

The common formula to estimate your maximum heart rate during physical activity relies on just one variable—your age. As a result, the estimate may not be very accurate.

If you are committed to keeping your heart in good shape, perhaps you already know how much heart-pumping aerobic exercise you should be getting each week. (For the record, it's at least 150 minutes of moderate-intensity exercise, or 75 minutes of vigorous-intensity exercise, or an equivalent combination).

But just how high should your heart rate rise during exercise? Should you aim for a specific target—and is it dangerous to go above your "maximum" heart rate? For answers to these and related questions, we consulted Dr. Sawalla Guseh, director of the Cardiovascular Performance Program at Harvard-affiliated Massachusetts General Hospital.

Maximum and target heart rates, explained

The term maximum (or peak) heart rate refers to the upper limit of what your cardiovascular system can handle during physical activity, measured in beats per minute (bpm). Accurately determining this number requires a cardiopulmonary exercise test, which tracks how your lungs, heart, blood vessels, and muscles react during an exercise challenge. However, it's more practical to estimate your maximum heart rate. The usual formula is 220 minus your age.

Be aware, though, that this just gives you a ballpark figure. "We know the ability to raise your heart rate tends to decrease with age. But using age alone really isn't the best metric for determining your maximum heart rate," says Dr. Guseh. Created in the early 1970s, the formula was based on testing done on men and tends to overestimate peak heart rates in women. In addition, he notes, estimates for all individuals may be off by as much as 15 bpm.

Target heart rates are expressed as a percentage of your maximum heart rate. For example, if you're 65, your estimated maximum heart rate is 220 minus 65, or 155 bpm. For moderate-intensity exercise, your target heart rate range is 64% to 76% of that (99 to 118 bpm). For vigorous-intensity exercise, your target range is around 77% to 93% (119 to 144 bpm). Of course, popular wrist-worn devices can do these calculations for you. But these gadgets have limitations (see "Heart rate tracking: The good, the bad, and the uncertain," page 193) and aren't really necessary.

Try the talk test

Remember that heart rate targets are simply guides, and there's no medical evidence that healthy people need to exercise at specific heart rates. But knowing the range that's considered moderate or vigorous for you can help determine whether you're meeting the recommended exercise goals and can be used to guide training to enhance your fitness or performance, says Dr. Guseh. Another option is to simply use the "talk test." If you're breathing faster than usual but can still

Heart rate tracking: The good, the bad, and the uncertain

Most smart watches and wearable fitness trackers use your age to estimate your target heart rate zones (see page 192). These devices periodically measure your heartbeat throughout the day, using optical sensors that detect light bouncing back from the blood flowing beneath the skin of your inner wrist.

For some people, working hard to reach their target heart rate motivates them to exercise more and further boosts their fitness levels, says Harvard cardiologist Dr. Sawalla Guseh. But if you're worried about your heart rate for whatever reason, checking the number too often might make you even more anxious, he says.

In addition, some studies suggest that the heart rate estimates from wrist-worn devices may be less accurate in people with darker skin compared with people whose skin is lighter. If you have one of these devices, you can check its accuracy by taking your pulse manually,

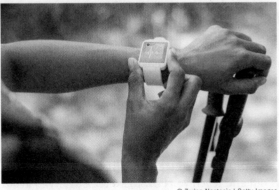
© Zorica Nastasic I Getty Images

ideally at rest as well as during activities of different levels of intensity. Press your index and middle fingers together on your wrist, just below the base of your thumb. Count the number of beats in 15 seconds and multiply by four to get beats per minute.

carry on a conversation, you're exercising at moderate intensity. If you have trouble finishing a sentence, you're doing vigorous-intensity exercise.

If you're new to exercise, start slowly and build up to more vigorous exercise gradually. If you're already an avid exerciser, it's usually not a problem to reach or even exceed your maximum heart rate for short periods of time. However, people who have or are at risk for heart disease should be more cautious and check with their clinician about how to exercise safely.

What else affects heart rate?

A normal resting heart rate is between 60 and 100 bpm. The best time to check yours is first thing in the morning, before you even get out of bed. Other than exercise, factors that can elevate your heart rate include hot weather, dehydration, being at a high altitude, or feeling nervous or excited. Certain drugs (such as stimulants)

and some medical conditions (anemia, asthma, infections, and fevers) can also cause your heart rate to rise.

Your heart rate usually dips during sleep, sometimes dropping as slow as 40 to 50 bpm, especially if your resting heart rate is on the low end. Medical problems that may lower your heart rate include heart disease, low thyroid function, and high blood levels of potassium. Beta blockers, a class of medications used to treat high blood pressure and other heart conditions, also slow down the heart; examples include metoprolol (Lopressor, Toprol) and carvedilol (Coreg).

Highly trained athletes often have low resting heart rates, sometimes in the 40s or even 30s, says Dr. Guseh. "After years of training, their hearts undergo what's known as exercise-induced cardiac remodeling. Because their hearts are bigger, each beat pumps more blood, so the heart doesn't have to beat as often to supply the body with blood," he says. ▼

How a personal trainer can enhance your workouts

Many people seek motivation, but working with a trainer can also help you avoid injuries and make exercise more enjoyable.

If your New Year's resolution to start exercising more has fallen by the wayside, hiring a personal trainer can be a good way to hold yourself accountable. Because exercise is such an important part of cardiovascular health, the cost is worthwhile—especially when you consider the added benefits of working with a professional trainer.

"A good personal trainer will create a balanced workout and teach you how to exercise safely to avoid injuries," says certified personal trainer Vijay A. Daryanani, a physical therapist with Harvard-affiliated Spaulding Outpatient Center. He always has his clients start with a dynamic warm-up, such as marching in place or sidestepping and doing arm swings, which helps loosen up the major muscle groups. "I'll also have them do some heel-to-toe walking to help fire up some of the smaller muscles," he says.

People focused on heart health often prioritize exercise that raises their heart rate (cardio or aerobic exercise). But strength training builds lean muscle mass, which helps burn body fat, keeps blood sugar in check, and may help reduce cholesterol levels.

Injury prevention

Using the proper form during strength-building exercises is key. The weight machines at gyms and fitness centers can be a good option for beginners because they target specific muscle groups within a limited range of motion, says Daryanani. But when you use free weights (dumbbells, barbells, and kettlebells), you use a much wider range of muscles, including core muscles and others that help with stability and balance. A trainer will help you choose the correct type and size of free weight based on your abilities and goals. Because free weights allow a greater range of motion, you need good body awareness to stay safe.

Always make sure to stand up straight and tall before starting any standing strength moves, says Daryanani. Most gyms and health clubs have mirrors that you can use to get feedback on your form as you exercise. Even a basic body-weight exercise like a squat requires careful attention to body alignment to avoid straining your joints (see "The right and wrong way to do a squat").

Choosing a personal trainer

Some gyms and fitness centers have personal trainers on staff or hire them as contractors. But many will come to your house and can devise an at-home workout

---

The right and wrong way to do a squat

Proper form is crucial to protecting yourself from injury and getting the most benefit from an exercise. A squat is a classic body-weight exercise that strengthens the lower body and core muscles in addition to improving your balance and posture. Here's the correct way to do this exercise without stressing the joints in your hips, knees, and ankles.

▶ Bend at your hips to work your gluteal (buttocks) muscles.

▶ Lean forward about 45° to keep your balance.

▶ Check that your knees are aligned and not rolling inward or outward.

▶ Keep your feet flat, with your heels on the floor.

▶ Don't let your knees go farther forward than your toes.

▶ Try not to let your thighs sink lower than parallel to the floor.

▶ Don't round your back; try to keep your spine in a straight line.

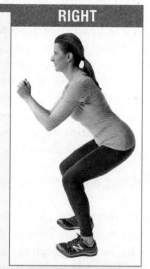

RIGHT

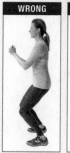

WRONG

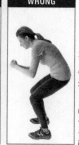

WRONG

Photos by Thomas MacDonald

plan for you, even if you don't own any machines or special equipment. Look for one who's accredited by one or more of these organizations:

▸ American Council on Exercise (ACE)

▸ American College of Sports Medicine (ACSM)

▸ International Sports Sciences Association (ISSA)

▸ National Academy of Sports Medicine (NASM).

Ask about the person's training background, experience working with clients your age, and approach to designing client programs. Consider asking for references, especially from clients like you. Sign up for a few sessions at first to gauge how well you and the trainer work together before you commit to something longer.

Prices vary widely, depending on where you live and possibly gym affiliations, and may range anywhere from $75 to $125 per hour. You might be able to save a little money by hiring a trainer to do small group sessions with you and one or several of your friends who have similar fitness levels and goals.

Another advantage to working with a trainer: a good one can make exercise feel like a fun challenge instead of a repetitive chore. "Getting someone in the right mindset is essential, and I find that positive energy can be very infectious," says Daryanani. 🛡

IN THE JOURNALS

Does tai chi beat aerobics to lower blood pressure?

If you had to guess which exercise is most effective at lowering blood pressure, you might not choose tai chi, known for its flowing motions and deep breathing to calm the mind and improve balance, strength, and mood. But a small randomized trial published in 2024 by *JAMA Network Open* found that tai chi was better at lowering blood pressure than aerobic activity (the kind that works your heart and lungs). Researchers divided about 340 people with elevated blood pressure—a precursor stage to high blood pressure—into two groups. One group practiced tai chi for an hour four times a week. The other group did an hour of aerobic exercise (stair climbing, jogging, brisk walking, or cycling) four times a week. After one year, systolic blood pressure (the top number in a measurement) had dropped by an average of seven points for people in the tai chi group, compared with about four points in the aerobics group. The researchers speculate that tai chi might have the edge because

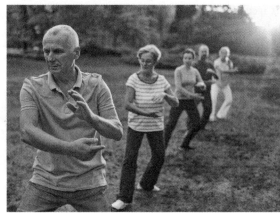
Westend61 | Getty Images

Tai chi lowered blood pressure more effectively than aerobic exercise for participants in a recent study.

it triggers the body's relaxation response, which helps lower blood pressure. But don't give up aerobic exercise; it's still crucial for many aspects of health. Just think of tai chi as another helpful tool.

3 strategies for safer home workouts

Create a safe exercise space, get safety gear, and practice smart workout habits to reduce your risk of injury.

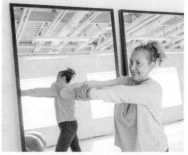

© kate_sept2004 | Getty Images

Use a mirror during a home workout so you can make sure you're maintaining the proper form.

Working out at home is convenient, but it comes with risks (especially if you exercise alone) such as muscle strains, falls, and injuries. This was evident during the first year of the pandemic, when COVID-19 risks led many people to exercise at home, and exercise injuries resulting in emergency room visits were up about 50% from the year before, according to some insurance company estimates.

To reduce your injury risks when exercising at home, focus on three strategies.

1 Create a safe workout space

Your exercise environment is the foundation for exercise safety. Make sure it's well lighted (to prevent falls), well ventilated (to keep the air fresh), and not too hot or humid (so you don't get overheated or dehydrated). Adding a dehumidifier (about $30 for one that handles a small room) to the space may help dry out humid air, if necessary.

A safe workout space should also have a level floor and plenty of room to move. "Your workout space should be wide enough that you can move your arms freely, without touching anything when you're standing, and long enough to accommodate your whole body when you're on the ground for floor exercises," says Janice McGrail, a physical therapist at Harvard-affiliated Spaulding Rehabilitation Hospital.

Keep the floor free of clutter and throw rugs, and remove any nearby furniture with sharp corners.

2 Stock the space with safety essentials

The following items can boost the safety of your workout.

A large mirror. Maintaining the proper form during exercise is crucial to avoiding muscle strains and sprains. A framed full-length mirror (about $10 at a big-box store) will enable you to see how you're doing. Secure the mirror to the wall to keep it from falling and shattering.

An exercise mat. A little cushioning underfoot will reduce pressure on your joints and provide a safer landing spot than a hard floor. The mat should be nonslip and about half an inch thick. A set of interlocking exercise foam floor tiles are perfect for the job. Prices for a set start at about $25. (Note: Don't exercise on thick carpet, which may cause your sneakers to get stuck and cause a fall.)

Supportive sneakers. The most comfortable sneakers you own might not be the safest for exercising. Wear a pair that fits snugly around your heel and midfoot and has a roomy toe box, good support, and soles that aren't too cushioned or beveled (as running shoes are), which may lead to a fall.

Water. Keep a water bottle nearby, so you can take a few sips in between exercises to stay hydrated.

A smart speaker. If you exercise alone, you'll need to call for help in case of emergency. A smart speaker that you can call out to is a great option (starting at about $30). Just make sure your workout space has a good Wi-Fi signal. Note: You can also use a smart watch or an alert button, but those can be pricey (hundreds of dollars). Your smartphone can also do the job.

A carbon monoxide monitor. Carbon monoxide is an odorless, colorless, potentially deadly gas emitted from combustion engines. If your workout space is in a garage, along with a car, install a carbon monoxide monitor (starting at about $20).

3 Practice safe exercise habits

Remaining aware of exercise risks and practicing safe exercise habits should be part of your routine—just like putting on a seat belt in a car. Here are some suggestions.

Get your doctor's okay. Make sure you have a green light for your exercise routine if you've been inactive recently, or if you have a chronic condition such as heart disease or poor balance. Start with a simple routine, and increase the difficulty gradually.

Warm up first. Strained muscles are common exercise injuries. Doing a 5- or 10-minute warm-up first—such as marching in place while swinging your arms—will prime your muscles and body for the demands of your workout.

Don't push yourself too hard. "In general, exercise should feel like a challenge or make you feel fatigued, but it should not cause sharp pain. It is okay and even expected for your muscles to feel tired and a bit sore after you exercise, but the soreness should go away in about a day. If you are still sore several days later, that's a sign that you did too much. Next time, use lighter weights or do fewer repetitions," McGrail says.

Carry weights carefully. "Grasp any weight, even a lighter one, in the middle of the handle to keep it steady so you don't drop it," McGrail says. "When picking up heavy dumbbells or kettlebells from the floor, bend at your knees and keep your back straight. When standing up again, use your legs rather than your back, so you don't strain it."

MOVE TO TRY: ARM CURLS

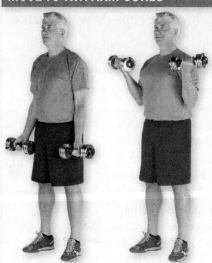

Stand with your feet about shoulder-width apart, your chest lifted, and your shoulders back and down. Hold a dumbbell in each hand with your arms down at your sides and palms facing forward. Slowly bend your elbows, lifting the dumbbells toward your shoulders. Hold. Slowly lower the dumbbells to the starting position. Repeat 8 to 12 times, take a break for 30 to 90 seconds, and repeat the process again.

Numbers © molotovcoketail | Getty Images

Tread lightly with treadmills. Treadmill accidents at home are common causes of broken bones, head injuries, and friction burns. If you have a treadmill, don't set the speed too fast or raise the incline too high, and change difficulty levels gradually. Take advantage of any safety mechanisms your treadmill has, such as a tether you can wear that automatically stops the machine if you fall. Keep the treadmill unplugged when you're not using it, to protect children who might want to play on it.

Stretch after a workout. Post-exercise, muscles are warm and ready for stretching. Don't bounce during a stretch, which can cause injury; hold each stretch for about 30-60 seconds at a time. This will help keep your muscles long and supple and prevent them from being injured during your next workout and your daily activities. 🛡

IN THE JOURNALS

About 20 minutes of exercise may offset risk of sitting all day

Just 22 minutes of brisk walking or similar activity daily may offset the risk of prolonged sitting, recent research suggests.

The study was based on health and activity tracker data on nearly 12,000 people ages 50 and older. Researchers linked the participants' data with death registry information over a median of five years.

People who spent more than 12 hours a day sitting were 38% more likely to die during the study period than people who sat for just eight hours a day. But that increased risk of death was only seen in people who got less than 22 minutes of moderate-to-vigorous physical activity each day. The findings were adjusted to account for confounding factors such as smoking, alcohol use, and disease. The 2023 study appeared in the *British Journal of Sports Medicine*.

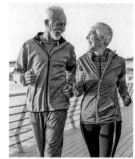

© filadendron | Getty Images

Push past your resistance to strength training

For a heart-healthy workout, include reps as well as steps.

If weight training (also called strength or resistance training) makes you think of body builders hoisting heavy weights in a gym, think again. You can tone and build muscle in the privacy of your home—no special equipment needed. Consider making it a regular habit: resistance training is good for your entire body, including your heart.

"Many middle-aged and older adults are aware that heart health is extremely important. But they tend to connect cardiovascular fitness mainly with aerobic exercise, such as brisk walking, jogging, and cycling," says Dr. Beth Frates, a clinical assistant professor in the Department of Physical Medicine and Rehabilitation at Harvard Medical School. However, combining both aerobic and resistance training offers the best protection against early death in general, she says, and from heart-related causes in particular.

A scientific statement from the American Heart Association (AHA), published in 2024 by the journal

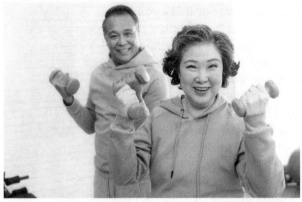

© ViewStock | Getty Images

You can do muscle-building exercises at home with small, inexpensive hand weights.

Circulation, details the heart-related benefits of resistance training. (Also see "Two workout strategies that reduce cardiovascular disease risk," page 200.) Doing

Muscle-strengthening activity: Types, terms, and examples

Anything that makes your muscles work harder than usual counts as a muscle-strengthening activity—something all adults should aim to do at least two days a week, according to the federal Physical Activity Guidelines.

Often referred to as strength training, this type of exercise works by harnessing resistance—that is, an opposing force that muscles have to strain against. It's also known as resistance training or weight training. You can use many different things to supply resistance, including your own body weight, free weights (such as dumbbells), elastic bands, or specialized machines. Other options include medicine balls, kettlebells, and weighted ropes.

Muscles grow stronger by exerting force through these three actions:

Concentric. Muscles move joints while shortening. Think of what happens when you flex your arm to show off your upper arm (biceps) muscle. It's the same type of motion you would use when raising a dumbbell or lifting a bag of groceries off the counter.

Eccentric. Muscles move joints while lengthening. As you slowly lower a dumbbell or grocery bag, your biceps muscles lengthen while producing force to lower the object in a controlled manner rather than simply letting it drop.

Isometric. Muscles don't shorten or lengthen much, and joints do not move. If you push against a wall, for example, or try to lift an object that is far too heavy for you, your arm muscles will tense. But since your muscles can't generate enough force to lift the object or shift the wall, they stay in the same position instead of shortening.

Muscle-strengthening exercise that include both concentric and eccentric movement is known as "dynamic" or "isotonic" strength training. Examples include push-ups, biceps curls, and squats. Examples of "isometric" or "static" strength training include doing wall squats (also called wall sits), planks, or an overhead hold.

resistance training on a regular basis can improve your blood pressure, blood sugar, blood lipids, and body composition. It's especially beneficial for older adults and people with an elevated risk for heart problems.

Bonus benefits of resistance training

Resistance training has also been shown to improve other factors closely tied to cardiovascular health. For example, it enhances blood vessel function, in part by keeping your arteries flexible. Resistance training also appears to lower levels of inflammation, which ignites the damaging, bodywide process that contributes to clogged arteries. But while you won't be able to feel those effects, you may experience noticeable improvements in both your sleep and your mood after adding strength-building exercises to your workout, says Dr. Frates. Both inadequate sleep and stress can contribute to cardiovascular problems.

Resistance training also supports weight loss because it burns calories both during and after your workout. When people lose weight, they usually lose muscle mass along with fat, while weight training helps preserve muscle mass. Given the popularity of effective weight-loss medications known as GLP-1s, such as semaglutide (Wegovy) and tirzepatide (Zepbound), it's important to recognize that muscle wasting (loss of muscle mass) is a possible side effect of these drugs, says Dr. Frates. That means resistance exercise is especially vital for people taking these medications.

Getting started

If you're new to this form of exercise, keep an open mind, says Dr. Frates. A good first step is visit a fitness center

Sample exercises for all major muscle groups

The following examples are from the AHA's scientific statement on resistance training. You don't need to do all the exercises in each training session—just try to rotate through the different major muscle groups and work all or most of them over the course of a week or two. For additional examples that don't require any equipment, see Harvard Health Publishing's Special Health Report *Body-Weight Exercise* (www.health.harvard.edu/BWE).

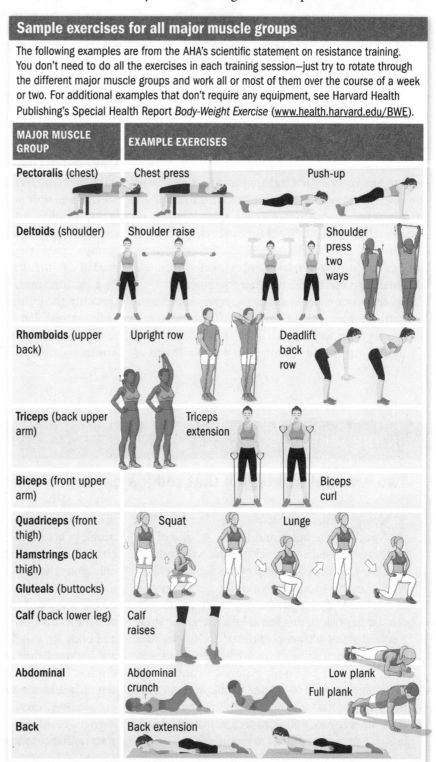

MAJOR MUSCLE GROUP	EXAMPLE EXERCISES
Pectoralis (chest)	Chest press · Push-up
Deltoids (shoulder)	Shoulder raise · Shoulder press two ways
Rhomboids (upper back)	Upright row · Deadlift back row
Triceps (back upper arm)	Triceps extension
Biceps (front upper arm)	Biceps curl
Quadriceps (front thigh) **Hamstrings** (back thigh) **Gluteals** (buttocks)	Squat · Lunge
Calf (back lower leg)	Calf raises
Abdominal	Abdominal crunch · Low plank · Full plank
Back	Back extension

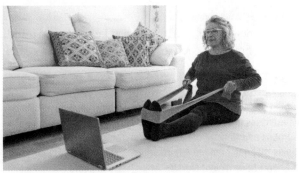

© Westend61 | Getty Images

Stretchy bands (also called resistance bands) can be used for a seated row, which strengthens the upper back muscles.

or gym and meet with a trainer, just to get a sense of the range of options for building strength. You can use machines, resistance bands (see photo), hand weights, or your own body weight. "Take time to explore them all as a curious child might explore the outdoors," says Dr. Frates. Consider a trial membership to see how it feels to use the machines and other equipment.

Another option is to seek out a supervised program at a senior center with a certified instructor who can teach you proper form, which is key to avoiding injury. If you have any mobility limitations due to arthritis or other health conditions, consider getting a referral to a physical therapist who can create a safe regimen tailored specifically to your needs.

While the camaraderie of in-person classes can be motiving and fun, you can't beat the convenience of exercising at home on your own, Dr. Frates says. You can find free online exercise videos on YouTube. Use a search term like "older adult strength training," and look for videos that clearly demonstrate the proper form, like those from the National Institute on Aging; see www.health.harvard.edu/exerciseforseniors.

How much, how often?

Aim for two strength-boosting sessions per week, which need only last about 15 to 20 minutes each. The AHA recommends focusing on eight to 10 different exercises (see "Sample exercises for all major muscle groups," page 199) to get a balanced workout. Set a goal of completing eight resistance training sessions in a month, marking the days on a calendar and tracking the number of repetitions (reps) you do of each exercise, Dr. Frates suggests. And it's often more motivating—and fun—if you can enlist a friend or family member to join you, she adds. ♥

IN THE JOURNALS

Two workout strategies that reduce cardiovascular disease risk

Doing regular aerobic exercise—the kind that works your heart and lungs—is one of the best ways to reduce your risk of cardiovascular disease. Now, findings published by the *European Heart Journal* in 2024 suggest that doing a combination of aerobics and strength training might reduce cardiovascular risk factors just as effectively. The study involved about 400 people (ages 35 to 70) classified as overweight or obese who also had high blood pressure. They were randomly assigned to one of four exercise programs: a 60-minute aerobic workout three times a week, a 60-minute strength training workout three times a week, a 60-minute combination of aerobics and strength training (30 minutes of each) three times a week, or no exercise at all. After one year, people in both the aerobics-only group and the combination exercise group (but not the strength-training-only group) had a significant reduction in a combined measure of cardiovascular risk factors, compared with people who didn't exercise. These risk factors included blood pressure, LDL (bad) cholesterol, blood sugar, and body fat. People doing the combined workouts also improved their muscle strength. What this means: it might be equally healthful to replace half of your aerobic workout with strength training, without adding additional exercise time. (For more on how to add strength-based moves to your routine, see "Push past your resistance to strength training," page 198.)

An easier way to do high-intensity interval training

HIIT might be more doable—and fun—if you try it in a pool.

By now, you're probably familiar with high-intensity interval training (HIIT), a popular workout strategy that alternates bursts of strenuous exercise with rest or lower-intensity activity. The technique helps you get fit faster than a traditional moderate-intensity workout. HIIT also produces equal or greater improvements in blood pressure, blood sugar, weight loss, and functional ability (such as walking quickly or getting out of a chair), compared with moderate-intensity exercise.

But what if you have an old sports injury, a chronic disease, or a sedentary lifestyle that makes HIIT seem too challenging? The answer might be to perform the powerhouse workout in a pool.

Aquatic HIIT

An analysis of 18 studies published in 2023 by *BMJ Open Sport & Exercise Medicine* found that people with chronic conditions who took part in high-intensity interval training in the water—called aquatic HIIT or AHIIT—experienced a similar boost in endurance (their maximum sustained physical exertion) as people who took part in land-based HIIT.

Almost 900 people were involved in the studies. Conditions among participants included arthritis, low back pain, lung or heart problems, peripheral artery disease, diabetes, obesity, a history of stroke, and spinal cord injury.

Getting started

While the benefits of AHIIT make it doable for people who are deconditioned or weak, it's still important to talk to your doctor before giving this strenuous workout a try, especially if you have a heart condition.

Once your doctor gives you the green light, take a gradual approach to AHIIT, depending on your current activity levels.

If you're not used to exercising: Work with a physical therapist or personal trainer to ease into an exercise routine, building up to 30-minute workouts on most days of the week. This can be a combination of working out in a pool on some days, and brisk walking on others. "For a pool workout, try leisurely swimming, walking in the pool, jumping up and down, using a kickboard and kicking across the pool, or wearing a flotation device and cycling your legs. Once your endurance improves, probably after two months, you'll be ready for AHIIT," says Brian Simons, a physical therapist and HIIT specialist at Harvard-affiliated Spaulding Rehabilitation Hospital.

If you're already a regular exerciser: Get used to exercising in a pool for a few weeks before trying AHIIT. Simons suggests seeing how well you do in different depths and trying the various pool activities mentioned above.

Diving in

You might find an AHIIT class at your health club or local YMCA. Or you can try an AHIIT program of your own making. Start with a warm-up, such as treading water for a few minutes to get your blood ▸▸

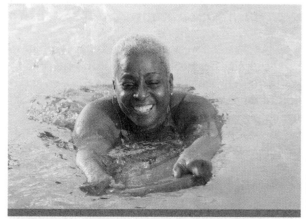

© kali9 | Getty Images

Water workout benefits

Exercising in the water is often easier—and more fun—than exercising on land. One reason is your body's buoyancy in water. "It reduces the load on your bones and muscles. You can move more easily, and you have less fear of falling than you do on land," says Brian Simons, a physical therapist and HIIT specialist at Spaulding Rehabilitation Hospital.

For more on making swimming a part of your exercise routine, check out the Harvard Special Health Report *Aqua Fitness* (www.health.harvard.edu/af).

▶▶ flowing and muscles ready. Then, alternate intervals of intense activity and rest or leisurely activity for a total of 30 minutes. For example:

Swim laps. Alternate periods of gentle swimming (such as swimming one very leisurely lap) with periods of intense swimming (such as swimming one or two laps as fast as you can). Repeat the process for 30 minutes.

Do a circuit. Alternate between periods of rest and a circuit of four or five exercises in a row that you do as fast as you can, for about a minute per exercise. While underwater, "you could jog in place or jump up and down on the floor of the pool, scissor your arms back and forth, scissor your legs back and forth, hang on to the edge of the pool and kick hard, and then rest for a few minutes," says Simons. Repeat the process until you reach 30 minutes.

Gradually increase the length of each high-intensity period. "Ideally, we want the rest break to be shorter than the working period. But if you have a chronic condition limiting your ability, take a longer rest break," says Simons.

If AHIIT still seems too challenging, Simons offers this observation: "I've noticed that people with chronic disease develop a high level of resilience that helps them push harder than other people," says Simons. "So don't be timid. With your doctor's approval, this is something that you can do." ▮

What makes water workouts so worthwhile?

Aquatic exercise is an effective, joint-friendly way to strengthen your cardiovascular system and muscles alike.

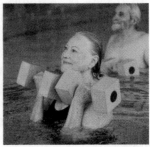
© wundervisuals | Getty Images

Summer's sultry weather often encourages people to spend time in a pool, lake, or ocean. Water can be both refreshing and relaxing—and it's also a great setting for doing a heart-healthy workout, whether that's swimming laps or doing water aerobics.

"Swimming is one of the best forms of cardiovascular exercise," says Dr. Aubrey Grant, a sports cardiology fellow at the Cardiac Performance Laboratory at Harvard-affiliated Massachusetts General Hospital. In fact, water-based exercise offers several unique advantages over aerobic exercise done on land, he notes.

Get into the swim of things

Swimming is a full-body exercise that uses nearly every muscle in your body to propel you forward. And because you're horizontal in the water, blood doesn't pool in your lower body like it does when you're exercising while upright, Dr. Grant explains. That, coupled with the pressure of water on your body (called hydrostatic pressure), increases blood flow from your extremities toward the center of your body and your heart. "This increases the amount of blood your heart pumps per minute, called cardiac output.

Your heart becomes more efficient, which means your heart rate is a little lower during swimming compared with other types of exercise," says Dr. Grant.

Moving your body through water provides far more resistance than moving through air, which means swimming strengthens your muscles and cardiovascular system simultaneously.

Water aerobics advantages

Still, swimming requires a certain amount of coordination and skill. If it doesn't come naturally to you, water aerobics can be a good alternative. Doing water aerobics (also called aquafit and aquarobics) also targets the heart and muscles together.

The simplest version is pool walking or jogging, done in water that's at least waist-deep (the deeper the water, the greater the resistance and effort). Added resistance translates to extra calorie burn compared with land-based exercise. For example, a 150-pound person burns about 250 calories jogging for 30 minutes on land. But jogging in water for 30 minutes burns about 350 calories. You can also do other moves like jumping jacks (see illustration) for a do-it-yourself water workout. For more examples, see the Harvard Special Health Report *Aqua Fitness* (www.health. harvard.edu/af).

An instructor-led class, which is often set to music, can be a nice introduction to water aerobics. To increase resistance and maximize strength gains, you can use equipment like foam dumbbells or paddles. Some classes include interval training, which alternates between lower- and higher-intensity exercises. In addition to those intensive workouts, there are more mellow alternatives that mimic other popular forms of land-based exercise, such as water-based Zumba, yoga, tai chi, and Pilates.

Aquatic therapy

Water can be an ideal setting for people with injuries or health conditions that make other forms of exercise painful or challenging. Aquatic therapy (which may be covered by insurance) features one-on-one exercises with a physical therapist or another licensed professional for a limited number of sessions.

"I see patients who tell me they want to exercise and lose weight, but they're unable to walk because of chronic lower back or knee pain," says Audrey Schmidt, a physical therapist at Harvard-affiliated Spaulding Rehabilitation Hospital. Doing gentle exercises while submerged in water takes stress off your joints, and the water's warm temperature (usually around 90° to 93°F) has a therapeutic effect. The conditions Schmidt treats most often include fibromyalgia, balance problems, and musculoskeletal pain in the lower back, neck, knees, or shoulder. Ideally, aquatic therapy serves as a bridge for people to be able to exercise on their own, says Schmidt, who urges her patients to find a nearby pool so they can maintain and build on their progress. ▼

Exercises to try in the pool

If you enjoy spending time at a pool, consider doing water workouts.

Pools are ideal spots for playing, cooling, and relaxing, and they're also great for exercising. Water resistance makes the heart and muscles work hard. Our buoyancy in water takes pressure off the joints, making movement less painful than it might be on land. And exercising in water always provides a soft landing if you lose your balance. Many people swim laps to take advantage of these benefits. You can also do a series of exercises as you would in a home workout routine.

We've provided some exercises to help get you started on a water workout. You'll find even more in the Harvard Special Health Report *Aqua Fitness* (www.health.harvard.edu/af).

Like any workout, you'll need to do a warm-up beforehand (such as walking in the water), and some stretches afterward (on land).

Keep these tips in mind for the pool exercises in between.

To make an exercise easier: "Go into slightly deeper water, where there's more buoyancy and support," says Jessica Hildebrandt, a physical therapist ▶▶

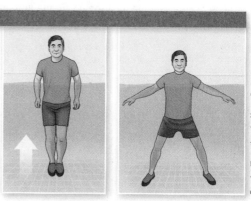

JUMPING JACKS

Stand with your feet together and your arms at your sides. Jump, separating your feet as you raise your arms out to the sides. Keep your hands below the surface. Jump, bringing your feet back together and your arms down to your sides. Repeat as many times as you can in 60 seconds.

Exercise illustrations by Alayna Paquette

▶▶ at Harvard-affiliated Brigham and Women's Hospital, and former competitive swimmer and water polo player.

To make an exercise harder: "Create more resistance: move faster or keep your fingers together like paddles. Or while water walking, hold a kickboard vertically in front of you to create resistance," Hildebrandt says.

To jog without touching the pool bottom: Wear a pool belt in deep water. The belt is a floatation device that lets you move your arms and cycle your feet as if you're jogging through the water.

To avoid soreness: Take it easy at first. "The water supports you, so you feel good and can do more than you're used to. But you can overdo it without realizing it," Hildebrandt says. "Start with easier exercises and shorter durations, or do less than you feel up to. If you're not sore the next day, you'll know it was the right amount of exercise for you. From there you can gradually increase the intensity." ▼

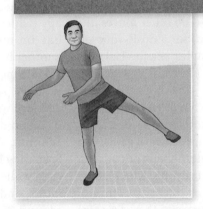

PENDULUM

Stand on your right leg with your left leg lifted out to the side. Extend your arms diagonally down and to the right. Jump off your right foot, swing it out to the side, and land on your left foot, while swinging your arms to the left. Repeat, swinging your arms and legs to the opposite sides. Continue jumping and alternating directions for 60 seconds.

DOUBLE KICKBACKS

Stand up straight with your feet shoulder-width apart and your arms at your sides. Jump up and bend your knees, bringing both feet toward your buttocks. Lower your feet back to the pool bottom. Let your arms swing naturally as you jump. Repeat as many times as you can in 60 seconds.

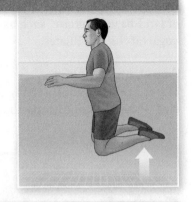

TWISTS

Stand with your feet together and your arms at your sides. Jump, while twisting your upper body to the right and your lower body to the left. Land with your knees, feet, and hips pointing diagonally to the left and your arms, shoulders, and chest pointing diagonally to the right. Jump again, twisting the other way

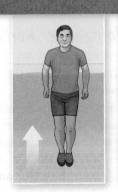 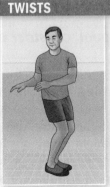 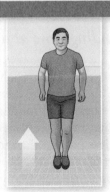 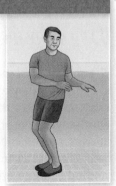

to reverse your landing position. Continue jumping and twisting in alternate directions for 60 seconds.

Power up your walking routine

Bored with looping the neighborhood? Add some kick to your stride.

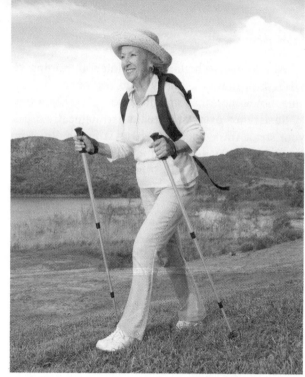
© IPGGutenbergUKLtd | Getty Images

Walking poles and weighted backpacks can boost the intensity of your walk.

Little can soothe us like the sound and feel of our feet hitting the ground, again and again, while we walk. Long the most popular form of movement among American adults, walking gained fresh appeal during the pandemic, when more than two-thirds of physically active adults reported it became their preferred exercise.

Several years downstream, however, maybe those endless loops around the neighborhood or track are feeling a little humdrum. Or maybe you need more than comfort from your walking routine. That's a sign to kick it up a notch, says Dr. Lauren Elson, a physiatrist (a doctor who specializes in physical medicine and rehabilitation) at Harvard-affiliated Spaulding Rehabilitation Network.

There's no question regular walks are better than staying in your chair, but stepping up your regimen can pay off in key ways—even if it just means you stick with it. "We know all the problems associated with sitting that walking counteracts, but anything that's not inspiring can be difficult to keep doing," Dr. Elson says. "There's almost no good reason not to walk."

Pace counts

A wealth of research supports walking's many health benefits, suggesting it improves circulation and heart health, strengthens bones and immune response, helps control weight, and lowers the risk of dementia. But a new analysis suggests it's not just the activity that matters, but the pace.

Published in 2022 by *JAMA Internal Medicine*, the study—which collected health data on more than 78,000 people (average age 61, 55% women) from 2013 to 2015—found that the risk of heart disease, cancer, and premature death dropped by 10% over the following seven years for every 2,000 steps participants logged each day, with the benefit peaking at 10,000 daily steps. But those who walked more briskly—about 80 steps per minute—reaped greater benefits, lowering their health risks more than slower-walking peers.

Walking can still fall short, Dr. Elson says, since it works primarily the legs but not many other muscles or body areas. "Adding a bit of oomph to your walking routine could make it more efficient and add some core strength," she says.

Ways to step it up

With a dash of creativity and flexible thinking, you can easily power up your walking routine. Dr. Elson suggests considering the following strategies:

Walking poles transform a legs-only activity into a full-body workout. There are multiple types, which go by such names as trekking poles and Nordic walking poles. Some are designed with rubber tips to grip the pavement, while others are pointed to add traction on trails. Using them works your arms, back, and shoulders, burning more calories in the process. "Walking poles can prevent stability problems and also help with lower-body discomfort," she says. "And because of that cross-body action, they add a little bit of core strength as well."

High-intensity bursts of speed increase heart rate, breathing, and muscle action for short, defined periods. Try alternating five minutes of your typical walking pace with 30-second intervals of speed walking, skipping, jogging, or sprinting. Repeat as desired. ▸▸

▶▶ Also known as high-intensity interval training, or HIIT, this pattern "definitely improves your cardiovascular fitness more than straight walking," Dr. Elson says.

Resistance exercise "breaks" strategically break your stride while boosting overall strength. Rotating five-minute periods of walking with squats, push-ups, or other resistance exercises "is a great way to not quite do HIIT, but to supplement cardiovascular exercise with strength and power work," she says. These types of activities are best saved for a park or backyard, as they're more difficult to squeeze in on a sidewalk.

Music, podcasts, or books on tape engage your brain while you add to your step count. Cranking up your favorite tunes can motivate you to walk to the beat, and exercise can also seem easier when you're focused on your playlist. Dr. Elson makes her walks perform double duty by listening to audiobooks. "It's a chance to kill two birds with one stone," she says. "If I don't have time to sit and read, I can at least get in some 'reading' while I exercise." Pay extra attention to cars, however.

Weighted backpacks enable you to firm up your leg muscles and give your heart and lungs an extra workout while walking. Fill a well-padded backpack with light weights—between five and 10 pounds to start—of dumbbells, books, or cans. But this tweak should only be attempted by seasoned walkers with no joint or muscle problems, which might be aggravated by the extra load. "Don't start a walking regimen doing this right away," she says. "View this as a higher-intensity option." ▊

Large study finds the sweet spot for daily step goals

Are you a step counter, aiming for 10,000 steps per day to stay healthy? Many studies have suggested you don't need to hit that mark to maintain good health and live longer. And now the largest study to date backs up that theory. The research, published in 2023 by the *European Journal of Preventive Cardiology,* evaluated 17 high-quality studies from around the world, including a total of almost 227,000 people (ages 18 and older) who wore fitness trackers for a week and were then followed for about seven years. Taking at least 3,900 steps per day (not quite two miles) was linked to significantly lower risks of dying from any cause during the study period. A reduction in death specifically from cardiovascular disease appeared with an even smaller number of daily steps—about 2,300. The data also showed that each 1,000-step increment was associated with a 15% decreased risk of dying, and each 500-step increment was tied to a 7% decrease in death from cardiovascular disease. In addition, the findings were consistent across varied climate zones in countries that

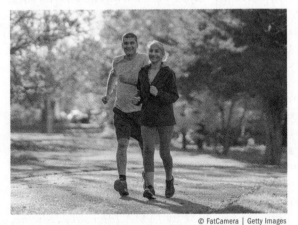

© FatCamera | Getty Images

The sweet spot: just under two miles of walking per day.

included the United States, the United Kingdom, Japan, and Australia. This study was observational and can't prove definitively that the number of steps people took lengthened their lives. But the findings underscore two common health messages: even a little movement makes a difference, and more is better.

Step up your running and walking workouts

Here's how to make your regular sessions more interesting and motivating.

Running and walking are two of the best exercises—not to mention among the easiest to adopt—for almost everyone. But let's face it: they're not always fun, and at times they get downright boring. Sometimes you need a nudge to stay motivated.

How can you put some pep in your steps? Here are some suggestions from Dr. Aaron Baggish, director of the Cardiovascular Performance Program at Harvard-affiliated Massachusetts General Hospital.

Change locations. It's easy to get into a rut when you cover the same ground over and over. Explore different locations and even commit to trying a new route once a week or once a month. "There are loads of websites and apps that map popular routes for runners and walkers with a variety of distances and types of terrain and scenery," says Dr. Baggish.

Tweak your regular route. Even making minor changes to your usual routine can be stimulating. For instance, go at an earlier or later time, or walk or run in the opposite direction.

Enlist a workout buddy. If it has become easier to blow off workouts, invite someone to join you. "We are 10 times more likely to commit to a workout if we know someone is waiting, as we don't want to disappoint them," says Dr. Baggish.

Join a running or walking club. Besides offering another way to show accountability, clubs offer organized group runs and walks where you can work out with others at your same level. Inquire about such clubs at your local specialty running store or senior community center.

Set regular goals. "People who choose small, incremental, achievable goals and write them down are more likely to get them done," says Dr. Baggish. For example, focus on covering a certain number of miles per week or month or gradually increasing your speed or distance for each workout. "Signing up for a 5K race or similar event also can be a useful carrot," says Dr. Baggish. "You will more likely follow through because you don't want to waste your entry fee."

Race against yourself. A self-challenge is also a great motivator. Try this: Time how long it takes to walk or run for a specific distance, like a mile around your neighborhood or local track. Then try to meet or beat that number. When you have achieved it, reset the challenge and start anew.

Create a cue. If you need help sticking to a routine, schedule your run or walk around a regularly scheduled activity, like when you first get up in the morning or before lunch or dinner. "Many daily habits are created when something signals you to do them," says Dr. Baggish

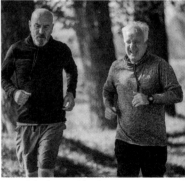

© South_agency | Getty Imagess

Enlisting an exercise buddy can help both of you stay motivated and committed to regular workouts.

Listen to an audiobook. Make a rule that you can listen to an audiobook only during your outing. Always keep the volume low and use only one earbud, so you remain alert for trouble in your surroundings.

Combine running and walking. Devote a regular outing to a run/walk routine. For runners, it helps break up the intensity by offering a brief recovery period, which may help you run farther with less struggle. For walkers, it's a great way to increase cardio output.

For example, run for one to two minutes and then walk for four to five minutes until you fully recover. (Walkers would speed walk for one to two minutes and then walk at a normal or slower pace for the recovery.) Repeat the pattern five times or until you have covered your usual workout time or distance. Adjust the times to make it easier or more challenging.

Take exercise "breaks." Break up your regular routine with two minutes or so of body-weight exercises. Stop and do 10 squats, walking lunges, or push-ups (on the ground or against a tree or bench).

Treat yourself. Accessories can make you feel confident. Invest in new workout shirts, shorts, hats, shoes. Treat yourself to a new water bottle, or upgrade to a hydration pack that carries water in a rubber bladder and offers handy pockets for snacks, phone, and keys.

Walkers also can try using walking poles, which are available with pointed tips for trails or rubber tips for sidewalks. They come in fixed or adjustable heights and are readily available online, as are videos on how to use them.

Putting your best feet forward

Here's how to treat and prevent common foot ailments.

A person who lives to age 80 may walk an estimated 110,000 miles, equivalent to more than four times around the Earth at the equator. That long journey can take a toll on your feet.

"Aging can affect all areas of the body, but the foot is particularly vulnerable, as it's home to so many bones, muscles, and joints," says orthopedic foot and ankle surgeon Dr. Chris Chiodo, who, with podiatrist Dr. Joseph Hartigan, served as medical co-editor of the Harvard Special Health Report *Healthy Feet: Preventing and treating common foot problems.*

In addition, older adults also are subject to natural foot changes, as feet widen and arches collapse. "All of this can increase the risks for foot problems that prevent many older adults from staying active and healthy," says Dr. Chiodo.

Proper foot care and maintenance can help avoid everyday problems and keep your feet strong and healthy as you age (see "Check your feet," page 209). However, some foot ailments common among older adults require special attention.

Plantar fasciitis

The plantar fascia (the ligament on the bottom of the foot) can become inflamed, leading to sharp heel pain called plantar fasciitis. It tends to occur if you overdo high-impact exercise or wear poor-fitting or poorly padded shoes. The pain is often most intense when you first get out of bed in the morning.

Plantar fasciitis often goes away on its own, although it can last for many weeks. To ease symptoms, apply ice to the painful area and take an over-the-counter anti-inflammatory pain reliever, such as ibuprofen (Advil) or naproxen (Aleve), as needed. In addition, use a gel insert that supports the arch and cushions the heel.

Gentle stretches can also help. Sit in a chair with one foot on the floor and the other ankle on your knee. Grasp the toes of the raised foot with your hand and gently pull them back until you feel a stretch in the foot's sole. At the same time, gently massage the stretched plantar fascia with your other hand. Hold for 10 seconds. Do this 10 times on each foot, three times per day. If you continue to have pain or discomfort after six weeks, see your primary care clinician or a podiatrist.

Flat feet

Flat feet occur when tendons, ligaments, and soft tissues that support the arches lose their elasticity, weakening the arch

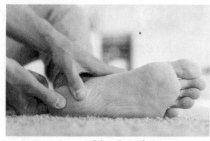

© Dima Berlin | Getty Images

Foot-related issues can keep you from staying physically active.

until the sole of the foot comes in contact with the ground or close to it. While this is often the result of many years on your feet, it also may run in your family.

Flat feet can make your feet tire easily and cause painful arches. The inner sides and bottoms of your feet can become swollen or develop bony prominences. You could also experience back or leg pain as your body compensates for the pain of standing or walking.

To see if you have flat feet, wet your feet, stand on a flat surface that shows your footprint (like concrete), and examine your footprint. Flat feet typically reveal an outline of the entire bottom of the foot. Flat feet are not preventable, particularly when there's a family history. If the problem is caused by aging, there are ways to support your arches and keep the problem from worsening.

"Using over-the-counter or custom orthotic inserts and good supportive shoes, or even molded braces, can provide extra arch support," says Dr. Hartigan. You may also reduce the pressure and load on your arches by performing calf muscle stretches. In addition, monitor your activities to determine when you most often experience arch pain. You may have to limit higher-impact or repetitive movements and switch to lower-impact exercise, like walking or cycling instead of running or hiking.

Osteoarthritis

Osteoarthritis is one of the most common diseases affecting adults ages 65 and older. Although the hips, knees, hands, and spine are more common sites for arthritis, your ankles and feet are also vulnerable due to their many bones and joints. "While age can increase the risk of osteoarthritis, people who have had repeated ankle sprains also may develop arthritis in their feet as they get older," says Dr. Chiodo.

Osteoarthritis can't be reversed, so the best approach is to manage the condition. Topical pain relievers (such as lidocaine-containing products) and anti-inflammatory agents like diclofenac (Voltaren gel) are effective. Or you might get more relief with an oral over-the-counter or prescription drug. Using orthotic inserts and arch supports can also help.

For more severe flare-ups, your doctor may suggest a corticosteroid injection to reduce inflammation and pain. Injections sometimes provide months of pain relief, even though they do not work for everyone. If these treatment options don't help and the pain becomes severe enough to cause disability, surgery may be offered. Depending on the location and type of osteoarthritis, the surgery may involve removing loose cartilage and inflamed tissues around the diseased joint(s) or even realigning, fusing, or replacing the joints in certain circumstances. ▼

Check your feet

Do a thorough foot check every week. Examine the tops and soles of your feet, the spaces between the toes, and the toenails. Newly formed calluses, blisters, and wounds suggest you may need updated footwear. (Get a professional fitting from a specialty running store to ensure proper shoe size and arch support.) Thick, discolored, or spotty toenails could indicate a fungus that may be treated with an over-the-counter remedy or, in severe cases, a prescription drug. Foot swelling or color changes could indicate poor circulation or even a fracture that requires immediate medical attention.

IN THE JOURNALS

Will walking faster reduce your diabetes risk?

A study published in 2023 by the *British Journal of Sports Medicine* suggests that picking up the pace of your daily walk—the faster, the better—is linked to a lower risk of developing diabetes. Researchers pooled the data of 10 studies from the past two decades, representing more than 508,000 adults (most of them middle-aged) from around the world. Participants were followed for three to 11 years. Compared with "casual" walking (at less than 2 mph), walking 2 mph to 3 mph (brisk walking) was associated with a 15% lower risk of diabetes, no matter how long people walked each day. Walking 3 mph to 4 mph was associated with a 24% lower diabetes risk. And going faster than 4 mph was tied to a 39% lower diabetes risk. The study was observational and doesn't prove conclusively that lively stepping keeps you from getting diabetes. But we already know that brisk walking, like any aerobic activity that works your heart and lungs, helps you control blood sugar levels, weight, and cardiovascular health, which are all important for avoiding diabetes and many other chronic diseases.

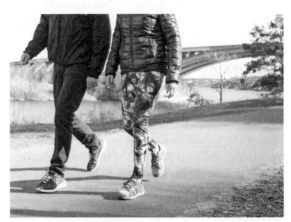

© Maskot | Getty Images

The right shoe for walking and running

Here's how to choose the proper footwear for your activity.

Walking and running are the most accessible types of exercise; the only equipment you really need is a good pair of shoes. But not just any footwear will do.

"While walking and running share similar movements, how your foot is supported differs, which is why most walking and running shoes are designed differently," says Dr. Adam Tenforde, director of the Running Medicine Program at Harvard-affiliated Spaulding Rehabilitation Hospital.

Taking steps

Walking involves less stress on the feet than running, absorbing about 1.5 times a person's body weight with each step compared with three times for running. When walking, your heels hit the ground first before your foot rolls forward to begin the next step. Because of this rolling motion, walking shoes are designed to have soft, flexible soles, which help you push off with each step. Also, because the heel strikes the ground first when you walk, walking shoes have an angled heel to absorb most of the shock and reduce pressure on the ankles.

In comparison, a runner's feet strike anywhere from the heel to the midfoot or forefoot. Therefore, running shoes are designed to have thicker soles that act as shock absorbers. They are also lighter than walking shoes to help with fatigue over longer distances. "Because of these differences, ideally running shoes can be used for walking, but you should not run in walking shoes," says Dr. Tenforde.

Proper protection

The right shoe for your activity can help you avoid foot and ankle pain. For example, plantar fasciitis, also known as heel pain, is caused by inflammation of the fibrous band of tissue on the bottom of the foot. Achilles tendinitis—inflammation of the tendon connecting the calf muscle to the heel—causes pain above the heel or along the back of the leg.

Proper footwear can also protect against knee pain. "Footwear can contribute to changes in your mechanics, and some shoes may cause pain,

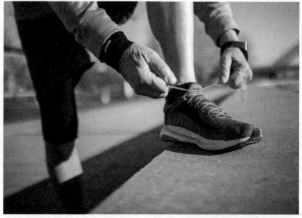

© Zorica Nastasic | Getty Images

Walking and running shoes are designed to support different kinds of foot movements.

suggesting these shoes place extra stress on your knees," says Dr. Tenforde.

Remember that while the right shoes can protect against pain and injury, they can't fix existing problems. "If you have any type of foot pain or impairment that makes walking or running uncomfortable, consult a physician or physical therapist to properly address the issue," says Dr. Tenforde. "Changing shoes won't help."

Get fitted

Because feet come in so many shapes and sizes, it's impossible to recommend a specific walking or running shoe that suits everyone. (Some people, though, may benefit from minimalist shoes; see "The big impact of minimalist shoes.") Still, you should follow some basic guidelines for shoe shopping and wearing. For example:

▸ Visit a specialty running store, as it will offer a variety of styles and have hands-on fitting experts.
▸ Have your arch and gait evaluated to find out whether your foot rolls inward (pronation), rolls outward (supination), or stays neutral. Many running stores provide this service.
▸ Feet tend to expand during the day, so shop in the early evening when your feet are at their largest.
▸ Bring your own socks. The thickness of your socks will affect how your shoes fit, so wear ones you like when trying on shoes. (When walking or running, always wear synthetic or cotton-synthetic blends to wick away moisture.)

- Your athletic shoes will usually need to be a half-size larger than your regular shoes to accommodate any swelling during activity.
- Bring along any orthotics or other shoe inserts you usually use. Many shoe brands do not accommodate them, so you may need to go up an additional half-size.
- Feet naturally widen with age, so make sure your shoes have adequate width. To do so, remove the shoe's insole and step on it. If your foot goes over the edges, the shoe is too narrow.
- There should be some wiggle room in a shoe's toe box. Aim for about a half-inch (or one finger's width) between your longest toe and the front of the shoe.
- Test a shoe's flexibility. Grab the toe and heel of a shoe and pull them toward each other. The shoe should bend easily at the ball of the foot. Flexibility offers a greater range of motion and an easier push-off.
- Shoes should feel right when you step into them and not need to be "broken in."
- Experts recommend replacing shoes every 300 to 500 miles. Walking or running for 30 minutes daily, five days a week, translates to a new pair every six to 12 months. ♥

The big impact of minimalist shoes

One popular type of walking and running shoe is called the minimalist shoe, which more closely mimics how people naturally walk or run barefoot. They're characterized by minimal cushioning in the midsoles and heel. "Less cushioning and a lower heel-to-toe drop may encourage you to land more on your midfoot or forefoot rather than your heel," says Dr. Adam Tenforde, director of the Running Medicine Program at Spaulding Rehabilitation Hospital. A 2021 study published in *Scientific Reports* found that people who wore this type of shoe daily for six months improved the strength of their foot muscles. Minimalist shoes also may help reduce the risk for knee and foot pain and improve balance. They are not suitable for everyone, such as people with peripheral artery disease or diabetic neuropathy. If you'd like to give them a try, Dr. Tenforde suggests easing into the shoes. "Wear them around the house for short periods and see how your feet feel," he says. "Then increase the duration and do your usual walk or run in them, and re-evaluate."

Yoga skepticism

Resisting yoga's pull? Consider bending your beliefs.

Yoga pants. Yoga mats. Yoga bolsters, blocks, and straps. You'd be forgiven if the first things you think of when contemplating yoga are the accessories it seems to require—or pervasive images suggesting people devoted to the ancient practice are all slender, flexible, and preternaturally zen.

None of it is imperative, however—neither the equipment nor the image. So if you've held back from trying yoga for these reasons, you may want to reconsider, says Dr. Darshan Mehta, medical director of the Benson-Henry Institute for Mind Body Medicine at Harvard-affiliated Massachusetts General Hospital.

"People think they have to be super-flexible and thin to do it, and that's just not true," Dr. Mehta says. "I also don't think people realize how many varieties of yoga can be adapted to the individual." (See "Which yoga style suits you?" on page 212.)

Yoga offers broad benefits

More than 300 million people worldwide practice yoga, which originated in India more than 5,000 years ago. In the United States, the number reached 38 million in 2022—1.7 million more than just six years earlier—and 74% are women, according to a 2022 global survey by the nonprofit Yoga Alliance.

But despite its growing popularity, a slice of humanity remains yoga skeptics. What stops people from trying it? Yoga seems too "touchy-feely" for certain ▶▶

folks, Dr. Mehta says, while others may erroneously believe its spiritual origins conflict with their own religion or faith tradition. Yet more feel it's too costly, once classes and gear are factored in.

But the pluses outweigh any perceived drawbacks, Dr. Mehta says. Scads of recent studies indicate yoga is a boon for physical and mental health, easing depression, boosting sleep quality, improving chronic pain, and reducing cardiovascular disease risks by lowering blood pressure and blood sugar levels. As they reap these advantages, some practitioners are also motivated to reach for other wellness goals, such as drinking less alcohol, eating more fruits and vegetables, and quitting smoking, according to the National Center for Complementary and Integrative Health.

"Well into the thousands of studies support yoga's benefits," Dr. Mehta says. "There's a whole host of medical conditions where yoga has been shown to be helpful."

Plunging in

If you're still reluctant to try yoga, Dr. Mehta offers several suggestions to overcome any misgivings:

Join a class. It shouldn't be difficult to find one, since essentially "every single fitness studio or gym has yoga classes now," he says. In-person is preferable to online formats so the teacher can guide you through your first poses. "Just like any activity, if you don't have proper guidance, you can get hurt," he says.

Take a friend along. It will be easier to dip your toe in if you do your first yoga postures alongside a buddy. Plus, "people like being in community with others," Dr. Mehta says. "There's a group effect."

Ask for modifications. If you have physical limitations, such as pain or joint problems, ask your teacher to help you modify poses to accommodate them. You may also want to try what's often called chair yoga, in which you stay seated or use a chair for balance.

Be patient with yourself. It's okay if your poses don't immediately resemble those done by longtime practitioners. "One of the things that's so beautiful about yoga," Dr. Mehta says, "is it allows you to understand the edges of yourself—how you can gently push yourself but not overdo it." ▾

Which yoga style suits you?

Yoga isn't a monolith. Indeed, the practice is as flexible as we try to become when practicing its poses, or asanas. Some yoga approaches are more soothing and others more physically demanding. Here are six of the most common yoga styles:

Ashtanga requires strength and endurance, making it ideal for experienced yoga fans.

Hot yoga is ideal for building flexibility. It's practiced in humid rooms generally heated to about 90 degrees, though temps can vary by style and studio (Bikram yoga, for example, is practiced at 104 degrees). But the high temperatures may be dangerous for people with certain conditions or taking certain medications, so check with your doctor before taking any hot yoga class.

Hatha combines basic poses with simple breathing techniques and is considered more relaxing.

Iyengar often integrates props such as blocks or straps to help you get into poses. The precision focus helps to

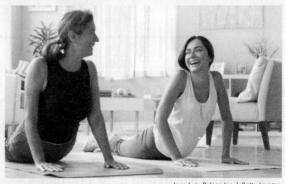

Jose Luis Pelaez Inc | Getty Images

Doing yoga with a friend makes it easier to start the practice.

strengthen key muscles that support joints, making it a good choice if you have injuries or pain issues

Kundalini offers a more spiritual experience, emphasizing chanting and breathing.

Vinyasa is more fast-paced and requires continuous movement. It's a good option if you hope to gain cardio benefits from yoga.

Do more for your core

A strong core is vital to staying active. Here are three exercises that can help keep it in shape.

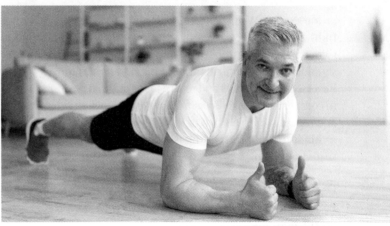

© Prostock-Studio | Getty Images

The plank pose is one of the best exercises for strengthening most core muscles.

Practically every move you make originates from one area of your body: your core.

When you mention the core, most people think of the "six-pack" of abs, a muscle called the rectus abdominis. But the core is made up of abdominal, pelvic, and back muscles.

Beside the rectus abdominis, the other main muscles include the external abdominal obliques, located on the side and front of your abdomen, and the internal abdominal obliques, which lie under the external obliques. A deeper layer called the transverse abdominis lies under the obliques and attaches to your spine.

"The core is vital for your body, as it serves as the foundation for upper- and lower-body movements," says Shawn Pedicini, a physical therapist with Harvard-affiliated Spaulding Rehabilitation Hospital. "Your core musculature must have a good combination of endurance, stability, and power for many activities."

Everyday moves

Your core is in action every day. For example, when you take a walk, your core muscles provide the support and endurance to maintain a healthy posture. Core strength allows you to transfer power during rotational movements, like swinging a golf club or tennis racket. Your core also generates stability around your spine to prevent back injuries, like when you lift and carry heavy objects.

In addition, core strength is essential for preventing falls. "Our bodies constantly have to adapt to ever-changing surfaces and environments," says Pedicini. "Adequate core stability and strength can assist you in reacting to sudden changes and prevent falls."

Strengthen weak muscles

Like any other muscles, your core muscles weaken with age. A sedentary lifestyle can also cause a person to lose core muscle strength faster over time compared with an active individual. "This is why it's important to maintain exercise habits as you age and give regular attention to building and maintaining core strength," says Pedicini.

He suggests doing core exercises two to four times per week. "Include them in your regular workouts," he says, "or perform them independently." And always get approval from your doctor, a physical therapist or a certified personal trainer if you have any physical limitations or health issues related to doing these movements.

The best core exercises are movements that activate many core muscles at one time. Here are three exercises to do just that.

Plank

To get into the starting position, kneel on all fours with your hands and knees directly aligned under your shoulders and hips.

Movement: Tighten your abdominal muscles and lower your upper body onto your forearms, clasping your hands together and aligning your shoulders directly over your elbows. Extend both legs with your feet flexed and toes touching the floor so that you balance your body in a line like a plank. Hold. This is one rep. Aim to hold for 30 to 60 seconds, doing as many reps as needed to reach that total. For example, if you can hold a plank for 15 seconds, you would do four reps.

Modifications: Do the exercise with straight arms (harder) or while leaning against a counter or table at a 45° angle (easier).

Diagonal chops

Stand and hold a lightweight medicine ball or dumbbell by your right side with both hands.   ▶▶

Movement: While keeping your abdominal muscles tight and your feet grounded, twist at the waist and swing the ball or dumbbell up until it's just past your left shoulder. Only your arms and midsection should move. Reverse the movement and return to the original position to complete one rep. Repeat five to 10 times, switch sides, and repeat. Complete two or three sets on each side.

Modification: If standing is a challenge, do this in a seated position.

Deadbugs

For this floor exercise, lie on your back with your feet off the floor and knees bent at 90°. Extend your arms toward the ceiling with your hands directly above your shoulders. Squeeze your abdominal muscles and maintain this tension throughout the movement.

Movement: Extend your right leg, holding it six inches above the floor, while at the same time you lower your left arm, extending it over your head, parallel to the floor. Pause and return to the starting position. Repeat with the opposite arm and leg to complete one rep. Do 10 reps to complete one set. Rest and then repeat the movements to complete two or three sets.

Modification: Make the movements less challenging by not lowering your arm and leg as close to the floor. ◗

Stay safe playing pickleball

How to avoid injuries playing America's fastest-growing sport.

Pickleball continues to skyrocket in popularity. According to the Sports and Fitness Industry Association, the number of pickleball players in the United States increased from 3.5 million in 2019 to 8.9 million in 2022, a 154% surge.

"Unfortunately, more playing leads to a higher incidence of injuries, especially among older adults," says Linda Murray, an orthopedic clinical specialist with Harvard-affiliated Spaulding Outpatient Center Malden. In fact, a study published in 2021 in *Injury Epidemiology* found that more than 85% of pickleball injuries involved players ages 60 and older.

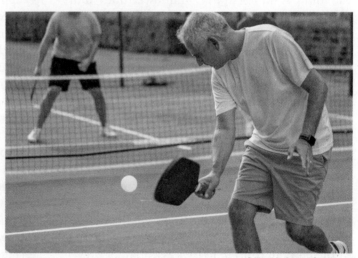
© Visual Art Agency | Getty Images
Pickleball injuries in the lower body are more common among men.

Types of injuries

Because pickleball uses a lighter ball that needs less force and requires no overhead shots, it rarely causes shoulder injuries like those common to other racquet sports.

"With pickleball, most injuries are strains and sprains in the legs and knees," says Murray. "And research has found that men are 3.5 times more likely than women to have these types of injuries." The wrist is another common site of injury, with sprains and fractures caused by falls.

Pickleball injury prevention is threefold: performing lower-body strength exercises at least twice a week, doing a dynamic warm-up before playing, and working on agility and balance. Here's a look at each.

Lower-body exercises

Murray recommends squats, lunges, and heel raises. "They target all major muscle groups in the legs and incorporate movements that you would be performing while playing pickleball," she says. "Plus, you can do them at home using body weight or light dumbbells."

Squat. "Squats use multiple muscle groups at the same time," says Murray. "Although you may seldom perform a full squat on the court, you want to strengthen and tone your leg muscles through a greater range of motion. This will enhance leg power, improve mobility, and reduce joint stiffness and tendon injury."

Lunges. Lunges work the muscles in the thighs and buttocks. There are numerous variations of lunges—reverse, forward, side—that can train your muscles and joints to function in all directions. "Lunges also challenge your balance and leg strength," says Murray. "This is a powerful training approach for pickleball, as it will enhance your ability to get to the ball no matter which direction it's moving."

Heel raises. This exercise helps build calf muscles. Pickleball courts are smaller than other racquet-sport courts, and there is much less long sprinting involved, especially when you play doubles. "Instead, you need quick foot action and the ability to lunge for the ball, which requires power from calf muscles," says Murray.

Warming up right

Performing a dynamic warm-up before playing can cut down on injuries.

"Warming up increases heart rate, loosens up joints, and increases blood flow to your muscles," says Murray. "Priming your muscles with a good warm-up will get your body ready for the explosive movements of the sport." Do each of the following 10 times before stepping on the court: squats, forward lunges, side lunges, arm circles, and jumping jacks.

Agility and balance

For improving agility and balance, Murray recommends carioca exercises. Carioca is the Portuguese name for anything related to Rio de Janeiro, Brazil. The exercises are called carioca because they resemble the Brazilian samba dance. "Carioca exercises activate

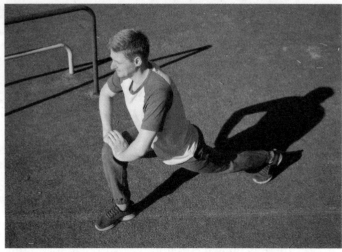

© AIDa.team | Getty Images

Lunges offer a deep stretch, improving flexibility and balance, and bolster strength in the legs.

the muscles in our hips, knees, and ankles in a way that will prepare your body for the quick directional changes and lateral movements required of pickleball," says Murray. There are different variations of carioca. One that she suggests for beginners is carioca walking. It works like this:

1. Start with your feet hip-width apart, knees and arms slightly bent.

2. Push off with your right foot and cross your right foot behind your left foot, touching it to the ground.

3. Next, step with your left foot to the side so your legs are uncrossed and you're back in the starting position, with your feet hip-width apart.

4. Push off again with your right foot, and this time cross your right foot in front of your left, touching it to the ground.

5. Step again with your left foot to the side so you're again back in the starting position.

6. Repeat this cross-cross motion with your feet, gradually increasing the tempo as you feel comfortable, moving to the left for a specified distance or number of steps.

7. Reverse direction, moving to the right until you reach the starting point. Repeat the sequence two times. ◗

by **HOWARD LeWINE, M.D.,** Editor in Chief, *Harvard Men's Health Watch*

What is considered a healthy body fat percentage as you age?

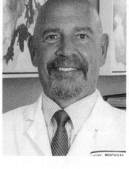

Q *I had a body fat measurement done at my gym. The reading was 17% body fat. I am 62, and aside from high blood pressure, I consider myself healthy. Is that a good reading? What is the best way to measure body fat?*

A There is no agreed-upon normal range for body fat, just as there is no ideal body weight. According to the World Health Organization, men ages 40 to 59 should aim for 11% to 21% body fat and women of the same age should aim for 23% to 33% body fat, while for men ages 60 to 79, the range is 13% to 24%, and for women of the same age, 24% to 35%. However, the "right" weight and fat percentage for an individual depend upon multiple factors, such as the following:

General health. A very low percentage of body fat and low body weight in someone not exercising regularly can indicate a medical problem.

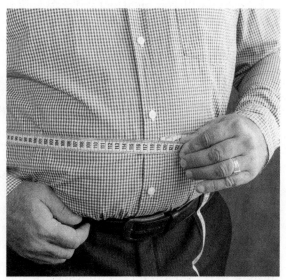

© Olga Trofimova | Getty Images

Comparing the sizes of your waist and hips reflects how much fat you have inside your belly.

Distribution of body fat. Even if your weight is close to the normal range, a large waist size may mean you have an unhealthy amount of belly fat (visceral fat). Higher amounts of belly fat increase the risk of diabetes and heart disease.

Metabolism. How an individual's body handles excess calories significantly affects whether those calories get deposited in fat or turn into energy used for physical activity and body heat.

Amount, type, and intensity of physical activity. You not only burn calories during exercise, but also continue to burn calories afterward as muscles replenish their energy stores. In addition, regular strength training can add a bit of muscle weight that is healthy.

Rather than relying on just one measurement to assess your body composition, I suggest using one or both of these measurements:

Waist size. There is no consensus on normal for this measurement either. Generally, men should strive for a waist size of no more than 36 inches. For men under six feet tall, I like to use a ratio of waist size to height: waist size should be less than one-half of your height.

Ratio of waist size to hip size. This is another way to evaluate waist size. Use a measuring tape to find your waist size just above your belly button. Then measure the size of your hips around the widest part of your buttocks. Divide the waist size by the hip size. The goal waist-to-hip ratio for men is no more than 0.9.

Both numerical waist size and waist-to-hip ratio offer a window into whether you are carrying too much dangerous visceral fat.

Chapter 9

Women's Health

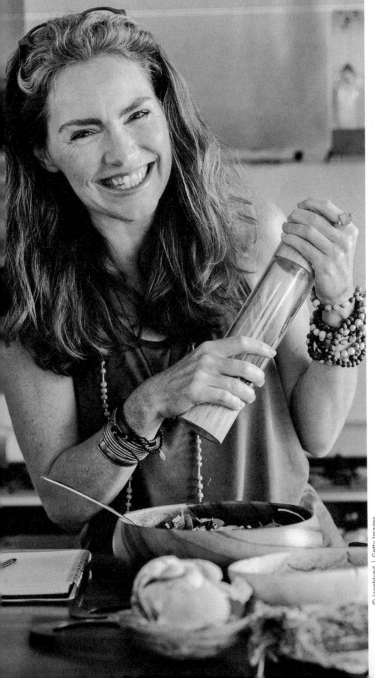

© jacoblund | Getty Images

Healthy Habits!
5 Things You Can Do Now

1 **Tackle hot flashes.** Among other treatment options, a first-of-its-kind drug can significantly reduce this hallmark symptom of menopause. (page 218)

2 **Check your protein intake.** Needs change as we age. Make sure you're getting enough. (page 223)

3 **Eat more magnesium-rich foods.** Nuts, seeds, whole grains, legumes, and leafy green vegetables are linked to brain health. (page 230)

4 **Consider your alcohol intake.** Do you really need that drink? (page 235)

5 **Ask for help.** If you're a caregiver, it's easy to neglect yourself—but assistance is available. (page 238)

New help for hot flashes

A daily pill joins a variety of nonhormonal options to treat menopause's highly disruptive hallmark symptom.

"Do you have your private summers?" In generations past, women knew exactly what this question alluded to: menopausal hot flashes and night sweats far more awful than their alluring "private summers" nickname would suggest.

Yet there's nothing singular about this phenomenon, known medically as vasomotor symptoms. Hot flashes and their nighttime iteration, night sweats, affect an estimated 80% of women and last an average of seven to nine years. For a third, these bursts of intense warmth, sweating, and flushing last more than a decade, according to the Menopause Society.

Hot flashes are also the symptom women in the menopause transition most often talk about and seek treatment for, Harvard experts say. That's why they're hailing a new nonhormonal medication designed specifically for hot flash relief as a game-changing advance.

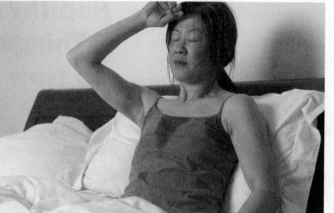

Hot flashes can make sleep elusive.

© Peter Dazeley | Getty Images

"Hot flashes are certainly in the top five symptoms women bring up in my office multiple times a day, every day," says Dr. Tara Iyer, who heads the Menopause and Midlife Clinic at Harvard-affiliated Brigham and Women's Hospital. "I see the entire spectrum, ranging from the mild end all the way to women who are debilitated by them and can't get anything done. Some even consider quitting their jobs and going on disability."

Indeed, the workplace toll of vasomotor symptoms only adds to the drag on sleep, mood, and thinking skills. Menopause symptoms cost American women about $1.8 billion each year in lost work time, according to a 2023 study.

"Getting hot flashes in the middle of an important task can really throw off a woman's concentration," Dr. Iyer says. "You can't really think about anything else but how you're burning up from the inside."

Cracking the code of hot flashes

The first-of-its-kind daily pill, fezolinetant (Veozah), was approved by the FDA in May 2023 for moderate-to-severe vasomotor symptoms from menopause. It works by targeting so-called KNDy (pronounced "candy") neurons—which regulate body temperature—in the brain's hypothalamus. Fezolinetant blocks these nerve cells when dips in estrogen cause them to behave erratically, triggering hot flashes.

The pill performed well in clinical trials, reducing vasomotor symptoms by 60%, says Dr. Jan Shifren, director of the Midlife Women's Health Center at Harvard-affiliated Massachusetts General Hospital.

"The reason this feels like such a game changer—and it's so exciting from a scientific standpoint—is that up until now we had this universal phenomenon going on for millennia and yet we still didn't know why it happened," Dr. Shifren says. "This drug was developed because we've finally figured out the basic biology of hot flashes."

Like nearly every drug, fezolinetant comes with a few caveats. It may cause mild side effects such as belly pain, diarrhea, or insomnia. Additionally, women need to have blood tests to check for liver damage before taking it. The tests are then repeated three more times at three-month intervals.

Fezolinetant is also costly: an estimated $550 for a 30-day supply. Since it's new, insurance coverage may vary. But the medication still represents great progress, Dr. Iyer says. "Frankly, we don't have enough nonhormonal options for hot flashes," she says, "and it's an area in which we've been failing women for a long time."

Hormone therapy alternative

Hormone therapy is still considered the gold standard for treating vasomotor symptoms, since it replenishes diminished estrogen levels and can help control other menopause symptoms as well.

Generally, hormone therapy is considered safe for healthy women under 60 who are within 10 years of their final menstrual period, Harvard experts say. But some women can't take estrogen or don't want to. Those who shouldn't include women who've had breast cancer or certain other cancers, blood clots, heart attack or stroke, unexplained vaginal bleeding, or liver disease.

"For women who choose not to take hormones, have not done well on them in the past, or can't because of a medical reason, this new drug is very exciting," Dr. Iyer says. "The more tools we have in our toolbox, the better."

Other choices

Fezolinetant joins a variety of other nonhormonal medications that have long been prescribed for hot flashes. But there's a key difference: fezolinetant is designed specifically for this use, while the rest are primarily meant to treat other conditions and prescribed off-label to lessen hot flash frequency and severity. They may also lead to troublesome side effects.

In June 2023, the Menopause Society updated its recommendations regarding nonhormonal hot flash remedies for the first time in eight years. In addition to fezolinetant, the group said these three options are also effective:

Selective serotonin reuptake inhibitors (SSRIs). These antidepressants, especially paroxetine (Paxil), have been a mainstay of treatment for women who opt not to take hormone therapy. "They may be effective in reducing hot flashes, but might cause weight gain or ▸▸

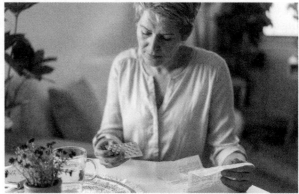

© Vladimir Vladimirov | Getty Images

A variety of medications can tackle hot flashes.

Lifestyle measures can also turn down the heat

While medications can tamp down hot flashes and night sweats, they're not the only game in town. Certain lifestyle measures can also spell relief.

In newly updated 2023 recommendations on nonhormonal interventions, the Menopause Society pointed to three evidence-backed options. Harvard experts explain why they appear effective.

Weight loss. "Data show that women who are at a healthier body mass index will be less bothered by hot flashes than women who aren't," says Dr. Jan Shifren, director of the Midlife Women's Health Center at Massachusetts General Hospital.

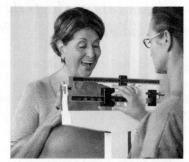

© Terry Vine | Getty Images

Maintaining a healthy body weight can help keep hot flashes at bay.

Cognitive behavioral therapy (CBT) and hypnosis. Scientists aren't certain why these mind-body approaches help ease hot flashes, but research shows a consistent benefit from each. "Vasomotor symptoms start in the brain, so it's not surprising that CBT and hypnosis have effects on brain activity," Dr. Shifren says. "We certainly know they can lower our heart rate and stress responses. And they're safe."

Dietary tweaks for hot flash relief aren't backed by science, according to the Menopause Society. But Harvard experts say each woman's own experience counts more. If you've noticed your hot flashes or night sweats flare after a glass of wine, a sugary treat, or a caffeinated drink, avoid that trigger.

"People feel so helpless when hot flashes happen," Dr. Shifren says. "Anything that makes you feel more empowered, regardless of the data, is a good thing."

▶▶ sexual dysfunction," Dr. Iyer says. "We may be helping some things and hurting others."

Oxybutynin (Oxytrol), which is typically prescribed for overactive bladder.

Gabapentin (Neurontin). This drug is usually prescribed for seizures or nerve pain. One of its side effects "is sleepiness, which is a real benefit for women with insomnia," Dr. Shifren says.

Aside from side effects, another possible downside of these nonhormonal drugs is that two or more are often needed to reduce hot flash frequency or severity. "Certainly we have options, but they're far from ideal," Dr. Iyer says. "With a condition such as menopause that can cause 40-plus symptoms, we have to be careful not to provoke new ones or cause some symptoms to be worse."

Seeking help

If you're interested in nonhormonal hot flash relief, Harvard experts offer this guidance:

Be bold. If your vasomotor symptoms are truly disruptive, make sure you tell your clinician and advocate for treatment. "Really, you should be the one to decide if your symptoms are bothersome—the clinician can't decide that for you," Dr. Shifren says.

Consider your other symptoms. Certain medications may seem more appropriate if hot flashes aren't your only issue. "If you're also dealing with symptoms of depression or anxiety, SSRIs could take care of both issues," Dr. Shifren says. "If you've got overactive bladder, oxybutynin could help. And if you're sleep-deprived, gabapentin can make a difference." ▌

Menopause marketing: Hype vs. truth

Some skin care products claim to meet women's specific midlife needs. But is it just smoke and mirrors?

Nestled just inches apart in the cosmetics section of a big-box retailer are two little pots of night cream, both made by the same manufacturer. One label is magenta, the other teal. "Wake up to skin that looks refreshed and less tired," promises the magenta version, labeled "menopause skin care." Meanwhile, the teal-clad "advanced overnight cream"—presumably meant for everyone else—pledges that "fine lines and wrinkles [will] appear visibly reduced."

A closer look reveals both night creams contain nearly identical active ingredients. But the menopause edition costs $5 more for the same amount—25% more than the standard anti-aging version. So what's the real difference? Aside from labeling and price, not much—meaning skin care brands may be quietly fleecing women at a vulnerable point, when worries over changing looks and vitality merge with hot flashes and hide-and-seek periods.

"If you're taking virtually the same product, changing the label's colors and wording to make it more appealing to midlife women, and selling it at a higher price, that's predatory," says Dr. Jan Shifren, director

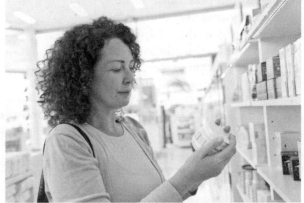

© izusek | Getty Images

Examine and compare ingredients, not promises, on skin care product labels.

of the Midlife Women's Health Center at Harvard-affiliated Massachusetts General Hospital.

"A brand could just be putting a 'menopause' label on a product when a lot of these products contain the same tried-and-true ingredients that are anti-aging for everyone," agrees Dr. Arianne Shadi Kourosh, a dermatologist at Massachusetts General. "There could be hype in the labeling."

Major spending power

It's no mystery why a plethora of "menopause skin care" products have popped up on store shelves in recent years. The trend coincides with a wave of aging women who may feel flush with extra cash as they burn their mortgages and finish paying children's college tuition. Nearly 63 million American women were 50 or older in 2021—roughly 20% of the U.S. population— and older adults are projected to outnumber children for the first time in U. S. history in 2034, according to the U.S. Census Bureau.

So, while anti-aging lotions and potions have been marketed for decades, the $49 billion beauty industry now sees dollar signs in midlife women at the height of their earning and buying potential, Dr. Shifren says. Women over 50 boast a combined spending power of $15 trillion and control 95% of household purchasing decisions, according to AARP.

"We're living longer, we're aging better, we're healthier, and we're wealthier," Dr. Shifren says. "Everyone has realized midlife women are a large group of consumers with money to spare, and it's caught the attention of these product makers."

"But midlife women need to know they're a target now," she adds. "We have to stay in a state of 'buyer beware,' or companies will try to take advantage of us."

Menopause skin basics

Staying ahead of potentially deceptive skin care marketing first requires understanding what happens to women's skin as we age. As the largest organ, the skin joins virtually every other body part in chronicling the effects of falling estrogen levels as menopause approaches.

Estrogen fuels the production of oil and other substances that moisturize and protect the skin. When levels drop, skin can't hold moisture as effectively, leading to dryness, dullness, and irritation. Estrogen decline also coincides with diminishing production of collagen, a type of protein that makes skin firmer.

Beyond that, many women in perimenopause and beyond develop new or worsening cases of rosacea, a chronic inflammatory skin condition marked by redness and rashes that usually arise on the nose and cheeks, Dr. Kourosh says. Why now? Because flushing related to hot flashes causes tiny blood vessels in the face to dilate or makes redness more obvious.

But over-the-counter skin creams typically can't make a big dent in rosacea symptoms, she says—only medications or in-office procedures such as laser treatments can. "Skin care is only going to take you so far," she notes.

This is also true for anti-aging products in general, since most of the changes our face registers over decades—wrinkles and sagging among them—are treatable but not preventable. "We can slow it down, but not stop it," Dr. Kourosh says. "Some of these forces are going to happen no matter what. Working with a trusted dermatologist through the process can help women navigate it more smoothly."

Beneficial ingredients

Nothing will turn back the clock. But certain active ingredients in beauty products can confront aging skin's biggest nemeses:

- Broad-spectrum sunscreen is a product in its own right but also is incorporated into many moisturizers and foundations. Sun exposure speeds up chronological skin aging and leads to age spots.
- Alpha-hydroxy acids exfoliate dead skin cells and reveal smoother skin underneath.
- Retinols and retinoids are forms of vitamin A. They ramp up skin cell turnover, combating fine lines and sun damage.
- Hyaluronic acid draws water to the skin and "traps" it in cells to retain moisture.
- Ceramides strengthen the skin's barrier to keep moisture from escaping.
- Moisturizers improve skin's smoothness, softness, and flexibility. Common individual ingredients include glycerin, shea butter, aloe vera, and various natural oils such as coconut, sunflower seed, jojoba, tea tree, and grapeseed.

While using these ingredients can't hurt, don't expect menopause miracles—no matter what a label says, Dr. Kourosh says. Unlike medications, the FDA doesn't approve over-the-counter skin care products before they're sold.

"I'm not aware of skin care products that are going to be game changers for the problems of menopause," she says. "They may help a little bit, but they contain the same anti-aging ingredients that people use throughout adulthood. And while certain skin care products, like retinols and moisturizers, can be helpful, they're not necessarily going to do the trick for everyone." ▶▶

►► Caveat emptor

If you're perusing skin care shelves and considering "menopause skin care" products, Harvard experts offer two main pieces of advice:

Cast a critical eye. Examine the product's ingredients rather than its claims. Does it contain something different from what you're already using? "Until someone proves that the needs of midlife women's skin are different and designs a product that meets those needs in a different way than for younger women—and no one has done that, to the best of my knowledge—you should probably stick with products you used in the past and not pay more for the same thing," Dr. Shifren says. "If you found a moisturizing cream that worked well for a long time, there's no reason to now buy one whose label says it's perfect for menopause."

Get back to basics. Including skin care in your self-care regimen is fine. But nothing is better for maintaining your skin and overall vitality than getting adequate sleep, staying hydrated, and working with a dermatologist to target your individual needs, Dr. Kourosh says. ▍

What does "clean beauty" really mean?

Are you more tempted to buy a beauty product if it claims to be clean? The notion of "clean beauty," ironically, is quite murky, a Harvard dermatologist says.

Consumers expect clean beauty products—part of a $7 billion global market that encompasses everything from lotions and soaps to hair care and makeup—to be free of harmful substances. But the "clean" moniker denotes nothing about the purity of the ingredients, says Dr. Arianne Shadi Kourosh, a dermatologist at Massachusetts General Hospital.

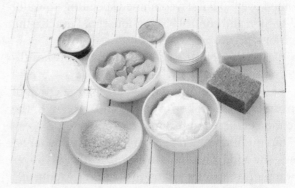

© S847 | Getty Images

Be wary of "clean beauty" claims.

"There is no legal or official definition of clean beauty," Dr. Kourosh says. "It's a term that's been used and misused by marketers from every section of the industry to the point where it has no meaning anymore."

The clean beauty movement came of age in recent years in parallel with "clean eating," but the latter has far more substance. "Clean eating has more structure to it, because people are trying to eat whole foods that are unprocessed and don't come in boxes," she says. "That's a little clearer."

Some beauty products claim they're "clean" when they're merely fragrance-free or hypoallergenic. But even fragrance-free products can contain pleasantly scented preservatives that legally skirt that definition. Other labels declare an item is "vegan," "cruelty-free," or "green." But while those individual claims might pass muster, often marketers are attempting to gain favor with various interest groups, Dr. Kourosh says.

"They're appealing to people's identity politics, using their sensibilities to sell products when the product isn't held to any standards," she add. "There's no accountability, because the FDA doesn't regulate skin care products."

If you're clear-eyed but still interested in what clean beauty products can offer you, drill down on what you're seeking—whether it's something hypoallergenic, for example, or sourced in an environmentally conscious way. "You need to be clear on your goals first," she says, "then do your research and consult with a dermatologist to get an idea of the ingredients you're looking for behind these nebulous and meaningless labels."

Building blocks

Women's protein needs change at different stages of life. Are you getting enough?

Dietitian Nancy Oliveira has noticed a theme among midlife women who are distressed at having gained weight: they blame menopause. But while hormone shifts may play a small role, Oliveira points out a surprising contributor to these women's weight woes—they often aren't prioritizing protein in their diets.

Since protein is at the heart of muscle growth and maintenance, skimping on this powerhouse nutrient can sabotage women's well-being. Indeed, every bodily function relies on protein, from building muscle and bone to producing blood, digesting food, and fighting off infections.

"Every cell in your body is made of proteins—your organs, muscle tissue, bones, and immune cells," explains Oliveira, manager of the Nutrition and Wellness Service at Harvard-affiliated Brigham and Women's Hospital. "I do think some women are eating mostly carbs and feeling tired. They're not protein-deficient, but could be mildly low in protein."

Weight gain can follow. "We look at menopause as a marker, but it may be that women are losing more muscle mass around perimenopause, and muscle maintains a healthy metabolism," Oliveira says.

Protein primer

Protein is one of the three macronutrients that we need in large amounts. (The others are fat and carbohydrates.) Protein requirements aren't based on sex, but on age, body size, activity level, and overall health.

How much do you need? Get out your calculator. The U.S. government's Recommended Dietary Allowance (RDA) is 0.8 grams per kilogram (2.2 pounds) of body weight, but that amount is a bit low, Harvard experts say. Instead, aim to consume between 1.2 and 2.0 grams of protein per kilogram of body weight.

"The RDA is based on the minimum amount you need to prevent disease," Oliveira says. "That doesn't mean it's all you actually need, because protein needs can go up for various reasons."

For a healthy 150-pound person, that means eating between 80 and 136 grams of protein each day. (See "Look to these foods to meet your protein needs,"

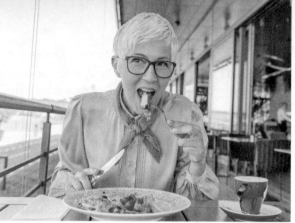

© RealPeopleGroup | Getty Images

Older people need sufficient high-quality protein.

page 224.) "People do well with round numbers," says Mary Ellen Kelly, a dietitian at Brigham and Women's Hospital. "If someone is 150 pounds, they need at least 90 grams of protein a day, with some variability."

When women need more

Despite sex-neutral protein requirements, women may need more for certain reasons men don't. These include pregnancy and breastfeeding, when growing and nourishing another human requires an especially rich supply of the nutrient.

Research is also beginning to illuminate that women are more prone to insulin resistance as years pass—when cells in our muscles, fat, and liver aren't as sensitive to insulin's blood sugar–regulating effects, Kelly says. Because of this, older women should "shift up" protein and fat intake and eat fewer carbohydrates.

"Our body's ability to metabolize carbohydrates begins to change as we age," Kelly says. "The answer is not to drastically reduce calories, but to fuel yourself adequately by eating more protein and unsaturated fat and less heavily processed carbohydrates."

As with men, women who are competitive athletes or trying to build muscle should also opt for higher amounts of protein. And for both sexes, aging alone increases protein needs as we become more vulnerable to diminishing muscle mass and bone-thinning osteoporosis, which strikes four times more older women than men.

"After age 40, we naturally start losing muscle and need to eat more protein to preserve that muscle," Oliveira says.

Consistent but flexible

Though it's ideal to keep protein intake consistent day to day, it won't hurt if you occasionally end up eating, say, 60 grams one day and 160 grams the next. ▶▶

"We don't want people to get caught up on eating the exact number of grams of protein on a daily basis," Oliveira says. "That can bring some anxiety."

But try to spread your protein intake throughout the day to keep your body humming. "Aim for 25 to 30 grams of protein at each meal, and at least 10 grams at each snack," Kelly advises.

Most people manage to eat enough protein without stringent measuring, Oliveira notes. "It's absolutely about your overall eating pattern," she says. "Learn what the protein-rich foods are and try to include some at every meal and snack, and then you don't have to worry so much about how much and what size. I do think you'll consume enough if you're mindful about it."

If you don't, your body may protest. Symptoms can include

- muscle loss
- persistent hunger
- fatigue or weakness
- moodiness
- dry, flaky skin
- brittle or damaged nails
- slow wound healing
- frequent or prolonged illness.

Without enough protein, "you may be more susceptible to colds and other viruses because your immune system is down," Oliveira says.

Look to these foods to meet your protein needs

Ask people where to find protein, and they're likely to answer "meat." While that's true, it's also found in poultry, fish, dairy products, and plant-based foods such as grains, nuts, seeds, vegetables, beans and other legumes, and tofu and other soy-based items.

Protein molecules are composed of smaller elements called amino acids, which support just about everything our bodies do. We produce some amino acids ourselves, but need to get the rest from our diet. These are called essential amino acids. Animal protein is known as a "complete" protein because it contains all nine essential amino acids; with a few exceptions, plant protein usually doesn't.

"I don't think people realize there are actually some plant foods that are considered complete proteins, such as soy foods, hemp seeds, and quinoa," says Nancy Oliveira, manager of the Nutrition and Wellness Service at Brigham and Women's Hospital. "Vegetarians who don't want to eat animal flesh can definitely get enough protein from plants, but you do have to be mindful about it to get those foods more regularly."

But animal products aren't the only foods people find polarizing. "The choice to consume dairy is probably the biggest debate," says Mary Ellen Kelly, a dietitian at Brigham and Women's. "But dairy can definitely provide high-quality protein, whether in milk, Greek yogurt, or cheese."

If you want to add up your daily protein intake, the Harvard T.H. Chan School of Public Health and USDA

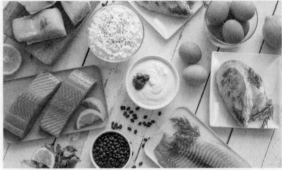

© Mike Kemp | Getty Images

Fish, Greek yogurt, poultry, and beans are among many foods rich in protein.

offer guidance on protein amounts in a smattering of common choices:

- broiled sirloin steak, 4 ounces: 33 grams
- grilled sockeye salmon, 4 ounces: 30 grams
- skinless chicken thigh, 4 ounces: 28 grams
- ham steak, 4 ounces: 22 grams
- cooked lentils, 1 cup: 18 grams
- plain Greek yogurt, 6 ounces: 17 grams
- cottage cheese, ½ cup: 14 grams
- cow's milk, 8 ounces: 8 grams
- cooked beans, ½ cup: 8 grams
- cooked pasta, 1 cup: 8 grams
- unsalted dry roasted almonds, 1 ounce: 6 grams
- one egg: 6 grams.

Supplement basics

If you're aware your protein intake could use a boost—whether you don't like to cook, have a poor appetite, or eat a fully plant-based diet—it's fine to use protein supplements or powders to fill the gap, Harvard experts say.

Widely available protein shakes, meal-replacement bars, and other commercial products make this an easy option. But don't rely on prepared versions too often, since many are ultra-processed and may contain a lot of added sugar, salt, and preservatives. "They're also lacking naturally occurring fiber, vitamins, and minerals," Oliveira says.

Want to whip up your own protein shakes? It's wise to know what you're putting in them. Whey- or casein-based protein powders (which are isolated from cow's milk) contain animal-based proteins, while pea, hemp, or rice protein powders are plant-based. And since dietary supplements aren't tightly regulated by the USDA or FDA, Kelly advises verifying that any protein supplements are labeled "NSF-certified for sport," which means they've met certain quality standards.

But aim to get the vast majority of your protein from whole foods. "They're called supplements for a reason—they supplement the diet," Kelly says. And people who get enough protein from their food don't need to take in more through supplements.

"Just use them as needed—a morning protein shake is fine," adds Oliveira. "I find them to be really helpful on days where you can't eat enough protein. They can be a useful tool to add to your diet."

IN THE JOURNALS

Hormone therapy linked to higher risks of GERD

Women who have used hormone therapy for menopausal symptoms may be more likely to develop gastroesophageal reflux disease, or GERD, a new analysis suggests.

The study, published in 2023 by the journal *Menopause*, analyzed data from five earlier studies involving more than one million women, none of whom had been diagnosed with GERD before the study's start. Researchers found that participants who were current or past users of hormone therapy for relieving menopausal symptoms were 29% more likely over all to develop GERD, which is characterized by heartburn, difficulty swallowing, and chest pain. Women who used estrogen alone had a 41% higher odds of GERD, while progesterone-only hormone therapy was linked to a 39% higher risk. Hormone therapy combining estrogen and progesterone was associated with only a 16% higher risk for GERD.

The study was observational, meaning it couldn't prove that hormone therapy causes GERD, only that an association exists. Female hormones are believed to relax the muscles that control the lower esophageal

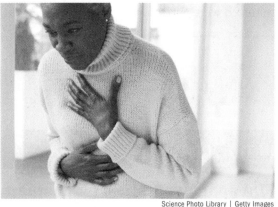

Science Photo Library | Getty Images
Female hormones are believed to relax muscles that allow stomach acid to flow upward.

sphincter (the valve between the bottom of the esophagus and top of the stomach), allowing stomach acid to flow back into the esophagus. Women considering hormone therapy should review their other risk factors for GERD and make necessary lifestyle changes to prevent it, including quitting smoking, maintaining a healthy weight, and not lying down after eating heavy meals, the study authors said.

Ovary removal before menopause may pose health risks

Women who have both ovaries removed before menopause face far higher odds of several chronic health conditions decades later, according to a 2023 study published in the journal *Menopause*.

The study involved 274 women (average age 67) whose ovaries had been removed before menopause for a noncancerous condition—either with or without a hysterectomy. An average of 22 years after their surgery, the women underwent comprehensive physical exams to assess the presence of any chronic conditions and measure their strength and mobility. Compared with women of the same age who still had their ovaries, women who were under age 46 when their ovaries were removed were 64% more likely to

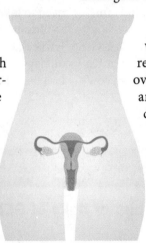

© Dmytro Lukyanets | Getty Images

have arthritis, twice as likely to have obstructive sleep apnea, and nearly three times as likely to have had a bone fracture. They also performed worse on a six-minute walk test. Women who'd undergone ovary removal between ages 46 and 49 also had higher odds of arthritis and sleep apnea than same-age women who didn't have the surgery. However, researchers didn't find a link between ovary removal before menopause and an array of other conditions, including cancer, diabetes, dementia, high blood pressure, high cholesterol, irregular heart rhythm, osteoporosis, or kidney, liver, or thyroid disease.

Women who have their ovaries removed before menopause should consider going on estrogen therapy until about age 50, the study authors said.

FDA approves first pill for postpartum depression

The FDA has approved the first pill for postpartum depression, which affects an estimated one in seven new mothers in the months after giving birth and can make it difficult for them to bond with their babies.

The fast-acting drug, zuranolone (Zurzuvae), received approval in August 2023 and is taken for just two weeks. The only other medication approved specifically for postpartum depression is brexanolone (Zulresso), which requires a hospital-based intravenous infusion. Like other forms of depression, postpartum depression includes symptoms such as intense sadness, lethargy, loss of interest in everyday activities, and thinking and memory problems. In severe cases, women may have thoughts of harming themselves or their child.

The pill's introduction should reduce the stigma of postpartum depression, encouraging more women to seek help, according to the FDA.

After the baby grows up, how will your heart fare?

Certain pregnancy complications can heighten a mother's cardiovascular dangers decades later. Find out who's at risk and why.

Pregnancy is seldom a walk in the park. But if yours was marked by complications such as high blood pressure or diabetes, you probably hoped those hurdles were behind you after your baby was born.

Hope isn't a strategy, however, when it comes to protecting your health. And it's becoming increasingly evident that certain pregnancy and reproductive factors raise red flags about your cardiovascular health years or even decades down the line. The Society for Maternal-Fetal Medicine equates pregnancy to a "cardiovascular stress test," noting that certain complications point toward higher risks for heart attack or stroke later in life.

"We now understand that pregnancy is a window into a woman's future health," says Dr. Brett Young, an OB/GYN and maternal-fetal medicine specialist at Harvard-affiliated Beth Israel Deaconess Medical Center.

For example, women who had high blood pressure or pre-eclampsia (a condition marked by high blood pressure that can impair function of the heart, kidneys, and other organs) while pregnant later develop chronic high blood pressure at least twice as often as women whose blood pressure remained normal in pregnancy. Women who had these blood pressure problems also have 70% higher rates of diabetes and 30% higher rates of elevated cholesterol later in life, according to a Harvard-led 2018 study in the *Annals of Internal Medicine*.

Diabetes or blood pressure complications, estimated to affect 5% to 10% of pregnancies, are on the rise as obesity rates climb and more women decide to have babies later in life.

"While they often resolve soon after, those conditions can translate into long-lasting increased risks for heart disease for these women," says Dr. Nicolas-Sonny Nguyen, a Boston-area family medicine doctor and clinical instructor at Harvard Medical School. "Once you've finished having children, years or decades may go by where these health issues may not come up."

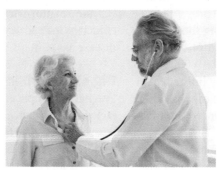
© andreswd | Getty Images
Your pregnancy history is important to your future health.

Common disease features

New research magnifies these revelations. Pregnancy and childbirth complications can pose deadly implications as long as 50 years later, according to a 2023 study published by *Circulation*.

The analysis, which used long-term data from more than 46,000 women who gave birth between 1959 and 1966, tracked participants' deaths from any cause until 2016. Pregnancy-related high blood pressure, gestational diabetes, and preterm delivery were all linked to a greater risk of death in the decades following childbirth.

Meanwhile, problems such as infertility, miscarriage, and stillbirth may be associated with greater stroke risks later in life, according to an analysis published in 2022 by *The BMJ*. Researchers reviewed data on nearly 619,000 women ages 32 through 73 from seven countries. Infertility was associated with a 15% higher risk of stroke, while repeated miscarriages were linked to a 37% higher risk. Women who'd had recurrent stillbirths were 44% more likely to die of a hemorrhagic stroke, characterized by uncontrolled bleeding in the brain.

What's the link? Pregnancy and reproductive difficulties can share common features with cardiovascular disease, including blood vessel problems and fat deposits in blood vessel walls, Dr. Young says.

"Pre-eclampsia is a systemwide condition that affects many organs," she says. "We think of it as a disease of the placenta, but the consensus is that it's actually a blood vessel disease that also affects the kidneys, heart, and brain."

Similarly, diabetes during pregnancy may signal simmering problems with a woman's insulin production or how efficiently her cells use energy. "Even if you had gestational diabetes for only a few months of your life in a span of five, six, or more decades, those few months may have made a difference in your risks," Dr. Nguyen says.

The need for check-ups

The mounting research drives home the importance of preventive care and screenings for women who ▸▸

▶▶ had complicated pregnancies and deliveries—especially at midlife and beyond, when heart disease risks already increase.

"The risks become less silent when women who had these pregnancy conditions reach menopause or beyond," Dr. Nguyen says.

But even younger women—including those whose pregnancies weren't marked by complications—shouldn't skip regular primary care visits. A 2022 study in the journal *Hypertension* suggests that limited medical follow-up in the year after childbirth may miss high blood pressure in one of 10 new mothers whose blood pressure wasn't elevated during pregnancy.

If you've dealt with pregnancy or reproductive difficulties, tell your primary clinician and your other doctors. Your blood pressure, cholesterol, and blood sugar levels should be monitored regularly, and any irregularities should be "treated aggressively," Dr. Young says.

"Even if a woman had problems during only one of her pregnancies many years ago, that history is very important. It should be part of a conversation for the rest of her life," Dr. Nguyen says.

Also don't ignore even mild symptoms that might be heart disease trouble signs, such as chest pain, unusual fatigue, neck or jaw pain, or shortness of breath.

"Talking about symptoms that pop up is important because early recognition is key," Dr. Nguyen says. "Create a platform to have these conversations with your clinicians instead of waiting years, when coronary artery disease has perhaps been brewing for a while."

Big-picture risks

Pregnancy complications, of course, are far from the only factor that influences a woman's future pregnancy risk. Also important are family history, race, diet, weight, and physical activity levels.

"It's important to know that heart disease affects one in five women, regardless of age," Dr. Nguyen says. "Some women may think, 'I'm 35 and had my kids, I'm healthy, and there's no way for me to get heart disease.' But that's not true. I emphasize this to encourage women to optimize their lifestyle."

"When you see your health care providers, be honest and thorough about your medical history, especially relating to your pregnancies," says Dr. Nguyen. ▮

High blood pressure during pregnancy also endangers the brain

Cardiovascular health isn't the only thing that might suffer in the aftermath of pregnancy-related high blood pressure. A new analysis suggests this complication is linked with later cognitive problems as well.

The study, published in 2023 by *Neurology*, involved more than 2,200 women (average age 73), 83% of whom had at least one pregnancy. Every 15 months over an average of five years, participants took nine tests of memory and thinking that evaluated aspects such as processing speed, executive function, language, and overall cognition.

After assessing the women's medical records for pregnancy-related data, researchers found that those who'd had high blood pressure during pregnancy experienced a greater decline in many aspects of thinking skills compared with women who maintained normal blood pressure while pregnant. The effects were even more pronounced among women who'd had pre-eclampsia, a more severe pregnancy-related blood pressure disorder.

The findings aren't surprising, given that blood vessel problems that may contribute to pregnancy complications can also affect vessels that carry blood to the brain, says Dr. Brett Young, an OB/GYN and maternal-fetal medicine specialist at Beth Israel Deaconess Medical Center. The results also suggest monitoring and managing blood pressure during and after pregnancy could pay important dividends for brain health later in life.

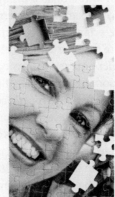
© Plattform | Getty Images

The findings are consistent with the understanding that pregnancy can illuminate a woman's future health risks, including many conditions that affect the blood vessels, Dr. Young says. "The brain," she says, "requires healthy blood vessels just like the placenta does—it's a system based on blood vessels."

by **TONI GOLEN, M.D.,** Editor in Chief, *Harvard Women's Health Watch*

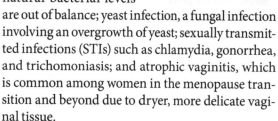

What's causing my vaginal symptoms?

Q *For the past week I've been dealing with vaginal itching, burning, and discharge. What might be causing these symptoms?*

A Vaginitis, inflammation of the lining inside the vagina, sounds like the culprit. But vaginitis—which can also include vaginal odor and soreness inside and around the vagina and vulva—is an umbrella term encompassing several distinct conditions that inflame or infect the vagina, all with different causes and treatments.

These include bacterial vaginosis, when natural bacterial levels are out of balance; yeast infection, a fungal infection involving an overgrowth of yeast; sexually transmitted infections (STIs) such as chlamydia, gonorrhea, and trichomoniasis; and atrophic vaginitis, which is common among women in the menopause transition and beyond due to dryer, more delicate vaginal tissue.

See your primary care clinician or gynecologist to get to the root of your symptoms. Treatments may include antibiotics, antifungal medications, or vaginal moisturizers. To keep vaginitis at bay, avoid products such as douches, vaginal wipes, or sprays; don't wear damp underwear or bathing suits; limit your sexual partners; and avoid STIs by asking male sex partners to wear condoms.

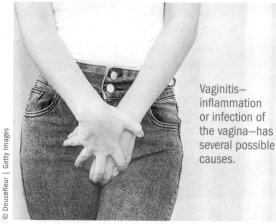

Vaginitis—inflammation or infection of the vagina—has several possible causes.

© Doucefleur | Getty Images

Why do I bleed after sex?

Q *I've noticed blood on my sheets after sex. Why might this happen?*

A If you're not menstruating at the time, bleeding after sex can be alarming, though some of its possible causes are minor. A top contributor is vaginal dryness, which is common among women after menopause due to declining estrogen levels and can also cause the vaginal walls to become thinner and more fragile. But bleeding after sex can also stem from inflammation from yeast or other vaginal infections, including sexually transmitted infections such as chlamydia or gonorrhea. Cervical polyps—small, typically noncancerous growths on the cervix—can also bleed from the chafing of vaginal intercourse.

Far less likely to cause bleeding after sex are gynecological cancers affecting the cervix, uterus, ovaries, or vagina, or postsurgical bleeding after a pelvic procedure. (You should get your doctor's okay before resuming sex after surgery.) See your doctor about any unusual or unexpected vaginal bleeding, whether it occurs after sex or at other times.

Physical activity may lower Parkinson's risk in women

Regular physical activity, including walking, climbing stairs, gardening, and cleaning, may help prevent or delay the onset of Parkinson's disease in women, a new study suggests.

The analysis, published in 2023 by the journal *Neurology*, tracked nearly 99,000 women (average age 49) who didn't have Parkinson's disease at the beginning of the study. Researchers compared participants' activity levels over nearly three decades using regular questionnaires, assigning each woman an activity score based on how often and how long she engaged in recreation, sports, and household

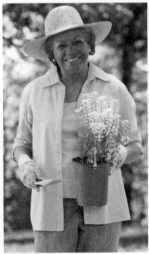

© Jose Luis Pelaez Inc | Getty Images

Staying active may help prevent Parkinson's disease.

activities. As women's activity levels increased, their risk of developing Parkinson's—a movement disorder marked by tremors, muscle stiffness, and gait and balance problems—dropped. Over the study's duration, women with the highest physical activity scores had a 25% lower risk of Parkinson's when compared with the least-active women.

Preventing Parkinson's disease appears to be another reason to stay physically active throughout adult life. The disease, typically diagnosed in people over 60, remains incurable, with treatments aimed only at reducing symptoms.

Magnesium-rich foods might boost brain health, especially in women

Eating more magnesium-rich foods is linked with better brain health as we age—especially in women—potentially lowering the risk of dementia, a new analysis suggests.

The 2023 study, published by the *European Journal of Nutrition*, involved more than 6,000 adults ages 40 through 73 in the United Kingdom. Participants completed an online questionnaire five times over 16 months, which researchers used to calculate their average daily magnesium intake based on how much participants ate of 200 specific foods. These included magnesium-rich choices such as leafy

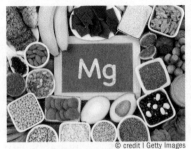

© credit | Getty Images

Feed your brain with magnesium-rich dietary choices.

green vegetables, legumes, seeds, nuts, and whole grains. MRI imaging measured participants' brain volumes. People whose diets included more than 550 milligrams (mg) of magnesium each day had higher brain volumes—which researchers equated with a brain age approximately one year younger by age 55—than participants who consumed about 350 mg of magnesium daily. These effects were greater in women compared with men.

Less age-related brain shrinkage is associated with better brain function and a lower risk of dementia in later life, the researchers said.

The pain gap

Scientists are still teasing out why women deal with more chronic pain than men. In the meantime, here's how to find the help you need.

When you're hurting, you want to know why—especially when pain returns day after day. So the frustration is real when a diagnosis is elusive, piling on to a cryptic but persistent gender gap in chronic pain.

The lopsided prevalence of chronic pain between the sexes has long been recognized. Women deal with the problem at rates 6% higher than men do. That's true for back, hip, and knee pain; migraine headaches; arthritis; lupus; and fibromyalgia, among other problems. And some chronic pain conditions strike only women, such as endometriosis; the bladder condition interstitial cystitis; vulvodynia (which affects the vulva); and pelvic girdle syndrome, which involves pain around the pelvic joints and lower back.

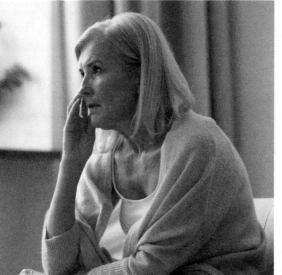
Hormones are just one possible factor contributing to pain.

© fizkes | Getty Images

What's still not clear is why. "We know this disparity exists, but the question is what drives it," says Dr. Christopher Gilligan, chief of the Division of Pain Medicine at Harvard-affiliated Brigham and Women's Hospital.

Estrogen's role

Evidence suggests that hormones are one contributing factor. A 2022 study found that women who got their first period (a time known as menarche) at a younger age are more likely to have chronic pain in adulthood. The analysis, published in the journal *Pain*, evaluated data on more than 12,000 women (average age 55). Across the full range of reported ages at menarche—9 through 18—the risk of chronic pain dropped 2% for each one-year delay in menstruation.

The findings add to earlier evidence suggesting exposure to increased estrogen levels from early menstruation may contribute to pain—and to overall sex differences in pain, the study authors said. Even so, genes and other biological factors may also be responsible.

Paths to pain relief

Adding to the burden of chronic pain is the difficulty many women have getting a firm diagnosis. This can delay effective treatment. Dr. Gilligan offers these strategies to get the help you may need:

Be persistent. If your primary care doctor can't pinpoint a cause for your pain, ask for a recommendation or referral to another medical professional. "Also, if you feel you're not being listened to, seek a second or third opinion until you find a provider who does," he adds.

Stay flexible. Before turning to medications, be open to trying different treatment approaches, including physical or occupational therapy.

Consider CBT. Cognitive behavioral therapy can help alter your perception of pain and teach you coping skills.

Seek support. Online and in-person support groups can link you with others to share pain relief strategies. Additionally, some hospitals offer so-called functional restoration programs—rehabilitation programs for chronic pain sufferers—that involve group support. ▉

Why women fall

Intriguing reasons explain why women fall more often than men, but there are simple ways to lower your risk.

In the friendly competition between the sexes, women face a hefty disadvantage in a distinctly dangerous arena: falling.

Falls are the leading cause of injuries and accidental deaths among American adults 65 and older, but women fall more often than men indoors. We're also 50% more likely than men to show up at an emergency room due to a fall, according to a large 2021 study in the *American Journal of Lifestyle Medicine.*

This disparity doesn't surprise Dr. Suzanne Salamon, clinical chief of gerontology at Harvard-affiliated Beth Israel Deaconess Medical Center. But she believes most people aren't aware of the myriad ways they can prevent an ill-fated tumble as they age.

"A lot of people know someone who has fallen and broken a bone, or had a parent who did, so they know it's possible in their future," Dr. Salamon says. "But it's definitely not inevitable."

Why we're vulnerable

Regardless of sex, balance tends to become more tenuous with age due to factors such as greater medication use, mounting vision and inner-ear problems, weaker muscles, and health conditions that can lead to numbness in the feet, such as diabetic neuropathy.

But women are particularly vulnerable. Here's why:

Our bones are weaker. Bone-thinning osteoporosis is linked to poorer physical performance and

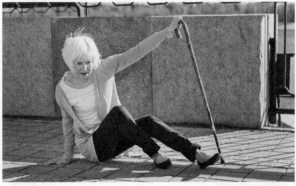

© Zinkevych | Getty Images
Balance can decline with age due to many factors.

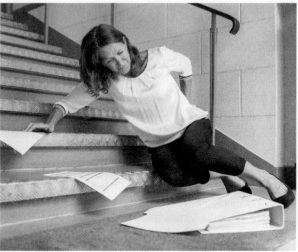

© AndreyPopov | Getty Images
Women are disproportionately injured by falls.

worse balance compared to women with normal bone density.

Our muscle mass is lower. This relative lack of strength can make it harder to avoid falling if we get off-balance. "The loss of estrogen due to menopause really does a number on bones and muscles to make them more fragile," Dr. Salamon says.

We deal with incontinence more often. Rushing to the bathroom can make a fall more likely, Dr. Salamon says, and some women slip on urine they've leaked onto the bathroom floor before they get to the toilet.

We take more antidepressants. Twice as many women as men take depression-fighting medications, whose side effects can make you dizzy and less alert—both of which increase your fall risk.

We have a penchant for multitasking. Efficiency is great until you tip over because you bend to pick up one more thing while carrying a teetering pile of laundry. "When in doubt, take two trips to the laundry room instead of one," Dr. Salamon says.

Prevention tips

Despite these sex-related differences, there's much you can do to reduce your fall risk. Dr. Salamon suggests these tactics:

Stay alert. Be mindful of transition points while walking such as curbs, thresholds, and other seemingly minor hazards.

Exercise with strength and balance in mind. Activities such as tai chi strengthen legs, while yoga can shore up core muscles that help you stay steady when you're upright. Even in people with osteoporosis, resistance and impact exercises such as weight lifting and jumping rope improve balance and eventually reduce fall rates, according to a 2023 report in the *Journal of Bone Metabolism*.

Consider physical therapy. Your therapist can recommend a regimen geared just toward improving balance. "The only problem is that some people go to physical therapy for a few weeks and then stop doing the exercises," Dr. Salamon says. "They need to become part of your daily routine."

Get regular eyesight and hearing checks. Treat any conditions as they arise and update your glasses and hearing aid prescriptions as needed.

Review your medications. Certain drugs, including over-the-counter remedies, have side effects such as dizziness or sleepiness. Ask your doctor if you can take another type of medication instead or change your dosing schedule.

Make your home safe. Keep floors and stairs clutter-free and make sure all areas are well lit.

Don grippy soles. Don't wear socks around the house unless they're coated with rubber on the bottom, and avoid slippers without treads.

Go hands-free. "I see so many women walking around with big handbags, but wearing a backpack is a better option because it leaves your hands free to hold onto railings," she says. 🛡

Fibroids: Not just a young woman's problem

These uterine growths can crop up even as menopause looms, and beyond.

For many women, the approach of menopause is cause for celebration. After decades of monthly bleeding, periods will finally be a thing of the past, as will pregnancy worries. But some of us eagerly anticipate the transition for another reason: waning estrogen levels often improve fibroids, noncancerous growths in the uterine wall that affect up to eight in 10 of us by age 50.

Women in their 40s or early 50s whose fibroids cause only mild problems may be told to be patient, since fibroids rely on estrogen to thrive. But for those with more distressing signs—including heavy bleeding, pelvic or lower back pain, bloating, frequent urination, or painful sex—there's a chance menopause won't bring relief. Stealthy growth over the years can lead fibroids to become even more problematic during perimenopause and beyond, not diminish as expected.

"The message women get is if you can hang on until menopause, the fibroids will get better," says Dr. Elisa Jorgensen, a minimally invasive gynecologic surgeon at Harvard-affiliated Massachusetts General Hospital. "But many women can't wait that long, because

© Veronika Zakharova/Science Photo Library | Getty Images
Menopause may not always bring relief from fibroids.

symptoms become overwhelming. And some women get to menopause but still have the bulk of them."

Factors influencing growth

Also known as uterine leiomyomas, fibroids can be as small as the tip of a sewing needle or as large as a grapefruit. While their cause is unknown, the growths can run in families.

While conventional wisdom holds that fibroids are a younger woman's problem, recent research indicates it's possible for them to become newly apparent as menopause approaches. About one-third of newly diagnosed fibroids occur in women in their mid-to-late 40s, according to a 2020 paper published in *Menopause* that cited a 2009 study involving nearly 1,800 women.

"A woman may have small fibroids earlier and not notice them, but with time—as she gets into her late 40s—the fibroids may be reaching the size where she does," Dr. Jorgensen says.

Another *Menopause* article, from November 2021, suggested small fibroids can keep growing after menopause is in the rearview mirror. The study tracked ▸▸

active fibroid growth in 102 postmenopausal women over five years using vaginal ultrasounds every six months. Researchers were surprised to observe that small fibroids grew more often than larger ones in these women. Additionally, fibroids grew faster and larger in participants who were overweight or obese.

Hormone considerations

Hormone therapy is another factor that increases the likelihood fibroids will develop or worsen with age, Dr. Jorgensen says. Because fibroids are sensitive to estrogen, women who take the hormone to allay menopausal symptoms may face this trade-off. On the other hand, doctors may prescribe combination estrogen-progestin birth control pills for pre- and peri-menopausal women with symptomatic fibroids. "They disrupt the body's natural hormone cycle, so they're not stoking the fire," she explains.

Treatment options after menopause

Treatments for other health conditions may also influence older women's fibroid symptoms. Abnormal bleeding, for example, usually eases as menopause arrives, even if other symptoms linger. But it often won't for women who need to take an anti-clotting drug.

"Even if bleeding goes away," Dr. Jorgensen says, "fibroids may still be pressing into the bladder, so women will still experience symptoms like urinary frequency, incontinence, and back pain, among others. Fibroids can take up space that prevents the bladder from expanding, so you need to go to the bathroom more frequently and are more likely to leak urine."

Beyond the consequences of intense symptoms, fibroids that continue to grow noticeably after a woman reaches menopause raise the possibility of cancer, she notes. "For these expanding fibroids, I would monitor their growth and may recommend surgically removing them," she says. "It's very uncommon for a fibroid to develop into cancer, but I'd want to make sure."

Surgical removal of fibroids, called myomectomy, joins hysterectomy as the two procedures doctors often advise for women seeking fibroid treatment after menopause, Dr. Jorgensen says. While an array of other techniques are available to treat fibroids, most don't work as well in women who have reached menopause because of the complex interplay between hormone levels and fibroid growth.

"If you're past menopause, you're generally not going to be able to take advantage of most other treatments that shrink fibroids," she says. That's because post-menopausal fibroids will presumably have done any possible shrinking once the body's estrogen production drops, so additional therapies aimed at blocking estrogen won't make a difference. 🛡

IN THE JOURNALS

Alcohol-related deaths rising faster among women

Alcohol-related deaths in the United States are rising faster among women than men, a recent analysis suggests.

For the study, published in 2023 in *JAMA Network Open*, researchers evaluated CDC data tracking underlying causes of death from 1999 to 2020. In that period, about 606,000 Americans died of alcohol-related causes, which included alcohol poisoning, liver disease, and heart problems, among others. The researchers found that while men still die of alcohol-related problems in far greater numbers than women, deaths among women are growing at a faster rate. Between 2018 and 2020, alcohol-related death rates among men increased by an average of 12.5% per year; for women, the annual average increased nearly 15%.

Several biological factors make women more susceptible to alcohol's effects, the study authors said. For example, women have lower levels of enzymes that metabolize alcohol, which means it takes our bodies longer to break down alcohol before it can damage organs. Women's bodies also have a lower proportion of water than men's do, allowing alcohol to become more concentrated.

The latest thinking on drinking

If you're confused about how alcohol affects your health, there's good reason. But women can't afford to tune out the noise.

If your Dry January quickly turned damp and later splashed into nightly cocktails on the patio, you probably weren't enthused by a recent analysis suggesting women's risks of dying early rise markedly when we drink an average of just under two alcoholic beverages a day.

But perhaps another recent study made you nod with satisfaction—one suggesting alcohol lowers the risk of heart attack and stroke by improving stress signaling in the brain.

What to believe? Not what the headlines blare, since most scientific evidence surrounding alcohol's health effects is decidedly weak, Harvard experts say. Tracking it—and gleaning useful insights into how we should shape our drinking habits—is not unlike watching an annoying ping-pong match. One day, drinking is touted as beneficial; the next, it's terrible. Back and forth, back and forth, until you want to ignore it all.

"Everything that comes out seems to capture our attention, but the evidence has always been prone to being misunderstood or misinterpreted," says Dr. Kenneth Mukamal, an internist at Harvard-affiliated Beth Israel Deaconess Medical Center who studies how alcohol and other lifestyle factors affect health. "With this yo-yo effect, every new study seems important, because we don't have strong evidence. It makes people's heads explode."

Research holes

For context, here's how drinking levels are categorized. A standard drink equals 1.5 ounces of distilled spirits, a 12-ounce beer, or a 5-ounce glass of wine. The CDC defines moderate drinking as one standard drink or less per day for women and two drinks or less for men. Heavy drinking is eight or more drinks a week for women and 15 or more per week for men.

But while those amounts seem clear, the related research is anything but. Part of the problem is that alcohol's health effects have never been studied in what's considered a scientifically rigorous way.

"There's never been a large-scale randomized controlled trial that's tested how reducing or increasing alcohol intake affects health," says Dr. JoAnn Manson, chief of the Division of Preventive Medicine

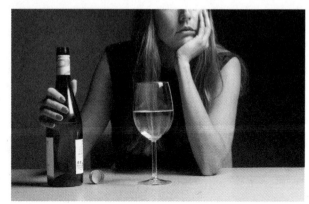
© Peter Dazeley | Getty Images

Rethinking drinking: much of the evidence surrounding alcohol's health effects is less than robust.

at Harvard-affiliated Brigham and Women's Hospital. This gold-standard study design would pit one scenario directly against the other, rather than rely on observations that could be influenced by extraneous factors. Another conundrum is that drinking and other lifestyle habits that influence health, like exercise, sleep, and social connectedness, can't easily be teased apart in study findings. The 2023 research review suggesting women's risks of dying early rise significantly from consuming just under two alcoholic drinks a day was intended to correct some of those design flaws. That study's authors said earlier analyses didn't point out that people considered light or moderate drinkers tend to have other healthy habits that improve their overall health—making it appear that alcohol contributes to good health outcomes. Conversely, "nondrinkers" in study comparison groups have often included people who once drank and quit because of addiction or other health problems. This factor skewed study findings to suggest drinking moderately was healthier than not drinking at all.

"We now understand those findings were likely spurious," Dr. Manson says.

Breast cancer caveat

One of the more robust findings involving alcohol's effects on health pertains specifically to women: drinking has been convincingly linked to developing breast cancer, as well as other cancers. ▶▶

A 2021 report from the International Agency for Research on Cancer estimated that alcohol accounts for about 4% of newly diagnosed cancers globally—most commonly those of the breast, esophagus, and liver. And breast cancers accounted for almost half of the more than 23,000 new cancer diagnoses in Europe traceable to light-to-moderate drinking in 2017, according to a 2023 study in *The Lancet Public Health*.

While the number of women who develop breast cancer every year due solely to alcohol is small, it's something we should consider before we imbibe. "The alcohol–breast cancer link is among the strongest evidence we have," Dr. Mukamal says. "Women who drink alcohol have higher levels of sex hormones like estrogen. If you're prone to breast cancer, this feeds it in a way it wouldn't if you weren't drinking."

Any woman concerned about her breast cancer risk—or whose mother, sister, or daughter has had the disease—should consider reducing or eliminating alcohol, says Dr. Manson, who is also a professor of medicine and women's health at Harvard Medical School. "It would be a strategy to mitigate risk," she says.

The bottom line

Where does this leave us? There's no perfect answer. But if you're healthy and already drink lightly or moderately, it's probably fine to continue to do so, Dr. Manson says—with some caveats.

"If someone drinks moderately and they're doing well, I don't push them to stop. If, however, they ask whether they should *start* to drink, or should drink *more*, to improve their health, the answer would be an emphatic no," Dr. Manson says.

"Many people find that drinking moderately reduces their stress. It's something they enjoy," she adds. "But it shouldn't be perceived as a health-promoting activity."

How do you know if you need to quit drinking?

If you reach for a drink just to feel normal, alarm bells should be ringing. That's a clear sign alcohol is more than just an enjoyable pursuit—it's a problem, says Dr. Robert Doyle, a psychiatrist at Harvard-affiliated Massachusetts General Hospital.

But many warning signs that suggest you stop drinking are more subtle, and it's common to slide into alcohol misuse by gradually drinking more and more without realizing it's excessive, Dr. Doyle says.

"A person who develops alcohol use disorder tends to be someone who, early on, is able to handle their alcohol," he says. "They don't seem to get drunk so easily, but then they start to drink more and their body becomes accustomed to it. It tends to sneak up on them."

Watch for these other signs that suggest you are drinking too much:

You crave alcohol to feel relaxed. People with alcohol use disorder often say that's why they drink, but they're usually imbibing to avoid the physical symptoms of withdrawal.

You drink alone. "You're wanting to just drink instead of socialize," Dr. Doyle says.

Your job or relationships have suffered. "You might miss work because you pass out and oversleep," he says, "or you're not meeting your obligations because of your drinking."

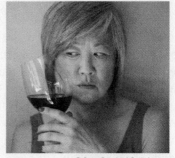
© Peter Dazeley | Getty Images

Some warning signs to quit drinking are subtle.

You hide your drinking. That might mean drinking in secret or concealing bottles around your home.

You drive after drinking. "The wake-up call is getting pulled over for a DUI or the threat of it," he says.

Your family tells you you've got a problem. "Pay attention to what they say, or ask your family, 'Do you think I overdo it?' Tell them you won't be mad at them for being honest," Dr. Doyle suggests. "Family members usually have your best interests at heart."

If you realize you need help to quit, ask your doctor how to get started. "Therapists and primary care doctors are all trained to recognize alcohol use disorder and help people find appropriate treatment," Dr. Doyle says.

Poor sleep linked to high blood pressure

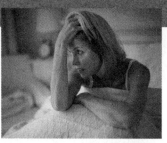

© credit I Getty Images

Prioritize sleep for heart health.

Sleep problems—including trouble falling asleep, staying asleep, and too little sleep—are associated with a greater risk of high blood pressure (hypertension) in women, according to a new study.

Published in 2023 in *Hypertension*, the study tracked the health of 66,122 women for 16 years. When the study began in 2001, the women ranged in age from 25 to 42 and didn't have hypertension.

After researchers accounted for various demographic and lifestyle factors, they found that, compared to women who slept seven to eight hours daily, those who slept six or five hours were 7% and 10%, respectively, more likely to develop hypertension.

Women who said they sometimes or usually had trouble falling or staying asleep were 14% and 28% more likely to have hypertension, respectively, compared to those who rarely had trouble sleeping.

The findings don't prove that sleep problems cause elevated blood pressure. However, as the authors suggest, one possible explanation for the link may be increased stress, which is associated both with poor sleep and high blood pressure.

Why does my back ache?

Pinpointing the cause can be challenging, but it can steer your next steps.

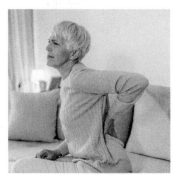

© Jelena Stanojkovic I Getty Images

Most cases of acute back pain will resolve within days to weeks.

You repeatedly lifted your 30-pound grandchild over the weekend, and today you're paying for it—your lower back throbs. Welcome to a very large club: an estimated 84% of Americans cope with lower back pain at some point in their lifetime.

While nearly every major movement we make involves our back, not all back pain is created equal. Symptoms can vary widely, ranging from a dull, ongoing ache to intense, shooting pain or spasms. Sometimes we can pinpoint exactly when back pain struck—like after falling or hoisting a heavy object—but more often, nothing specific happened to trigger the pain.

"It's a bit complicated, because in many cases of back pain, we don't really know exactly where the pain is coming from," says Dr. Joerg Ermann, a rheumatologist at Harvard-affiliated Brigham and Women's Hospital. "But an important message is that it's very common, and in all likelihood it will ease over the course of days to weeks."

Acute vs. chronic back pain

If your back pain started within the past month, it's considered acute (short-term). Doctors often categorize low back pain as nonspecific, meaning they haven't identified an underlying reason for why it's happening. Nonspecific back pain is often muscular in nature, however. It means you've pulled or strained muscles or other soft tissues, such as tendons and ligaments.

▶▶

Pulls and strains usually happen in a single moment, showing up as sudden, stabbing pain that worsens when you move or twist. You may also feel stiff and achy and have difficulty standing upright. If you've fallen or injured yourself in another way, bruising and swelling on a specific area of your back may be noticeable.

When it's not muscular in nature, back pain can be caused by a lengthy list of conditions that often stem from what are called mechanical problems with spinal discs (the shock absorbers between spinal bones) or, less commonly, inflammation in the spine. These conditions often result in long-lasting or recurrent pain. When the pain continues for more than three months, it's labeled as chronic. "It's an important distinction, because the types of problems that can cause acute or chronic back pain are different," Dr. Ermann says.

These non-muscular causes include
- herniated discs, which may press on surrounding spinal nerves
- osteoarthritis of a facet joint, which can narrow the space around the spinal cord
- degenerative disc disease, in which discs shrink and the spine becomes less flexible
- fractures of spinal bones (vertebrae)
- axial spondyloarthritis, an inflammatory condition of the spine, where back pain is typically worse in the morning and eases with movement.

"There are some bad things that can cause lower back pain, but in most cases, a sudden onset is from muscular strain or injury," he says.

Treatment approaches

Time and home-based treatments usually do the trick for most cases of acute back pain. While you may not feel like moving if you're in serious distress, short walks and gentle stretching can help keep muscles loose and speed your recovery. Other measures include taking anti-inflammatory pain relievers such as ibuprofen (Advil, Motrin) or naproxen (Aleve) and alternately applying heat and ice.

Consider seeing a doctor when back pain that came on suddenly just won't quit. "If after a couple of weeks it's still substantial, you need evaluation by a clinician," Dr. Ermann says.

After symptoms ease, your doctor may also recommend physical therapy involving stretches and exercises. "We don't often do the things that our spine deserves, which include strengthening the core muscles that support it," he says.

If your lower back pain is accompanied by additional symptoms, the problem may be more serious. Alarming symptoms include fever and chills, unexplained weight loss, pain that spreads down the legs, bowel or bladder problems, and weakness, numbness, or tingling in one or both legs. These signs should prompt an immediate medical evaluation.

"It depends on how bad your symptoms are, but you definitely don't want to wait it out," Dr. Ermann says. "If you can't pee, go to the ER. But if you have shooting pain down your leg, going to urgent care the next day may be appropriate." ▮

Caregiving crisis

Supporting loved ones often takes an overlooked toll on caregivers' own health.

If a traditional caregiving scenario were captured on time-lapse video, Katherine Lyman contends that early scenes would depict an adult daughter accompanying her aging parent to a doctor's appointment looking "put together" and on top of things. Just a few years later, however, the daughter would appear drastically different—"really disheveled, because she isn't taking care of herself."

"I cannot tell you how many times I've leaned forward, looked the daughter in the eyes, and asked, 'How are you coping with all of this? What are you doing to let off steam? It's great that you're keeping all these plates spinning, but it comes at a cost,'" recounts Lyman, a geriatric nurse practitioner at Harvard-affiliated Beth Israel Deaconess Medical Center.

Increasingly, that cost is caregivers' own health and well-being. Indeed, the story of caregiving in the United States is becoming something of a cautionary tale as troubling forces collide.

More caregivers are on tap than ever, with 43 million Americans providing unpaid assistance to a family member or another loved one. Nearly three-quarters are 50 or older themselves, while more than 75% are women, according to the Family Caregiver Alliance. Meanwhile, an estimated 73 million Americans will be 65 or older by 2030, potentially fueling the need for additional caregivers.

Longevity is perhaps the biggest contributor to the brewing storm, Harvard experts say. "A lot of us are living into our late years and living very well and independently, but not all of us," Lyman says. "Those years may come with increased infirmity or cognitive impairment, or both."

Spectrum of responsibilities

As people age, several core issues tend to prompt the need for spouses, adult children, or others to step in to help. Let's dub the problem areas the three M's: mobility, memory, and medications. Yet caregiving is far from a one-size-fits-all proposition, with duties falling on a spectrum from occasional to relentless and minor to suffocating.

"It runs the gamut from actually living with the person to living in a different state and putting cameras in different rooms to check on them," says Dr. Suzanne Salamon, clinical chief of gerontology at Beth Israel Deaconess Medical Center. "Some caregivers come periodically, fill pill boxes, take people to doctor's appointments, or take them shopping. But caregiving can also be financial: paying the bills, organizing the taxes, or taking over as power of attorney."

Whether they're popping in a few times a week or handling daily bathing, dressing, and toileting—or something in between—caregivers often wear many hats, Lyman notes. "You become not just their caregiver, but their confidante, psychiatrist, chef, grocery shopper, laundress, chauffeur, and pharmacist," she says.

Health fallout

Such comprehensive responsibilities can exact an underappreciated physical and mental toll—especially if your loved one's deterioration is prolonged—and create a downward spiral that affects both caregiver

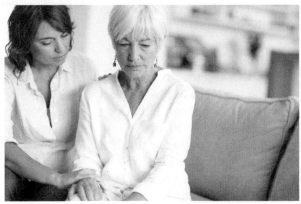
© laflor | Getty Images

Many caregivers neglect their own health due to their responsibilities.

and recipient. Six in 10 caregivers work part-or full-time, spreading themselves even thinner.

Copious research has focused on the mental health fallout. Between 40% and 70% of caregivers deal with significant symptoms of depression. And those who are women fare worse than men who take on such duties, reporting higher levels of depression and anxiety.

Similarly, a wide range of studies point to caregiving's physical consequences, especially pain. Caregivers are prone to headaches and often suffer back injuries or cope with arthritis, Dr. Salamon says.

A 2023 study published by *The Gerontologist* that gathered data from nearly 2,000 caregivers (average age 62) showed just over half suffered pain of some kind. About 30% said their pain limited the ways they could provide care.

Caregivers also face an increased risk of heart disease, and women caring for a spouse are more likely to report having high blood pressure, diabetes, and high cholesterol, according to the Family Caregiver Alliance.

"Many caregivers in their 50s, 60s, and 70s have their own health issues," Dr. Salamon says. "It gets more stressful as time goes on and the patient and caregiver both get older."

About 10% of caregivers acknowledge their own health has suffered as a result of their responsibilities. But that doesn't mean they're vigilantly attending to it. Nearly three-quarters reported not having gone to a doctor as often as they should, while more than half had missed medical appointments, according to the Family Caregiver Alliance.

"People start losing weight, not eating properly, and not paying attention to themselves," Lyman says. ▶▶

▶▶ "Their health takes a back seat, and so do their interests."

Finding help

Even as they feel the strain, caregivers are often loath to seek support. "They're good at giving help, but lousy at asking for it," Lyman says.

Still, it's crucial to make that leap. Harvard experts offer these strategies for caregivers to preserve body and soul:

Look into respite care. Some assisted living or nursing facilities provide temporary care so family members can take a vacation. Adult day programs can provide a daily break. "Sometimes they only run from 9 a.m. to 1 p.m., but that can be huge," Lyman says. "And some provide transportation."

Call your local Agency on Aging. Some offer housekeeping services to eligible older adults, while others coordinate volunteers who can pinch-hit and "stay for a few hours so the caregiver can get out and be free for a little while," Dr. Salamon says.

Sniff out informal help. "Ask friends who drive if they can pick Mom up and bring her to the senior center or to her hair appointment," Lyman suggests.

Explore houses of worship. Local religious groups may have cadres of helpers. "Some have volunteers who pick up people who want to go to their service and take them home afterward," Lyman says.

Consider therapy. Nearly four in 10 caregivers describe their responsibilities as emotionally stressful. Talking to a therapist can bring relief.

Tap into telehealth. Schedule virtual visits with doctors or therapists to get the care you need. "You don't have to leave Mom unattended," Lyman says. "You can go into the next room and shut the door for a half-hour or hour." ▮

How to rally the troops

Even in large families, the lion's share of caregiving responsibilities often falls to one sibling when Mom or Dad is declining. But family members should recognize that the caregiver isn't a hero—and shouldn't be expected to perform like one.

"I don't think a lot of family members realize how stressful caregiving is, and they don't offer to help," says Dr. Suzanne Salamon, clinical chief of gerontology at Beth Israel Deaconess Medical Center. "They leave it to the caregiver to ask them, and that's not right. They need to wholeheartedly offer."

To smooth that process—and the sometimes-fraught dynamic between caregiver and other relatives—Harvard experts offer these tips:

Call a family meeting. This can be held in person or over Zoom, ideally including the patient's doctor or a geriatric care manager. The best result: everyone gets on the same page about day-to-day problems and caregiving responsibilities that require attention.

Create a schedule. This might include setting up a shared online calendar for family members to sign up for tasks and time periods to chip in.

Rotate care. "Set up a schedule so every day 'belongs' to a different child," Dr. Salamon suggests.

Match people's tasks to their abilities. If your sister is a finance whiz, she's probably the right one to handle Dad's taxes. Your brother is a lawyer? Ask him to sort out the legal nuances of Mom's property sale.

Be specific. If you're the caregiver, you may want two hours to go to a social event or appointment. Say so. "It's very important to make your requests concrete, tell others exactly what you need, and do it in spite of any guilt," Dr. Salamon says.

Ask how you can help. If you're not the main caregiver, can you take over one evening each week or stay for a weekend? Or perhaps you can coordinate services such as housecleaning, yard work, or transportation to medical appointments. Be explicit about what you can provide. "Say, 'I can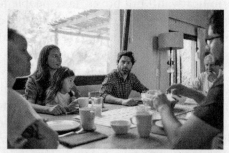

© FluxFactory | Getty Images

A family meeting about caregiving can help everyone decide on a shared path forward.

take Mom to the hairdresser on Wednesday afternoon,' or, 'I'm coming on Wednesday for two hours—why don't you take some time off?'" Dr. Salamon says.

Debunking common wellness myths

Let's tease out the truth of health advice touted as "facts."

Some tried-and-true wellness guidance we can spot a mile away: get enough sleep, move your body regularly, and eat plenty of fruits and vegetables, for starters. But social media now pummels us with so-called health advice at such a rapid pace it can be difficult to know what to heed—and what to ignore.

Much of it is of dubious value. But the reason this counsel is confusing is that many wellness myths contain a grain of truth, says Dr. Leonor Fernandez, a primary care doctor at Harvard-affiliated Beth Israel Deaconess Medical Center.

"There's some good information out there," she says, "but the general problem with the Internet is that it's sometimes hard to distinguish what's reliable from what's being spread for commercial, political, or other purposes."

People can also be vulnerable to questionable advice because they're hungry for a quick fix, even when that's rarely possible.

"We're often looking for a one-pill type of solution, that one thing we can do to take care of a problem or simplify our lives to feel effective," Dr. Fernandez says. "But for most things in health, the solution lies in the balance between what you do and what you eat rather than one specific thing."

Fiction vs. fact

Dr. Fernandez dissects three common wellness myths and offers time-tested ways to improve your well-being.

1 MYTH: Thin is synonymous with healthy.

Truth: It's not that simple. "There's certainly not just one healthy body type, and I've seen many people with a low body weight who aren't healthy," Dr. Fernandez says.

Indeed, carrying extra weight is associated with higher risks of many health problems, including heart disease, diabetes, and some forms of cancer, "so it's not realistic to say that our weight has no impact on our health," she says. "But it's a distortion to think that body mass index alone gives us a good indicator of our current health."

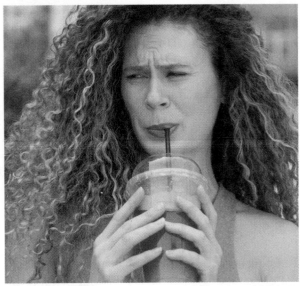

© Elisaveta Ivanova | Getty Images

Detoxes and cleanses are unnecessary and can prove dangerous.

What you can do: Stay physically and mentally active, regardless of your size. "What matters most, perhaps, is how much we move and how connected and engaged we are," she says. "Being sedentary is definitely a negative for our health, and being heavier is sometimes associated with being sedentary."

2 MYTH: Detoxes and cleanses make you healthier.

Truth: Your body doesn't need them, and they may do more harm than good. Maybe your sister swears that detoxes or cleanses help her feel and look better by removing toxins and jump-starting weight loss. But these tactics won't help you—and may harm you, according to the National Center for Complementary and Integrative Health (NCCIH).

These approaches often involve short-term diets and periods of fasting, and they may call for teas or juices, nutritional shakes, or specific supplements or herbs. Detoxes, in particular, are marketed on the premise that they help the liver "reset" and work more efficiently to remove toxins we're exposed to in food and the environment.

▸▸

▸▸ But these products haven't been proven to offer any health benefits and can be dangerous for older adults, women who are pregnant or breastfeeding, and some people with underlying health conditions, according to the NCCIH. They can lead to an excessive intake of vitamins and minerals; kidney problems from drinking juices of high-oxalate foods, such as spinach and beets; and bacterial infections from unpasteurized products.

Moreover, we naturally get rid of toxins through our breath, sweat, urine, and feces.

What you can do: "My advice isn't that thrilling: eating a balanced, highly plant-based diet with fewer processed foods is better for you than any particular cleanse or detox," Dr. Fernandez says.

3 MYTH: Eating before bedtime leads to weight gain.

Truth: **Timing doesn't count as much as what's on your plate.** Popular wisdom posits that our metabolism slows at night, automatically converting any evening snacks into fat. But chips or ice cream somehow tend to trump an apple while we're watching TV. It's no wonder we feel sluggish and doughy in the morning.

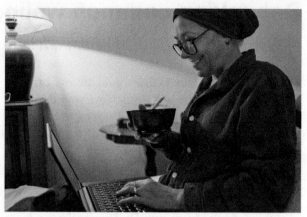

© playb | Getty Images

Opt for healthier choices before sleep, rather than sweets.

"There may be some truth that our metabolism and insulin secretion change at night because we're sleeping," Dr. Fernandez says. "But I suspect what you eat, and whether your eating is mindful, matter more."

What you can do: Incorporate more protein, fiber, and complex carbohydrates into dinner choices to keep you feeling full through the evening. If you still feel compelled to snack, keep healthy options available when the urge arises, such as Greek yogurt and berries or carrots dipped in hummus. ▮

Chapter 10

Men's Health

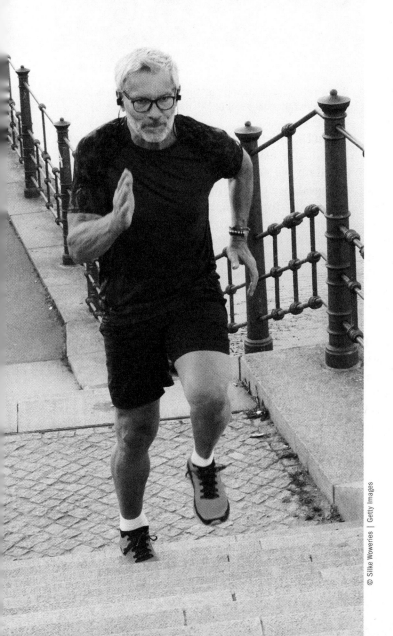

© Silke Woweries | Getty Images

Healthy Habits!
5 Things You Can Do Now

1 **Schedule time for health.** Block out exercise routines and preventative care—don't simply wait until a problem comes up. (page 244)

2 **Measure your waist and hips.** Doing so can help you keep tabs on visceral fat, the riskiest kind. (page 246)

3 **If you or your partner struggle with sleep quality, consider sleeping apart.** With the right preparation, it could bring you closer. (page 253)

4 **Keep expectations for testosterone therapy in check.** Ads you may see on TV are largely hype. (page 255)

5 **Step up your walking game.** Learn tips from an expert walker. (page 262)

Overcoming heart health obstacles

What do cardiologists tell their male patients about managing heart disease? Two Harvard experts share their experiences.

Prevention is the best medicine, but many men wait for a problem to arise before seeking help. For heart disease—the No. 1 cause of death among men—it could be runaway blood pressure, escalating cholesterol levels, or even a heart attack.

Yet, when faced with the reality of heart disease, men often encounter obstacles that keep them from managing their condition or lowering their risk. What can they do?

To find out, we asked two cardiologists—Dr. Haider Warraich and Dr. Dale Adler with Harvard-affiliated Brigham and Women's Hospital—what they hear from their male patients and the advice they offer.

Think about the future. During consultations, Dr. Warraich asks his patients about how they define longevity. "When they reflect on what they hope to achieve as they age, most say they value a high quality of life and independent living rather than simply living a few years longer than normal," he says. Getting men to focus on their future helps them define goals and then determine if they are on the path to meet them. "It helps them understand their shortcomings, like needing to be serious about weight loss or managing cholesterol, and can motivate them to make lasting changes," says Dr. Warraich.

Monitor your blood pressure. Men sometimes don't feel in control of their heart health, says Dr. Warraich. One way they can play an active role is to regularly monitor their blood pressure. "The heart health risks of high blood pressure are far-reaching, and even if men are not taking medication to manage high levels, keeping tabs on their numbers can be a proactive way to look out for potential problems," says Dr. Warraich. Men can easily do this by investing in a home blood pressure monitor. Record weekly readings and alert your doctor about sudden changes.

Confront suspicions about medication. Dr. Adler has found that many men who need blood pressure medicine, statins to manage cholesterol, or other medications are hesitant to take them. "They often focus too much on potential side effects and less on the benefits," he says. Much of this may reflect a general mistrust of medicine and the idea that they may have to take the pills indefinitely.

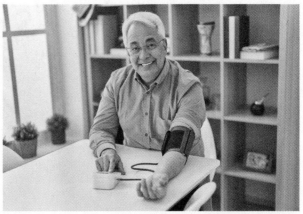

© AaronAmat | Getty Images

Taking regular home blood pressure measurements is one way to monitor potential heart health risks.

But Dr. Adler says men can overcome this resistance by realizing they have a say in how the drugs are used. "I tell my patients that by making diet and lifestyle changes, they can possibly take lower doses or even eventually stop taking them," he says. "When they understand their power, they are more open to taking medication they need for better heart health."

Schedule time for health. Consistency is vital for maintaining heart-healthy exercise. But one of the top complaints Dr. Adler hears is lack of time. "In general, men are receptive to routine and schedules, but they often don't do well when it gets disrupted," he says. Dr. Adler advises his patients to find a few blocks of time that work with their schedule and daily energy levels so they have multiple options for exercise. For instance, try scheduling a workout in the morning as soon as you wake up, or in the evening before dinner (exercise before a meal also curbs appetite).

Also, treat workout sessions as critical meetings, and always have a backup plan in place. "This way," Dr. Adler says, "if you miss your scheduled workout, you can automatically go to plan B." For example, take a quick walk, do five minutes of squats and push-ups, or stop by the gym.

Make weight loss a group effort. One of the greatest threats to heart health is weight gain. "Weight loss is not easy, but studies have found that sharing your weight-loss efforts through friendly competitions or online community forums is a tool for staying motivated and overcoming setbacks," says Dr. Adler. You could also enlist friends and begin your own weight-loss club, where you share your daily or weekly weigh-ins, exchange tips and strategies, talk about challenges, and encourage each other.

Learn portion control. "People are generally not great at estimating food portions," says Dr. Adler. This is one reason weight-loss programs like Jenny Craig and Weight Watchers are effective, he adds. "They give you the exact portions you are supposed to eat, which is what you need to feel satisfied."

He tells his patients trying to eat healthier or lose weight to always plan their meals in advance and get in the habit of measuring portions. "This way, you

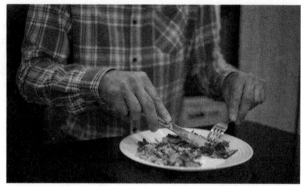

© Rockaa | Getty Images

Being mindful about food portions can prevent overeating and assist with weight loss.

can take the guesswork out of what to eat and avoid consuming extra calories."

Weighing the dangers of extra weight

Carrying a few seemingly innocent pounds invites serious health risks.

An estimated 70% of adults in the United States are overweight or obese based on body mass index (BMI), a calculation that takes into account both height and weight.

Standard definitions consider a healthy BMI as between 18.5 and 24.9, overweight as 25 to 29.9, and obese as 30 and higher. (Calculate your BMI using the online tool at www.harvard.health.edu/bmi.)

While far from perfect, BMI offers a simple gauge of whether someone's weight might pose a problem. Studies have found that a BMI higher than 25 increases your risk for heart disease, diabetes, and some types of cancer.

But what if you have put on only a little extra weight in

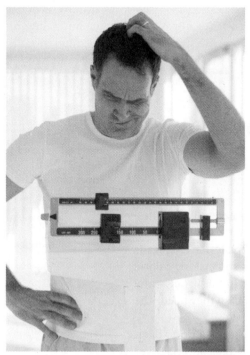

Tetra Images | Getty Images

Even a small amount of excess weight can increase the risk for many health problems.

recent years—say, five pounds or so—and your BMI doesn't fall into the category of overweight? Is that still cause for concern?

"Any excess weight can pose a health risk and affect one's daily life," says Dr. Walter Willett, professor of epidemiology and nutrition at the Harvard T.H. Chan School of Public Health. "When you carry extra pounds, you also are more susceptible to joint pain, low energy, and problems sleeping."

Yet the greatest threat is the potential for gaining even more weight. "It's easy for five pounds to quickly turn into 10 pounds and then 15 pounds, and as the weight increases, so do the health risks," says Dr. Willett. ▶▶

▸▸ Why do you gain weight?

It's common for men to gain some weight with age. Metabolism naturally slows, and lean muscle mass steadily declines, both of which cause the body to burn calories at a slower rate. In addition, most men consume more daily calories than they need. "When you take in extra calories and don't burn them off, they will be stored as fat," says Dr. Willett.

But where you accumulate that extra fat is the real issue with weight gain.

Based on its location, fat can be described as either subcutaneous or visceral. Subcutaneous fat is located just under the skin. Visceral fat lies deep within the abdominal cavity and pads the spaces between your abdominal organs.

Of the two, visceral fat is more dangerous, as high amounts are linked with heart disease risk factors like high blood pressure, elevated blood sugar, and high cholesterol levels. Do you have too much visceral fat? Check your waist size (see "Waist management," page 247). "Even a small change in your clothing, like pants that now feel snug or having to change notches in your belt, are signs of increasing visceral fat," says Dr. Willett.

What is your ideal weight?

There's no one-size-fits-all number for a person's ideal weight. The number depends on age, genetics, body frame, medical history, and average weight as a young adult.

"Your BMI can offer a clue about whether you need to lose excess weight, but consulting with your doctor can help determine your ideal healthy weight range," says Dr. Willett.

Still, you should not ignore even small weight changes. "A little weight gain may seem normal for many men, but that doesn't mean they should accept it and not do anything about it," says Dr. Willett. "It's easier to make modest adjustments now than to wait until you gain a lot more weight."

You can turn back those extra pounds with a combination of aerobic exercise, strength training, and a healthy diet.

Experts recommend at least 30 minutes of moderate-intensity aerobic exercise (for example, brisk walking, swimming, or cycling) most days of the week, plus at least two weekly weight or resistance training sessions to maintain muscle mass and strength. To avoid putting on more pounds, stick with a diet that prioritizes plant-based foods, like the Mediterranean or DASH diets. ▉

An inside look at body fat

Keep tabs on visceral fat, the kind you cannot see or feel.

As men age, their metabolism naturally declines, and they burn calories more slowly. While testosterone levels drop, they may also be less active, leading to potentially less muscle mass and making calorie burning even more challenging. In addition, many men consume more daily calories than they need. The typical outcome: too much body fat.

"When you take in extra calories and don't burn them off, they eventually get stored as fat and, over time, can accumulate," says Dr. Caroline Apovian, co-director of the Center for Weight Management

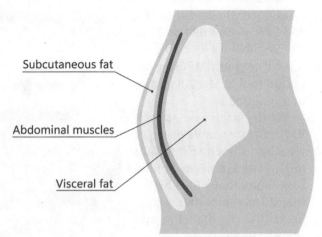

Subcutaneous fat

Abdominal muscles

Visceral fat

© Elena Pimukova I Getty Images

Visceral fat can be hard to measure because it lies deep within the body.

and Wellness at Harvard-affiliated Brigham and Women's Hospital.

But the real problem is where this fat ends up. Many people think of "bad" fat as the kind they can pinch around their waist. But the fat that collects just under the skin—called subcutaneous fat—appears to cause few health issues.

A more dangerous type of fat, called visceral fat, is stored at waist level, but inside the abdominal cavity and around vital organs like the pancreas, liver, and intestines.

Visceral fat makes up only about 10% of a person's total body fat. Still, research has found that high amounts can raise several heart disease risk factors, such as blood pressure, blood sugar, and total cholesterol levels.

How to measure

How can you measure visceral fat? The most accurate way is with an MRI, but that can be expensive (and the test is not covered by health insurance if ordered solely to assess visceral fat). Body mass index (BMI) provides a reasonable estimate using a person's height and weight. (Find your BMI at www.health.harvard.edu/bmi.) But BMI does not account for ethnic differences, nor does it consider extra weight from muscle and bone mass.

One of the best (and easiest) ways to gauge visceral fat is your waistline, according to Dr. Apovian. "In general, a man whose waist measures 40 inches or more has excess visceral fat." (See "Waist management," right.)

But what if you have only put on an extra three to five pounds that moves the belt buckle over one hole? Is that a problem? Not necessarily—but be careful, warns Dr. Apovian. "It's easy for five pounds to quickly turn into 10 pounds, and the more extra weight you carry, the greater the risk for high amounts of visceral fat."

Going deep

The best way to fight the fat you cannot see is the same as for fat you can see—aerobic exercise, strength training, and a healthy diet. But keep in mind that visceral fat can be slow to come off. "You first gain visceral fat, and then you gain subcutaneous fat," says Dr. Apovian. "But when you lose weight, only about one-third is visceral fat."

Dr. Apovian recommends a combination of 30 minutes to an hour of moderate-intense aerobic exercise, two or three days a week, plus two sessions a week of weight or resistance training to add muscle mass. "The combination helps to burn calories and tap into stored visceral fat," she says.

The kind of aerobic exercise doesn't matter as long as the intensity raises your heart rate enough that it is difficult to have a conversation. Some of your aerobic workouts should include high-intensity interval training, or HIIT, Dr. Apovian adds.

With HIIT, you run or walk at a higher intensity for a brief time, followed by a period at a slower pace to catch your breath. You repeat the cycle for the entire workout. You can enlist a personal trainer to help design a HIIT program and teach you how to perform the exercises correctly and safely.

Besides following a healthy, plant-based diet, make sure you eat enough daily protein to help build muscle mass. The recommended daily intake is 0.8 grams per kilogram of body weight. (You can convert your body weight from pounds to kilograms by dividing by 2.2.

So, for instance, 160 pounds is 72 kg; multiplying this by 0.8 equals about 58 grams of protein a day.) Fish, poultry, beans, and yogurt are good protein sources. You can also mix protein powder into smoothies, oatmeal, or a glass of water or milk. (For more on meeting your protein needs, see page 248.) ◗

Waist management

A tape measure is a simple way to keep tabs on visceral fat. Place the bottom of the tape at the top of your right hipbone, then pull the tape around at navel level (not the narrowest part of your torso). Do not suck in your gut or pull the tape tight enough to compress the area. A waist circumference of 40 inches or more is considered a sign of excess visceral fat for men. In addition, monitor whether your pants get snug, which also can be a sign you have gained visceral fat.

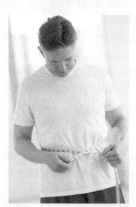

© tetmc | Getty Images

Are you eating enough protein?

Men need adequate protein in their diet to combat age-related muscle loss, but many don't get enough.

Age-related muscle loss, called sarcopenia, is a natural part of aging. After age 30, men begin to lose as much as 3% to 5% of their muscle mass per decade, and most will lose about 30% during their lifetimes.

Strength training and protein are two ways to build muscle mass and combat sarcopenia. With strength training, many experts recommend progressive resistance training, where you gradually amp up your workout volume—weight, reps, and sets—as your strength and endurance improve.

This constant challenge builds muscle and helps prevent plateaus where you start losing the gains. (Enlist a personal trainer to help you set up a detailed sequence and supervise your initial workouts to ensure you perform the exercises safely.)

Muscles also need fuel, and that's where protein comes in. The body breaks down dietary protein into amino acids, which it uses to build muscle. "Men need adequate protein in their diet to increase and maintain muscle mass as well as assist their body when it must recover from surgery or injuries," says Dr. Frank Hu, a professor of nutrition and epidemiology with Harvard's T.H. Chan School of Public Health.

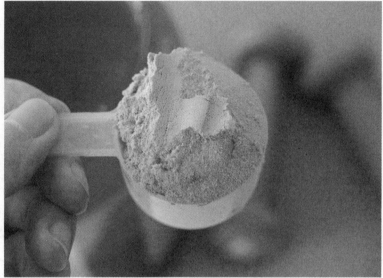

© Professor25 | Getty Images

Adding protein powder to your diet can help you attain your daily protein goals.

a 180-pound man, that is approximately 65 grams of protein per day. According to many experts, most Americans meet and even exceed this amount. Still, some estimates suggest that approximately 10% to 25% of older adults consume less than the RDA. And aging men—especially those trying to build muscle mass—may need more protein than the guidelines recommend.

In fact, a 2023 research review published in *The Journals of Gerontology: Series A* suggested older adults may benefit from consuming 1 to 1.6 grams of protein per kilogram of body weight daily (about 82 to 130 grams for a 180-pound man) to help increase muscle strength.

However, according to Dr. Hu, you should be careful about consuming very high amounts per day—2 grams per kilogram of body weight or more. "Some studies have shown that too much

Protein by the numbers

Despite this need, there's a good chance aging men don't get their optimal daily protein intake, especially if they also are cutting calories to lose weight. The Recommended Dietary Allowance (RDA) of protein is 0.8 gram per kilogram of body weight, or about 0.36 gram per pound. For

Timing your protein

Research suggests that the body can make use of only 20 to 40 grams of dietary protein at one time. "So there is no benefit from getting most of your daily protein from one meal," says Dr. Frank Hu with Harvard's T.H. Chan School of Public Health. Instead, try to evenly distribute your protein over breakfast, lunch, dinner, and snacks. Also, to maximize muscle growth and improve recovery, consume a portion of your daily protein within 30 minutes to one hour after your strength training workout, through either a drink or a meal.

protein is associated with an increased risk of chronic diseases and mortality," he says.

The best sources

The first step to merging protein with strength training is to get a realistic estimate of how much protein you consume daily. "People tend to over- or underestimate how much they actually eat," says Dr. Hu. He suggests tracking your protein intake with each meal for a week to get a daily average. "Make sure to read labels and assess your protein per serving as accurately as possible, and don't guess at amounts."

Once you have a general idea of your usual intake, you can increase it as needed. Dr. Hu recommends focusing on high-quality sources, like lean poultry, fish, dairy, and plant-based foods, such as soy, legumes, nuts, and whole grains. (Some people may need to avoid common high-protein food sources like meat, eggs, or dairy due to health concerns or dietary restrictions.)

Here are some examples of how much protein you can get from typical servings of high-quality protein sources:

- 3.5 ounces lean chicken (31 grams)
- 3.5 ounces salmon (24 grams)
- 1 cup cooked beans (about 18 grams)
- 6 ounces plain yogurt (17 grams)
- 1 cup skim milk (9 grams)
- ¼ cup nuts (7 grams)
- 1 egg (6 grams)

Another option is whey protein powder or vegan powders made from soy, peas, or brown rice. (The exact amount of protein per serving varies by brand.) Powders are a useful choice if you have trouble getting enough protein from foods. They can be added to oatmeal and smoothies or stirred into a glass of water. "Because powders come with measuring scoops, they can help you track how many protein grams you add to your daily diet," says Dr. Hu.

IN THE JOURNALS

Waist-to-hip ratio better than BMI in predicting future health issues

A person's waist-to-hip ratio may be a better tool than body mass index (BMI) for predicting chronic health problems, according to a study published in 2023 by *JAMA Network Open*.

Waist-to-hip ratio is the circumference of your waist divided by the circumference at your hips. For the study, waist circumference was measured at the smallest natural waistline (usually near the belly button) and hip circumference at the widest part of the hips. BMI is calculated by dividing your weight in kilograms by your height in meters squared.

Researchers collected measurements from 387,672 participants (59% men). Everyone's health then was tracked until their death.

Afterward, the researchers identified people who developed weight-related health problems like high blood pressure, heart disease, and type 2 diabetes and then cross-referenced with their measurements. They found that waist-to-hip ratio was a better predictor of a person's future health issues than BMI. The reason, they said, was most likely that waist-to-hip ratio better reflects levels of abdominal fat, including dangerous visceral fat. According to the researchers, a healthy waist-to-hip ratio for most men is below 0.95.

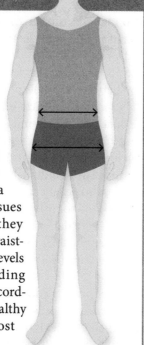

© chanakon laorob | Getty Images

The (almost) last word on alcohol and health

Is drinking alcohol healthy or harmful? It still comes down to how much you consume.

New information has again opened the debate about what role, if any, alcohol plays in health. Is a moderate amount good for your heart? Can you still enjoy the occasional beverage, or should you become a teetotaler as you age?

Like so much in life, it's complicated.

"There's good evidence that, in general, moderate drinkers who average one to two drinks a day tend to live longer," says Eric Rimm, professor of epidemiology and nutrition and director of the Program in Cardiovascular Epidemiology at the Harvard T.H. Chan School of Public Health. "Whether that is directly linked with alcohol, other lifestyle factors, or some combination is still being explored."

Different findings

Why might alcohol be healthy? It's thought that moderate intake helps raise levels of "good" HDL cholesterol, higher amounts of which are associated with a lower risk for heart disease. Alcohol also may discourage the formation of small blood clots that can lead to heart attacks and stroke.

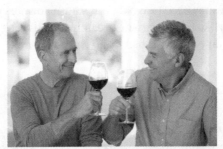
© Chris Ryan | Getty Images
Enjoy an occasional drink, but the evidence for health benefits is mixed.

Still, recent studies have cast doubt on the connection between alcohol and good health.

For instance, a meta-analysis (that is, a study based on data collected in multiple earlier trials) published in 2023 in *JAMA Network Open* concluded that low-volume drinkers (1.3 to 24 grams of alcohol daily, or less than two standard drinks) did not live longer than people who never drank.

Medium-volume drinking (25 to 44 grams, about two to three daily standard drinks) also didn't offer significant health protection. Rimm is quick to pump the brakes on this and similar conclusions based on data from multiple studies.

"New findings do not mean that everything else that came before is wrong," he says. "The problem with these studies is that they combine good and poor research. So, it's difficult to make a conclusion with information where alcohol is assessed so differently.

For many studies, they completely ignored measuring drinking patterns."

Another issue is that most alcohol-related studies are observational—that is, they can show an association, but not cause and effect.

Other factors linked with alcohol intake may contribute to drinkers' well-being. For instance, a study published in 2022 in *JAMA Network Open* found that moderate drinkers had the lowest heart disease risk compared with nondrinkers, suggesting that some alcohol intake may benefit heart health.

Yet the research team also discovered that light-to-moderate drinkers had healthier lifestyles than abstainers. They were more physically active, ate more vegetables and less red meat, and didn't smoke as much.

Glass half-full

What seems clear in most research supporting the health benefits of alcohol is that the amount is key. Light to moderate intake remains the best advice.

The CDC classifies moderate alcohol intake for adult men as two standard drinks or fewer on days when they drink. A standard drink is approximately 12 ounces of regular beer (5% alcohol by volume, or ABV), 8 to 9 ounces of malt liquor (7% ABV), 5 ounces of wine (12% ABV), or 1.5 ounces of 80-proof spirits (40% ABV). (See "What is a standard drink?" on page 251, and to more accurately analyze your drink's alcohol content per serving size, use this drink calculator from the National Institutes of Health: www.health.harvard.edu/size.)

Of course, most people don't drink daily, and some may go for long periods without alcohol. "But even occasional drinkers may still receive some benefits," says Rimm.

Does the type of alcohol matter? Not really. Your body reacts to alcohol the same way whether it comes from a California wine, Scotch whiskey, or craft beer. "The differences between beverages are the percentage of alcohol," says Rimm.

Your choice of beverage can have adverse health effects unrelated to the alcohol. For instance, a gin-and-tonic cocktail contains high amounts of sugar, and most beer is high in carbohydrates and calories.

One part of the alcohol debate everyone agrees on: not drinking too much.

"Studies have found that regularly drinking beyond the recommended amount can raise a person's risk for numerous health problems, like liver failure, high blood pressure, heart failure, and several types of cancer," says Rimm. Avoid regular excessive drinking and binge drinking (consuming five or more drinks on one occasion).

Last call
So what is the conclusion? According to Rimm, if you don't drink, there is no reason to begin. If you only occasionally drink, don't increase your intake for health reasons. But for the casual or regular drinker, it's fine to enjoy an alcoholic beverage—in moderation.

But you should also weigh your alcohol intake with your overall heart health, adds Rimm. For example, if you have high blood pressure, you may want to drink less or abstain from drinking and focus on getting your blood pressure under control.

"If you have any health issues, it's best to speak with your doctor about what is the proper amount of alcohol for you," says Rimm. ▌

What is a standard drink?

12 ounces regular beer
About 5% alcohol

8–9 ounces malt liquor (in a 12-ounce glass)
About 7% alcohol

5 ounces table wine
About 12% alcohol

1.5 ounces distilled spirits (gin, rum, tequila, vodka, whiskey, etc.)
About 40% alcohol

Source: National Institute on Alcohol Abuse and Alcoholism, NIH.

Stress at work takes a toll on the heart

Men who report specific types of job-related stress face a higher risk of heart disease than those without such stress, according to a recent study.

Researchers followed more than 6,500 white-collar workers for 18 years and identified two job-related conditions linked to higher cardiovascular risks. One was job strain, defined as high demands (such as having a heavy workload and tight deadlines) coupled with low control (for example, having little say in decision making). The other, called effort-reward imbalance, occurs when a person's effort is high but their salary, recognition, or job security are low.

Compared with people who didn't experience work stress, men who reported either of those stressors

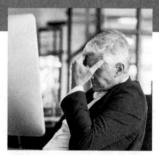
© Stígur Már Karlsson /Heimsmyndir I Getty Images

had a 49% higher risk of heart disease. But their risk doubled if they reported both types. Among women, the results were inconclusive, which the authors say might reflect the fact that women tend to develop heart disease later in life than men. The men were also more likely to have diabetes, high blood pressure, and other factors that raise heart disease risk. The study was published in 2023 by *Circulation: Cardiovascular Quality and Outcomes.*

Overcoming bedroom barriers

Here's how to manage common obstacles men and their partners may encounter in their sex life.

Every aspect of your life changes over time, and your sexual life is no exception.

"Partners in relationships face many challenges that can affect intimacy, whether those are health issues, physical changes, or fluctuations in desire," says Dr. Sharon Bober, director of the Sexual Health Program at Harvard-affiliated Dana-Farber Cancer Institute. "Older couples often have core beliefs, including that their sex life is bound to diminish or that individuals need to conform to a certain ideal as they age, but with communication, planning, and creativity, both partners can continue to enjoy a satisfying sexual relationship over time."

Here's a look at three common issues older couples often face and how to successfully navigate them.

Stuck in a rut

Eventually, most longtime partners get stuck in romantic ruts. Here are some ways to get back on track.

Start dating again. A satisfying sex life begins outside of the bedroom. Schedule regular dates with your partner and consider having experiences that are new for both of you, like participating in a local event, taking a class together, or going on a spontaneous overnight or weekend romantic getaway to a new place. "Doing something different and unexpected can offer a shared sense of excitement that increases desire and can bring you and your partner closer together, which also helps cultivate desire," says Dr. Bober.

Turn it around. Focus less on yourself and more on your partner's pleasure and satisfaction. "This can be a big turn-on for both people," says Dr. Bober.

Out of sync

Many couples go through phases where desire is not equally shared. "When one partner wants sex more often than the other, this can lead to frustration for both partners," says Dr. Bober. Getting back in sync relies on better understanding each other's needs and finding common ground. For example:

Try different ways to satisfy. You might focus more on "outercourse," which means directing your attention and energy toward foreplay and manual

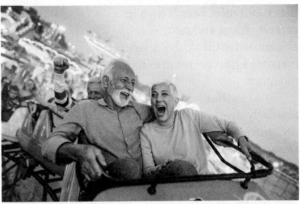
© skynesher | Getty Images

Going on regular dates and spontaneous trips offer ways for couples to reignite passion.

stimulation with your partner, like massages, sensual touch, kissing, or snuggling naked in bed. Another option is to share erotic fiction or watch videos. "Make the emphasis on intimacy, sensuality, and closeness without the pressure of having a romantic encounter always leading to intercourse," says Dr. Bober.

Plan time for intimacy. Sometimes, you need to make sex happen to get back in rhythm. "This way, neither partner needs to feel pressured to initiate, but rather, you can look forward to and anticipate a romance encounter together," says Dr. Bober. Desire can vary throughout the day and night and from one person to another, so communicate about what time is best, and try to find a compromise.

Low energy

Older women deal with the effects of menopausal symptoms like vaginal dryness, which can affect desire and sexual satisfaction. For men, it's usually low sexual energy caused by erectile dysfunction or low testosterone levels.

Erectile dysfunction (ED). Men with ED can experience low energy because the condition can be a blow to their self-esteem. "Men may feel embarrassed about not being able to get or keep an erection or worry they cannot perform as well as they once did, so motivation and energy for sex can diminish along with that worry," says Dr. Bober.

ED drugs can help by improving blood supply to the penis. Studies have shown that they can help produce an erection sufficient to start intercourse in about 70% of healthy men. The most commonly prescribed medications are sildenafil (Viagra), avanafil (Stendra), and tadalafil (Cialis). Speak with your doctor about which drug and dose may be best. If ED drugs don't work, or if you cannot tolerate side effects like headaches, flushing, upset stomach, or dizziness, other therapies may be an option. For instance, if sustaining an erection is a problem, consider a penile band, also known as an ED ring, or a vacuum pump.

Low testosterone. Levels of testosterone, the male sex hormone, drop about 1% each year beginning in a man's late 30s and can fall by as much as 50% by age 70. Fatigue is a common side effect. Increasing testosterone via topical gels, patches, injections, or absorbable pellet implants can help restore energy in men with low levels. Your doctor can check your testosterone levels with a blood test and then discuss testosterone therapy options. (For more on low testosterone and whether you need it, see "When to consider testosterone therapy" on page 255.) ▼

Sleeping apart: Good for your sex life?

More couples are sleeping in separate beds for various reasons, but the practice may strengthen their love connection.

A 2023 survey by the American Academy of Sleep Medicine found that one-third of respondents reported occasionally or regularly sleeping in separate rooms to accommodate a bed partner.

This may seem like a sign of a troubled relationship, but the practice is quite common and can lead to couples being happier and closer, according to Sharon Bober, associate professor of psychology at Harvard Medical School and founding director of the Sexual Health Program at Harvard-affiliated Dana-Farber Cancer Institute. "Just because you don't always sleep in the same bed doesn't mean that you feel separated as a couple," she says.

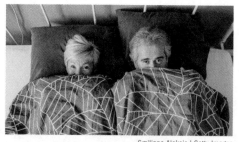

Smiljana Aleksic | Getty Images

Sleeping apart can help couples feel more rested and bring them closer together.

Contributing issues

The main motivation behind separate sleeping is not about lack of physical desire or emotional intimacy, but simply the need for both people to get a good night's rest.

"Sharing a bed means you share the other person's sleep behavior," says Bober. "If a person snores, grinds their teeth, thrashes and twitches, or gets up repeatedly at night, this can disrupt their partner's sleep, making partners more tired and irritable, which can strain the relationship."

Other issues that could contribute to sleeping apart include environmental factors (one partner needs the bedroom to be cooler or warmer) and sleeping schedules (one might like to stay up later reading or watching TV, or might need to get up early).

"Getting restful sleep is essential for good health and a good sex life," says Bober. "Sometimes sleeping in separate rooms, both people can sleep better and feel rested. Instead of resulting in something negative, this might allow for both partners to have more energy, better mood, and consequently more desire for sex."

Pillow talk

Sometimes just one person expresses the desire to sleep separately, which can make their partner feel rejected and worry about their relationship.

"If either partner feels concerned about not sleeping in the same bed, the couple needs to talk about what might feel worrisome," says Bober. "The ▶▶

conversation might reveal an issue not related to intimacy that has been lingering for a while."

Before sleeping apart, another option may be to consider compromises that address the issues of disrupted sleep and are acceptable to both people.

For example, if your partner's snoring wakes you up, wear earplugs, use a bedside sound machine, or wear earbuds and listen to a podcast as you fall asleep. The snoring partner could try sleeping on their side or see a doctor to find out whether there's an underlying health problem, like sleep apnea.

Even when a couple agrees to a new sleeping arrangement, Bober suggests several strategies to enhance and maintain connection while also making the transition smoother for both partners:

Set a schedule. At first, you might agree to sleep apart during the week or on specific days when partners need the most rest, but choose to sleep together on the weekends and make adjustments as needed.

Make both sleeping spaces cozy. "You both need a comfortable sleeping environment," says Bober. "Make sure both people are happy with their sleeping space."

Have a snuggle time. Before bedtime, spend time together in bed to snuggle, talk, read together, or have some romantic time; then, when it's time for sleep,

move to your separate beds. You can also do the reverse: get in bed together in the morning and connect with coffee and conversation. "This kind of flexibility can help couples continue to associate the bed with closeness, pleasure, and intimacy," says Bober.

Make a date for sex. Not sleeping together can interfere with spontaneous sex. If you and your partner are concerned about a declining sex life, schedule time for intimacy. "This can create a sense of excitement and allow for anticipation," says Bober. To enhance the experience, tie your get-together to a date night or a romantic evening at home.

Nap together. Another idea is napping together during the day. "Even a short nap together can help maintain the bedroom bonding and is something couples can do either on occasion or more regularly," says Bober.

Assess the arrangement regularly. Check in with each other every day to see what's working and what isn't. "It's not good enough if sleeping separately feels helpful only for one person in the relationship," says Bober. "You can always go back to the drawing board and come up with a revised plan. Sleeping apart, either once in a while or more regularly, can be beneficial, if both partners are happy with the setup, sleep well, and continue to feel connected as a couple."

IN THE JOURNALS

Erectile dysfunction drugs linked to lower Alzheimer's disease risk

Another benefit to taking erectile dysfunction (ED) drugs? They may help lower your risk for Alzheimer's disease, according to a study published in 2024 in *Neurology*. Researchers studied the health records of approximately 270,000 men who were diagnosed with ED between 2000 and 2017. The men's average age at diagnosis was 58. Over a median period of about five years after diagnosis, men who took any of the ED drugs known as PDE5 inhibitors— sildenafil (Viagra), tadalafil (Cialis), vardenafil, and avanafil (Stendra)—were less likely to have

an Alzheimer's diagnosis than those who didn't take one of the drugs.

How may these drugs help? These ED medications appear to increase brain blood flow, and they may reduce brain inflammation associated with developing Alzheimer's disease. While the results only show a link between taking PDE5 inhibitors and lower dementia risk, the findings align with similar studies, according to the researchers. While the potential for brain benefits is enticing, much more research is needed before concluding that any of these ED drugs might help maintain cognitive fitness.

When to consider testosterone therapy

Learn what it can and can't do.

You may have seen advertisements and various celebrity endorsements touting the wonders of testosterone replacement therapy (TRT). They claim that raising testosterone levels makes men feel younger and stronger, and boosts their sex life.

All that sounds wonderful, but is TRT really a potent anti-aging elixir? As with many miracle claims, don't believe the hype.

"For some older men, raising low testosterone levels can improve some aspects of their physical and mental well-being," says Dr. Michael O'Leary, a urologist at Harvard-affiliated Brigham and Women's Hospital. "But TRT won't suddenly turn back the clock."

Lowdown on low T

Testosterone is the sex hormone that gives men their manly qualities. Produced by the testicles, it helps to form traditional characteristics like a deep voice, facial hair, and muscle size and strength. It also fuels a man's libido.

Doctors define a normal blood level of testosterone as 300 nanograms per deciliter (ng/dL) and higher. According to the American College of Physicians, a man's testosterone level declines about 1.6% per year beginning in his mid-30s. About 20% of men ages 60 and older have low testosterone levels; that proportion rises to 30% for men in their 70s, and 50% for men in their 80s.

In addition to natural age-related decline, a significant drop in testosterone might also stem from medications (especially anabolic steroids) or damage to the testes, such as from an injury, an infection, radiation treatment, or chemotherapy.

Getting an accurate reading might require several blood tests, as your testosterone level fluctuates during the day. Tests are often done between 7 a.m. and 10 a.m., when testosterone is at its peak. Low levels can cause any of the following symptoms and conditions:

▸ depression
▸ reduced self-confidence
▸ difficulty concentrating
▸ disturbed sleep
▸ declining muscle and bone mass

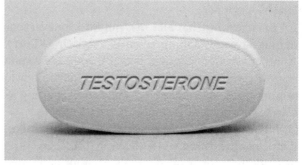

© Science Photo Library I Getty Images

Testosterone replacement therapy may help some men, but it's not a miracle drug.

▸ increased body fat
▸ fatigue
▸ swollen or tender breasts
▸ flushing or hot flashes
▸ lower sex drive
▸ fewer spontaneous erections
▸ difficulty sustaining erections.

Dr. O'Leary says you and your doctor might consider TRT if your levels drop below 300 ng/dL, but it's not automatic. "The first step is to determine if any symptoms attributed to low testosterone are related to something else that's treatable."

For example, symptoms like fatigue, trouble concentrating, and low sex drive could be caused by a poor diet, lack of exercise, and insufficient sleep. Stress, anxiety, and depression can be side effects of erectile dysfunction. "Raising low testosterone levels alone won't fix these problems," says Dr. O'Leary.

Trying TRT

If troublesome symptoms and low testosterone remain after these paths are explored, your doctor then may prescribe short-term TRT. TRT is usually given as a daily gel, cream, or patch applied to the skin (usually on the shoulder or thigh, which are easy to reach). TRT also can be taken as daily oral medication or weekly or biweekly injections. Another option is pellets implanted into the buttocks that slowly release testosterone over several weeks. "There is no advantage over the different applications," says Dr. O'Leary. "But injections may produce a faster change."

After you've been on TRT for about two months, your doctor will evaluate your symptoms. If ▸▸

there's no noticeable improvement, the dosage may be increased, continued at its current amount for a bit longer, or stopped.

"Keep in mind that TRT may not work for everyone or may have only a minimal effect," says Dr. O'Leary. Another aspect to consider is that if you have a good response, you may need to stay on TRT indefinitely to maintain the benefit, as your body stops making its own testosterone while you're on the therapy.

TRT can have short-term side effects, such as acne, disturbed breathing while sleeping, breast swelling or tenderness, or swollen ankles. "But for most men who qualify for treatment, the benefits of TRT usually outweigh these potential risks," says Dr. O'Leary.

Still, there are concerns about the long-term use of TRT. Although testosterone therapy does not cause prostate cancer, the hormone can stimulate faster growth of prostate cancer cells already present in the gland.

A recent clinical trial provided some reassurance that TRT in men with testosterone deficiency did not increase risk of cardiovascular events. However, older observational studies suggested a link between TRT and heart attacks. As a result, your doctor may want to be cautious if you are at increased risk of heart attack or stroke. 🛡

IN THE JOURNALS

Testosterone therapy may be safe for men at risk for heart attack and stroke

Does testosterone replacement therapy (TRT) raise men's risk for heart attacks or stroke? A recent study suggests not, although with some caveats. Researchers enrolled 5,246 men ages 45 to 80 with testosterone levels of less than 300 nanograms per deciliter (ng/dL). (Normal levels range from 300 to 1,000 ng/dL.) More than 50% had existing cardiovascular disease, while the others were considered at increased risk because of such factors as diabetes, high blood pressure, smoking, and an imbalance of lipids (total cholesterol, low-density lipoprotein, high-density lipoprotein, and triglycerides).

For an average of 22 months, the men applied a gel to their skin daily. For half of the men, the gel was a placebo (inactive). For the others, it contained enough testosterone to maintain their hormone levels between 350 and 750 ng/dL. At the three-year follow-up, the researchers found no difference in the rate of heart attacks, strokes, or death from cardiovascular problems between the TRT and placebo groups. However, compared with

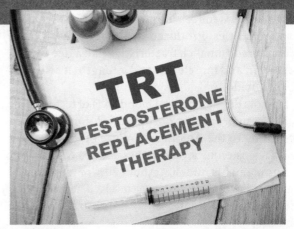

© airdone | Getty Images

the men using the placebo, those using TRT were more likely to have developed atrial fibrillation (an irregular heart rate that can increase the risk for stroke and heart failure) and pulmonary embolism (in which a blood clot travels to a lung artery and blocks blood flow).

The researchers pointed out that their findings do not apply to men who do not have a testosterone deficiency. Men considering TRT should discuss possible risks with their doctor, especially if they have any cardiovascular disease risk factors. The results were published in 2023 by *The New England Journal of Medicine*.

Several factors may cause testosterone levels to drop

Testosterone levels tend to slowly decline in middle-aged men, and often fall faster after age 70.

In an analysis of 11 studies involving about 25,000 men in total, researchers looked at the possible factors for this more rapid decline in testosterone levels later in life.

They found that having a body mass index higher than 27 and engaging in less than 75 minutes of weekly vigorous activity were each linked to lower testosterone levels. Other contributing factors were having ever smoked and health issues like high blood pressure, cardiovascular disease, cancer, and diabetes. Low testosterone levels can contribute to symptoms such as fatigue, weakness, and reduced sex drive.

While the findings only showed an association, the researchers stressed the need for older men to continue engaging in healthy lifestyle behaviors and managing chronic health issues, which could help maintain their body's testosterone production. Men also should address these areas before considering hormone therapy for low testosterone. The 2023 analysis appeared in *Annals of Internal Medicine*.

Aerobic activity may work as well as medication for helping erectile dysfunction

If you are concerned about the potential side effects of erectile dysfunction (ED) drugs and you're looking for an alternative treatment, try doing more aerobic exercise.

Researchers reviewed 11 randomized controlled trials involving more than 1,000 men with mild or moderate ED. They found that men who regularly exercised for 30 to 60 minutes three to five times a week saw more improvement in their ED compared with men who did not exercise. They also found that the worse a man's ED, the more exercise helped. The men participated in aerobic exercise like walking, running, and cycling.

The improvement in some men appeared to be similar to that provided by ED drugs like sildenafil (Viagra) and tadalafil (Cialis), as well as that from testosterone replacement therapy.

The researchers noted that aerobic exercise can help treat ED in many ways. For instance, it reduces inflammation, blood pressure, and excess weight,

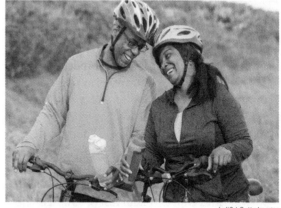

kali9 | Getty Images

Men who consistently do activities like cycling may see improvement in their mild or moderate erectile dysfunction.

all risk factors related to a higher risk for ED. Aerobic exercise also helps to improve blood flow and lower stress, which can help men obtain and keep erections. The 2023 study was published in *The Journal of Sexual Health*.

Rising up from a fall

Practice these movements to help you get up safely.

Prevention is the best protection against falls. Exercising, working on balance, and fall-proofing your home are essential. But if you take a tumble and you're uninjured, can you safely get back up?

"Your body requires certain movements to rise from the ground that we don't always practice or do as well as we age," says Janice McGrail, physical therapist and clinical specialist with Harvard-affiliated Spaulding Rehabilitation Network. "This is also why it's often difficult for older adults to get up and down in everyday life, like when they're kneeling in the garden, looking for something under the bed, or playing on the floor with the grandkids."

Exercises that can help you rise from a seated position and improve your daily up-and-down movements are the kneel-to-stand, crawling, and the sit-to-stand.

"Practicing these also can make you feel more confident about being active and able to live independently," says McGrail. "The moves also are a way to gauge your current fitness, flexibility, and mobility and identify areas where you need to improve."

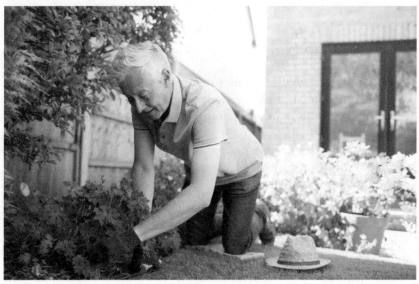
© Carruthers & Hobbs | Getty Images

The ability to safely kneel and rise also helps you perform many everyday movements.

Sit-to-stand
Muscles worked: *core, legs, hips*
This movement helps you practice rising from a seated floor position and is an excellent test of balance, coordination, and overall wellness, as it requires many physical skills.

Sit down on the floor with your legs crossed or straight out. Now stand up again. (This can be a difficult movement, especially for people with sore knees, arthritis, or poor balance, so practice with someone next to you for safety.) Note how you used your body for support.

Repeat the movement again, only this time, grade your effort. Beginning with a score of 10, subtract one point each time you do one of the following for support while sitting or standing:

▸ use your hand
▸ use your knee
▸ use your forearm
▸ use one hand on the knee or thigh
▸ use the side of your leg
▸ lose your balance at any time.

For example, take off one point if you sat with no problem but had to use either a hand or a knee to get up. If you had to use both hands and both knees, deduct four points (one point for each hand and knee). If you can sit on the floor and stand without assistance, you scored a perfect 10. If you cannot get up at all, your score is zero. Ideally, you want a score of eight or higher.

Kneel-to-stand
Muscles worked: *core, hips, thighs*
When you're on the ground, you often need to stabilize yourself in a kneeling position before you can stand. To practice this move, place a pillow, cushion, or folded towel on the floor. From a standing position, kneel so one knee is on the padding and the other leg is bent, so you are in a "marriage proposal" position. Stay there for one or two seconds, and then stand up.

If needed, push your hand against the bent knee for leverage, or do the exercise next to a chair or table and use it for assistance. Repeat the down-and-up movement five to 10 times. Then repeat, kneeling with the other leg, the same number of times.

Crawling
Muscles worked: *core, shoulders, hips*
If you fall, you might need to crawl to a couch or chair or another place where you can lift yourself up.

To practice crawling, get into a hands-and-knees position on the floor with your wrists under your shoulders and your knees under your hips. To crawl, move your right hand and left knee forward, then vice versa. Crawl in one direction for 10 counts, then turn around and crawl back. ◗

Plan for a soft landing

You can't always avoid a fall, but you may reduce injury by controlling how you fall. Falls happen quickly, and it can be challenging to think fast, but here are some strategies to help soften your landing.

▸ Lean forward into the fall, which gives you some control over direction.

▸ Fall sideways, if possible.

▸ Turn your shoulder into the fall to protect your head.

▸ Fall like a sack of beans—relax everything.

▸ Fall on the soft, fleshy places, like your buttocks and thighs. These areas have more protection and are lower to the ground.

▸ As you complete the fall, try to roll to your side in a ball. This will spread the impact to reduce injury and stop you from rolling farther.

IN THE JOURNALS

Study questions commercial men's health clinics services

When it comes to direct-to-consumer (DTC) men's health clinics, it's "buyer beware," as many offer costly treatments not supported by evidence and lack proper medical oversight, according to an investigative study published in 2023 by *Urology*.

Researchers identified 233 DTC men's health clinics. These clinics offered treatments such as testosterone replacement therapy (TRT) along with penile shock wave therapy and platelet-rich plasma (PRP) injections to treat erectile dysfunction. However, the researchers noted that the criteria for using TRT are still under debate and that most of the clinics did not follow standard protocols for testing and diagnosis of low testosterone levels. The effectiveness of penile shock wave therapy and PRP are still being studied,

they added, and should only be offered in clinical trial settings.

In addition, most of the clinics did not have a urologist or endocrinologist on staff. Instead, their primary providers were clinicians other than doctors, such as nurse practitioners and physician assistants. While such individuals have the skills to provide these treatments, it's not clear if they are supervised by physicians with expertise in men's health, according to the researchers.

The DTC clinics also charged high out-of-pocket costs. Among clinics that listed prices, TRT cost $80 to $500 monthly. PRP and shock wave therapy cost as much as $1,200 and $3,000 per treatment, respectively. The researchers concluded that these clinics should have more oversight and regulation from state agencies and medical associations.

No bones about it

Men get osteoporosis, too. Here's how to protect yourself from this common bone-weakening disease.

© Christopher Pattberg | Getty Images
Getting enough dietary calcium can help keep bones strong.

Although osteoporosis, the bone-weakening disease, strikes more women, men are not immune. In fact, estimates suggest about 6% of men ages 65 and older have osteoporosis, and about one in five will break a bone because of it. Research also has shown that, following a fracture due to osteoporosis, men are more likely to die than women.

"Looking out for your bones is equally as important as other aspects of your health as you age," says Dr. Harold Rosen, an endocrinologist with Harvard-affiliated Beth Israel Deaconess Medical Center. "There are many ways men can keep their bones strong to help prevent osteoporosis or slow its progress if it occurs."

Close to the bone

During your life, bones undergo a continuous maintenance cycle, called remodeling, in which they are simultaneously broken down and rebuilt. But, as you age, the body eventually loses bone faster than it can rebuild it. This is what causes osteoporosis, where bones become thinner, more porous, weaker, and more susceptible to fractures. Most men begin losing bone density around age 60, and, over time, they can get osteoporosis. Besides age, other factors can contribute to osteoporosis, including smoking, heavy alcohol use, family history, and chronic diseases of the kidney, lungs, stomach, and intestines.

When used over the long term, several medications can significantly increase the risk of osteoporosis. Chief among these are corticosteroids, such as prednisone, which are used to treat inflammatory bowel disease and other inflammatory and autoimmune disorders.

Other medications that may cause problems for bones include androgen deprivation therapy, used to treat prostate cancer; anticonvulsants for epilepsy; certain drugs given to organ transplant patients; and some chemotherapy drugs.

Slowing the loss

Trying to stop or at least slow bone loss is key to preventing osteoporosis and treating it if it occurs. "It's sometimes possible to slightly increase bone density, but the main goal is to preserve as much of your bone mass you have left," says Dr. Rosen. Here are some ways to help do that.

Calcium and vitamin D. Both calcium and vitamin D work together to keep bones healthy. Calcium is a building block of bone, while vitamin D helps the body absorb calcium. For older adults, the goal of adequate calcium intake is to limit bone loss.

"Consuming more calcium does not mean you are feeding your bones calcium. Instead, you are supplying your body with enough calcium so it won't pull calcium from your bones and thus weaken them," says Dr. Rosen.

The recommended daily calcium intake for men ages 50 to 70 is 1,000 milligrams (mg); for men ages 71 and older, it's 1,200 mg. Recommendations for vitamin D are 15 micrograms (mcg) or 600 international units (IU) daily until age 70 and then 20 mcg (800 IU) afterward. How can you tell if you lack calcium or vitamin D? Dr. Rosen says to examine your diet and outdoor exposure. "It's often easy to get enough calcium through a regular healthy diet." he says.

For instance, one cup of milk, yogurt, or calcium-fortified orange juice, as well as an ounce of cheese, all have between 300 and 400 mg of calcium each (along with 100 IU of vitamin D in fortified milk). "So, eating three or four servings can give people plenty of calcium," says Dr. Rosen. Other good calcium sources include one cup of soymilk (300 mg), ½ cup of tofu (138 mg), and ½ cup of cooked turnip greens (100 mg).

Sunlight exposure is the best way to improve your vitamin D level. One study found that eight to 10 minutes of sun exposure to 25% of the body (hands, face, neck, and arms) produces the recommended daily amount of vitamin D in people with light skin. People with darker skin may need 15 to 30 minutes of similar sun exposure.

But that can be a challenge in the winter or if you live in a northern climate, or if you're diligent about limiting sun exposure for skin care reasons. (While sunscreen blocks UVB light, few people put on enough to block all UVB, or they use sunscreen irregularly. As a result, sunscreen typically has a limited effect on vitamin D level.)

Therefore, Dr. Rosen recommends taking a daily multivitamin or a vitamin D supplement. For most people, a 1,000 IU dose is sufficient. (Most multivitamins also contain a decent amount of calcium—around 200 to 300 mg.)

Exercise. Research has suggested that weight-bearing activities (in which your bones support your weight) can help to slow bone loss and even increase bone density, although estimates suggest it's a modest 1% to 2% increase in adults.

Weight-bearing examples include speed walking, running, stair climbing, and elliptical training. These activities put stress on bones that, in turn, pushes bone-forming cells into action. Regular exercise also builds muscle and improves balance and agility, all of which helps lower your risk of falls.

Dr. Rosen suggests adopting an exercise program that includes weight-bearing activities, strength training, and balance, stretching, and flexibility exercises, such as yoga, tai chi, or Pilates.

Medications. Low testosterone levels can contribute to osteoporosis. Men with confirmed low levels of this hormone should consider a bone density test (see "Should you have a bone density test?" above).

Should you have a bone density test?

Osteoporosis is called a "silent disease" because there are typically no symptoms, and most people who have it don't know until they break a bone. One way to diagnose osteoporosis and determine future fracture risk is with a bone density test, which uses specialized x-rays to measure the thickness and strength of bones. The lower your bone density, the higher your risk of breaking a bone. While women age 65 years and older should be screened for osteoporosis, most experts do not recommend bone density testing in men based on age. Men who should ask their doctor about getting tested include those who have low testosterone levels, have lost more than 1.5 inches in height, or have risk factors for nutritional deficiencies.

"Replacing testosterone can help maintain and might even improve bone health," says Dr. Rosen.

A class of drugs known as bisphosphonates can treat osteoporosis in men by reducing the rate at which bones break down. Examples include alendronate (Fosamax), pamidronate (Aredia), risedronate (Actonel), and zoledronic acid (Reclast). Talk with your doctor about whether testosterone therapy or bisphosphonates are warranted. 🛡

Strength training tied to smaller risk of knee osteoarthritis and pain later in life

People who engaged in strength training were less likely than those who didn't to develop knee pain and knee osteoarthritis as they approached their senior years, according to a study published in 2023 by *Arthritis & Rheumatology*.

Researchers recruited 2,607 people (average age 64, 44% men) without arthritis and asked them if they did strength training and when they first began. Then, for eight years, participants submitted periodic questionnaires about how often they engaged in strength training. Every four years, they underwent knee pain assessments and knee x-rays to look for osteoarthritis. Over all, rates of knee osteoarthritis and pain were 20% lower among those who did strength training versus those who never tried it.

The researchers also found that engaging in strength training later in life, even if you begin after age 50, can help provide joint damage protection similar to those who began earlier.

While the findings of this observational study don't prove that strength training itself reduces your risk of developing knee osteoarthritis and having less knee pain, the results suggest another potential health benefit beyond the known improvements in muscle mass and strength as people age.

Walking advice from a master walker

A champion master-level racewalker shares tips on how to step up your walking routine.

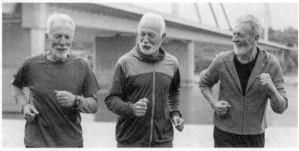
© credit | Getty Images

Make walking a part of your daily routine by starting slow and then stepping up duration and intensity.

Dr. Alan Poisner, 88, was a latecomer to the world of competitive walking. He took up racewalking at age 50, and over the past 38 years has become one of the country's most decorated master-level walkers. He has won five gold medals representing the United States in international competitions and has competed in 14 National Senior Games, where he holds several records. A medical researcher, Dr. Poisner also has a long career exploring the physiology of walking, especially among older adults.

It's safe to say, Dr. Poisner walks the walk. So, we asked him to share his advice and wisdom about walking for health and fitness—from beginning a routine, to staying motivated, to elevating your workouts. Here are his suggestions.

Choose a time. Like other new health habits, it's best to set aside a specific time and day(s) of the week to walk for fun or fitness. "Some prefer mornings to free up later hours, but I enjoy the afternoon, when my body has been warmed up by usual routine activities. Whatever you choose, you do not need to be obsessive. Make it part of your daily activity. You'll be surprised how much you miss walking if you have to skip a regular session."

Vary your settings. Dr. Poisner likes different locations depending on his workout goal. "For pleasure walks, I enjoy non-urban trail-like settings to experience new areas. For structured workouts, I often use a treadmill or an indoor or outdoor track that helps me better measure distance and pace."

Shake it up. Walks measured by time (20 to 30 minutes) or distance (1 to 2 miles) are ideal for most beginners, but you can eventually add structured workouts. Two of Dr. Poisner's favorite workouts are intervals and ladders.

For intervals, you first walk at a comfortable pace. Then, for a short period (for example, 30 seconds to two minutes) walk at a faster pace, where your breathing is a bit labored but you can still talk. Then slow to a comfortable pace to let your heart rate recover. Repeat the pattern of fast pace and recovery for 10 to 15 minutes.

For ladders, you begin walking at an easily maintained pace for a few minutes. Then, gradually increase the pace every one to two minutes until you reach a pace that is difficult to maintain. You then gradually slow the pace back to your starting speed. "This is most easily done on a treadmill, but it can also be done outside by monitoring your pace with a fitness watch or your breathing." (You can find more sample workouts for all levels at www.racewalking.org and www.racewalk.com.)

Hydrate. Approach walking as any other cardio activity, and take in enough fluid. "I hydrate before and after walking. If the walk is an hour or more, I carry a water bottle and drink regularly."

Take it slow. When beginning a walking program, don't be in a rush to increase speed or distance, which can lead to injury. "Focus on weekly, incremental increases in duration and intensity."

Join a group. There is often strength in numbers. "Walk on your own, but try to enlist some companions or join a local walking club to make it easier to maintain the discipline of daily walking."

Sign up for a race. "I entered many road races with no competitive walking division over the years. I did it just for the camaraderie, the chance to exercise, and often to support a charitable cause." To begin, look for races offering 5K (3.1 miles) or 1-mile "fun run" categories.

Get swinging. Walking can be a full-body workout if you engage your arms while you walk. "I focus on swinging my arms in a natural form so that the motion and location of my arms is the most efficient."

Have fun. "I tell new walkers that there are two rules: don't hurt yourself, and have fun. If walkers follow these rules, they will enjoy this activity for many years." ◗

Chapter 11
Advances in Health Technology

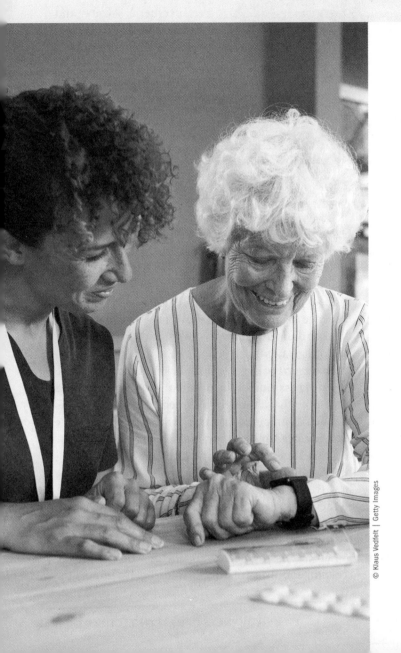

© Klaus Vedfelt | Getty Images

Healthy Habits!
5 Things You Can Do Now

1 **Shed extra pounds.** If you're overweight or obese, new weight-loss drugs could help. (page 264)

2 **Try a new health tool.** The PREVENT equation offers an earlier, more precise estimate of heart disease risk. (page 268)

3 **Get a flu shot.** While a one-and-done version may not yet be on the horizon, this winter-prep step still offers important protection. (page 270)

4 **Consider wearable health trackers.** Apps, smart watches, and other tools provide significant benefits. (page 271)

5 **Skip a new Alzheimer's test.** The screening tool cannot diagnose, and no accuracy data is publicly available. (page 287)

Understanding new weight-loss drugs

A class of drugs called GLP-1 receptor agonists can help with weight loss in people who live with obesity or type 2 diabetes. But are they suitable for other people?

Some people who struggle with weight loss have been able to find assistance from several FDA-approved weight-loss medications, such as bupropion plus naltrexone (Contrave), phentermine (Adipex-P), phentermine plus topiramate (Qsymia), and orlistat (Xenical, Alli). On average, such drugs can help people lose 5% to 7% of their body weight when paired with a healthy diet and exercise.

Now a newer class of medications used to treat type 2 diabetes has gained attention because of their impressive weight-loss results—in many cases, 10% to 20% of a person's body weight. They're called glucagon-like peptide-1 (GLP-1) receptor agonists.

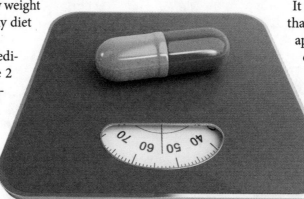

© 3dfoto | Getty Images

New drugs can help certain people lose weight, but they're not meant for modest weight loss.

Tale of two drugs

Two of these GLP-1 receptor agonists are FDA-approved in formulations specifically designed for weight loss in people without diabetes: liraglutide (Saxenda) and semaglutide (Wegovy).

Lower-dose versions of these same active ingredients, known respectively as Victoza and Ozempic, have been used for years to help people with diabetes control their blood sugar levels.

"They can lead to substantial weight loss when used in conjunction with healthy lifestyle changes in people who are overweight or have obesity with or without type 2 diabetes," says Dr. A. Enrique Caballero, an endocrinologist at Harvard-affiliated Brigham and Women's Hospital. "But whether they can be safely used for all people who simply want to lose an extra 10 to 20 pounds is questionable."

How the new drugs work

GLP-1 receptor agonists mimic the GLP-1 hormone that is naturally released in the gastrointestinal tract in response to eating.

"The drugs prompt the body to produce more insulin after eating, limiting the elevation of blood sugar levels after meals, something particularly crucial for people with type 2 diabetes," says Dr. Caballero. The drugs also regulate appetite by sending signals to the brain to tell the body it is full, which inhibits overeating.

It is important to remember that these medications are only approved for people who meet certain criteria. Wegovy and Saxenda are for adults diagnosed with obesity—a body mass index (BMI) of 30 or higher—or those with a BMI of 27 plus at least one weight-related condition, like high blood pressure, high cholesterol, or type 2 diabetes. The other versions of these drugs—Victoza and Ozempic—are for people with type 2 diabetes.

Still, that has not stopped some doctors from prescribing these medications "off-label" for weight loss, which means they are used for a different purpose than explicitly intended. "But there isn't enough evidence to know whether these drugs might be beneficial or dangerous for people who fall outside of the FDA criteria," says Dr. Caballero.

However, the larger issue is that many people see the new drugs as a quick-fix solution. "It is paramount to remember that all weight-loss medications are recommended as an aid in the overall strategy that centers around a healthy meal plan and regular physical activity," says Dr. Caballero. "In fact, people who stop taking these drugs will often regain the weight unless they have truly established a consistent and effective change in their eating and physical activity habits."

Know the downsides

When discussing with your doctor whether GLP-1 receptor agonists are worth exploring, it's important

ADVANCES IN HEALTH TECHNOLOGY

to understand their potential downsides. You might develop various gastrointestinal side effects, including gas, bloating, indigestion, nausea, or irregular bowel movements.

But these issues usually resolve within a few weeks, according to Dr. Caballero. "The lowest doses of these medications are usually given at first and then gradually increased so people have less chance of developing side effects," he says.

Another downside is the cost: the drugs are expensive—about $900 to $1,500 per month. Finally, be aware that the drugs are given via injection into the arm, stomach, or thigh using a pen-like device with a tiny needle the width of two human hairs. (Semaglutide is given weekly, while liraglutide injections are done daily.) Semaglutide prescribed for diabetes is also available as a daily pill called Rybelsus. You have to wait 30 minutes to an hour after taking it before you can eat or drink. ❦

Questions and answers about the new anti-obesity medications

They're the most effective drugs for weight loss to date. But they're expensive, scarce, and not right for everyone.

A blockbuster batch of anti-obesity drugs continues to grab headlines and dominate social media posts, and not just because the new year revs up our resolve to shed pounds. The medications—semaglutide (Wegovy), liraglutide (Saxenda), and tirzepatide (Zepbound)—are backed by science and stunning accounts of people losing as much as 20% of their body weight.

While that's remarkable, it's not the whole story. Many questions about the drugs remain, and some answers are complicated.

What are they?
The recently FDA-approved anti-obesity medications are in a class called GLP-1 receptor agonists (GLP-1s). They mimic a hormone (glucagon-like peptide 1) that helps the body slow stomach emptying, control blood sugar levels, and suppress appetite, a combination that leads to weight loss. One of the drugs, Zepbound, mimics GLP-1 as well as a hormone called a glucose-dependent insulinotropic polypeptide (GIP), believed to promote the effects of GLP-1.

"Many people say these anti-obesity medications have changed their lives," says Dr. Caroline Apovian,

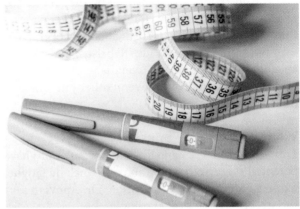
© CR | Getty Images

Most of the new anti-obesity drugs are daily or weekly injections that come in preloaded injector pens.

an obesity medicine specialist and co-director of the Center for Weight Management and Wellness at Harvard-affiliated Brigham and Women's Hospital.

The drugs also significantly reduce the risk of death from heart-related causes in people with overweight or obesity as well as heart disease (or both heart disease and diabetes, depending on the drug). Plus, they enhance the ability to exercise and boost quality of life. "The medications may even affect the reward center in the brain, the part that enables you to eat chocolate cake even though you're full. These drugs seem to dampen the reward response, which also may reduce addictive behaviors like cravings for alcohol, sugar, and nicotine," Dr. Apovian says.

Wait—aren't they diabetes drugs?
All three of the anti-obesity drugs were first approved by the FDA solely to treat diabetes, under the brand names Ozempic, Victoza, and Mounjaro.   ▸▸

▶▶ But people taking them noticed they were losing substantial amounts of weight. Studies confirmed this effect, and the FDA eventually approved the medications for weight loss under new brand names: Wegovy, Saxenda, and Zepbound. For overweight or obesity, the drugs are typically prescribed in higher doses than their diabetes counterparts.

There are older GLP-1s approved for diabetes, such as dulaglutide (Trulicity), but these treatments have less effect on weight.

How do you take the medications?

Most of these new drugs come in the form of injections that you give yourself daily or weekly. They are loaded in an injector pen (like an EpiPen for an allergic reaction) that you press against your abdomen or thigh.

A pill form of semaglutide (Rybelsus) is also available. It's FDA-approved to treat diabetes, but not yet approved for weight loss. Several other pill formulations are being tested.

What are the side effects?

Both the anti-obesity and diabetes formulations have potential side effects. Common ones include fatigue, nausea, vomiting, or constipation. Dr. Apovian says those tend to go away after a few weeks.

In rare cases, the drugs might cause an obstruction in the small bowel, gastroparesis (stomach paralysis), or inflammation of the pancreas (pancreatitis).

"As far as I know, side effects are not permanent. They go away if you stop taking the medications," Dr. Apovian says. But the very long-term effects of taking the newer medications are not yet known."

Who's a candidate for the drugs?

The drugs are approved for weight loss only in people diagnosed with obesity (a BMI of 30 or greater) or a higher range of overweight (a BMI of 27 to 29.9), as well as a medical problem related to excess weight, such as high blood pressure or high cholesterol. Of course,

that hasn't stopped some people who don't meet these criteria from using them.

Because these drugs are new and powerful and are the subject of intense study, it is expected that recommendations as to who should use them will change in the coming years. Researchers are likely to identify new groups of people who might benefit—or, conversely, people who may be at extra risk from their side effects.

How long do you take the drugs?

Taking one of the new GLP-1s is not a short-term solution. Once you go on the drug, you must stay on it indefinitely to keep getting the benefits. You regain the weight if you stop taking the medications.

"Overweight and obesity, like diabetes and hypertension, are serious conditions that often require ongoing, even lifelong treatment. There are no 'one-and-done' treatments," Dr. Apovian says.

Costs and coverage

Spectacular results don't come cheaply, and the new drugs range from about $900 to $1,500 per month. Don't expect your insurance to pay for them. Medicare does not cover the anti-obesity medications, and private insurance coverage varies depending on your plan.

Some manufacturers of GLP-1s offer coupons with steep discounts, but many pharmacies don't accept them. And beware of budget-friendly versions touted in online ads or offered by "med-spas." Dr. Apovian says these are compounded (custom-mixed) drugs brought in from other countries, with no oversight by the FDA, and no guarantee of what they contain.

The drugs' frenzied rise in popularity initially caused shortages, making them hard to find. "The shortage had to do with the manufacturers not anticipating this kind of demand," Dr. Apovian says. "Over 40% of Americans have obesity. The drug companies didn't anticipate how many of them would want to use the medications." ▮

Beyond appetite suppression

New evidence suggests blockbuster weight-loss drugs might also curb addictions and other types of compulsions. What does the future hold?

It's nearly impossible to miss the buzz surrounding the newest generation of obesity drugs, whose popularity is soaring alongside reports of jaw-dropping weight loss among people taking them.

Semaglutide—first marketed as Ozempic for diabetes and later as Wegovy for obesity—is heralded as a breakthrough drug for its ability to promote an average loss of 15% to 20% of a person's body weight. But it's becoming apparent that the medications, which include others in its class and mimic a naturally produced hormone called GLP-1, might offer additional benefits, dampening cravings for things other than food.

Some people taking GLP-1 drugs have reported less interest in addictive and compulsive behaviors such as drinking alcohol, smoking, gambling, shopping excessively, and even biting their nails. Dr. Caroline Apovian, co-director of the Center for Weight Management and Wellness at Harvard-affiliated Brigham and Women's Hospital, is hearing similar accounts from her own patients, especially about cravings for alcohol and sweets.

Why might this happen? GLP-1 drugs, which suppress appetite and help people feel full, appear to hamper activation of the brain's reward pathways. These are normally stimulated by substances such as food, alcohol, and nicotine as well as pleasurable activities such as gambling or shopping.

"We're not quite sure why, but they're doing something very positive for behavioral change," Dr. Apovian says. "It's a breath of fresh air."

Intense research

GLP-1 medications are already producing surprising long-term health benefits in areas other than weight loss. Wegovy may lower the risk of serious heart problems such as heart attack and stroke by 20%, the drug's manufacturer reported in 2023. The trial involving 17,000 people, published in November 2023, is the first to show that GLP-1 drugs can confer heart health benefits for people who are overweight but don't have diabetes.

Other research is beginning to unwrap the drugs' potential to quell alcohol abuse and smoking. A 2022 study of 127 adults published in the journal *JCI Insight* suggested that people with both obesity and alcohol use disorder who were treated with a GLP-1 drug called exenatide (Byetta, Bydureon) drank dramatically less than those who received only a placebo drug. Participants who received exenatide also displayed significantly less activation of the brain's reward centers when shown pictures of alcohol while undergoing functional MRI scans.

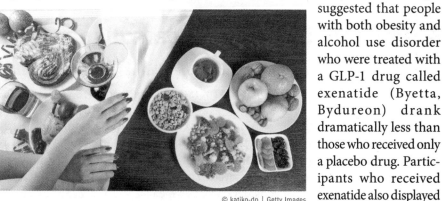

© katiko-dp | Getty Images

GLP-1 drugs might help drive people toward better habits.

Another small trial in progress is focusing on 48 people with alcohol use disorder who also smoke. It aims to determine if those who receive escalating doses of semaglutide over two months will drink and smoke less than participants who receive a placebo injection.

If further research confirms preliminary findings, Dr. Apovian believes the stampede to obtain these drugs will only increase. But FDA approval for uses other than diabetes and obesity will likely take several more years, after large clinical trials are completed. "I think there will certainly be more demand, which is already rising astronomically," she says.

Reaping advantages

The success of GLP-1 drugs for a range of cravings could offer proof that addictions and compulsions stem from brain-based disorders, not a lack of willpower, Dr. Apovian says. "A moral failing? We have to get rid of that stigma. The big punchline here is that all of these are diseases."

▶▶

▶▶ If you're intrigued at the thought of using one of these drugs to curb an addiction or compulsive behavior, Dr. Apovian suggests these tactics.

Pursue it. If you're struggling with obesity but aren't taking a GLP-1 drug, perhaps it's time to start. "Someone with obesity who also has compulsions for alcohol, gambling, or smoking could certainly obtain one of these medications for obesity and then potentially benefit from its other effects," she says.

Watch for cheaper options. Wegovy and other newer GLP-1 drugs can be costly and in short supply. But other first-generation GLP-1s approved for diabetes or obesity, including dulaglutide (Trulicity) and liraglutide (Saxenda), may be sold as generics before long. That should make them easier to obtain—and far more affordable. "Staying patient is tough to do," Dr. Apovian says. "But some GLP-1 drugs are less expensive or perhaps will be soon." ▼

A new tool to predict heart disease risk

The PREVENT equation—which takes kidney and metabolic health into account—estimates a person's risk of heart disease over the next 30 years.

In 2024, the American Heart Association (AHA) released a new online calculator to predict a person's odds of developing heart disease (to use it, go to professional.heart.org/prevent). Compared to previous calculators, the updated tool considers broader measures of health and a longer horizon of risk. The goal? To encourage earlier, more targeted strategies to help people avoid cardiovascular problems.

The PREVENT equation (its name is based on the phrase "predicting risk of cardiovascular disease events") was designed to capture an accurate picture of the American population. Researchers created and validated the model using data from more than 6.6 million adults in the United States from a variety of ethnic, racial, socioeconomic, and geographic backgrounds.

"It's a big step forward, particularly in terms of appreciating the role of kidney and metabolic health in cardiovascular disease," says Dr. Mark Benson, director of preventive cardiology at Harvard-affiliated Beth Israel Deaconess Hospital. The older, 2013 ASCVD risk calculator (health.harvard.edu/heartrisk) considers a person's age, sex, race, smoking status, and presence of diabetes. But the only clinical values considered in the calculation are blood pressure and cholesterol.

What's new?
The PREVENT calculator includes body mass index and another clinical value: estimated glomerular filtration rate (eGFR), which gauges kidney function based on blood levels of creatinine (a waste product filtered by the kidneys) along with age and gender. A normal value is 90 and above.

In a recent advisory, the AHA also highlighted several other biomarkers for cardiovascular-kidney-metabolic (CKM) syndrome (see box, page 267), including

▶ Urine albumin-to-creatinine ratio, which detects very small amounts of a protein called albumin in the urine. A normal value is 30 milligrams per gram or lower.
▶ Hemoglobin A1c (HbA1c), which is a three-month-average measure of blood sugar. A normal value is 5.6% or below.

New treatment options
The blood test most people get at routine health care visits (called a basic metabolic panel) includes the information needed to calculate eGFR, which is used to diagnose and determine the severity of kidney disease, says Dr. Benson. While doctors have known for decades that the risk of cardiovascular disease rises as kidney function drops, there weren't effective therapies to address the problem. "Now, we have several new medications that can improve kidney health and lower cardiovascular risk," says Dr. Benson.

These include SGLT-2 inhibitors, which were originally developed to treat diabetes. The drugs promote

Cardiovascular-kidney-metabolic (CKM) syndrome

A 2024 presidential advisory from the American Heart Association outlined four stages of CKM syndrome. The new PREVENT heart disease risk calculator includes biomarkers related to these stages to better define a person's risk.

Stage 0: None of the following risk factors.

Stage 1: Excess body fat or abdominal fat or prediabetes (defined as an HbA1c of 5.7% to 6.4% or fasting blood glucose of 100 to 125 mg/dL).

Stage 2: Type 2 diabetes, high blood pressure, high triglycerides, or kidney disease.

Stage 3: Stage 2 plus early cardiovascular disease (or a high risk of cardiovascular disease).

Kidneys

Stage 4: Stage 2 plus symptoms of cardiovascular disease (such as a heart attack, stroke, or heart failure). Stage 4 is further divided into Stage 4a (without kidney failure) or Stage 4b (with kidney failure).

weight loss, lower blood pressure, and help prevent kidney damage even in people who do not have diabetes. SGLT-2s such as dapagliflozin (Farxiga) and empagliflozin (Jardiance) also have cardiovascular benefits, especially in people with heart failure. Another class of diabetes drugs, known as GLP-1s, promotes even more dramatic weight loss. The best known of these, semaglutide (Ozempic), also lowers the risk of cardiovascular problems, even in people without diabetes. Finally, another medication, finerenone (Kerendia), also helps slow the progression of diabetic kidney disease and prevents heart-related complications.

Reducing risk

The progression toward cardiovascular disease starts early in life, and people often accumulate risks in a stepwise fashion, says Dr. Benson. The PREVENT calculator evaluates people's risk starting at age 30—a decade earlier than the older calculator. "What's important to recognize is that you can improve your score by addressing known risk factors on the CKM scale," Dr. Benson says. Losing weight (if needed) and keeping your blood pressure and cholesterol in a healthy range is a good start. But be sure to monitor your HbA1c and eGFR as well. ♥

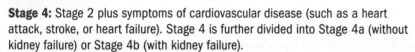

A smart watch may help detect early risks for certain heart problems

Smart watches can do more than just check texts and emails or track your steps and heart rate. Many of the devices measure the electrical activity of your heart, similar to an electrocardiogram (ECG) that you'd get in a doctor's office. Those tests in clinical settings measure electrical activity from different points on your chest and limbs for about 15 seconds. But smart watches measure activity from just one spot (your wrist). Is that enough to detect heart problems? Possibly, suggests an analysis published in 2023 by the *European Heart Journal: Digital Health*. Scientists asked 83,000 healthy people (ages 50 to 70) to undergo one-lead, 15-second ECGs that mimicked a smart watch ECG, and then followed their health for up to 11 years. After analyzing the recordings, scientists found that people whose ECGs showed a type of extra heartbeat called premature ventricular contraction were more likely to later develop heart failure; people with another type, called premature atrial contraction, were more likely to develop atrial fibrillation. Smart watches are expected to become increasingly useful in spotting early signs of heart problems.

© Nerthuz | Getty Images

© SergeiKorolko | Getty Images

by **ANTHONY L. KOMAROFF, M.D.,** Editor in Chief, *Harvard Health Letter*

When will we see a "one-and-done" flu shot?

Q *Why can't we get just one flu shot that protects us for a lifetime?*

A Many scientists are working to develop improved influenza (flu) vaccines. Our current vaccines are imperfect, but they still protect us.

The flu is much more serious than the common cold: globally, 300,000 to 500,000 people die from the flu each year—most of them unvaccinated. In the worst flu pandemic in history, 50 million to 100 million people died. Our current, imperfect flu vaccines saved 40,000 lives in the United States alone between 2004 and 2014. Imperfect protection is much better than no protection.

The perfect flu vaccine would protect against all different strains of the flu virus. A virus has a shape, with different parts. The parts of the virus that traditional vaccines attack are constantly changing, generating new strains. That's why a new flu shot is needed each year. Fortunately, scientists are finally having some success building vaccines that attack the parts of the virus that don't change—the "conserved" parts. A vaccine that targeted the conserved parts could theoretically protect against all strains of the flu virus, past and future.

A perfect vaccine also would prevent any symptoms. Our current flu vaccines don't guarantee you won't get the flu, but they do lessen symptom severity and are quite good at preventing hospitalization and death. One reason they are only partially effective is that, with current technologies, it takes at least six months to manufacture the vaccine.

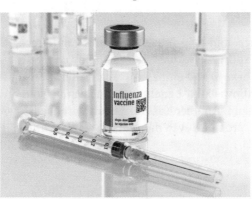

© Sergii Iaremenko/Science Photo Library | Getty Images

That means scientists must decide each winter which strains of the virus will be circulating eight to 10 months later when the next flu season begins. Unfortunately, sometimes the virus fools us: the strains that are circulating in the winter are replaced by other strains before the next flu season arrives. Scientists are working on new types of vaccines that can be produced much more quickly, such as the extremely successful mRNA vaccines developed for COVID-19.

Finally, a perfect flu shot also would offer protection for a lifetime. A special kind of mRNA vaccine is in development that would cause the body to keep attacking the virus for a long time, if not a lifetime.

Although the COVID pandemic led to a greater investment in vaccines against the flu and other viruses, in my opinion the investment still is not great enough, given the potential return from investing in vaccines. For example, in the United States alone, by early 2023 COVID vaccines had prevented 19 million hospitalizations and over three million deaths, saving the economy $1.2 trillion. It cost only a small fraction of that to develop the vaccines.

Will we ever see a perfect flu vaccine? Probably not in my lifetime or yours. But we almost surely will see improved, less imperfect, vaccines. And, to repeat myself, imperfect protection is very much better than no protection.

The latest on wearables for finding atrial fibrillation

Several smart watch brands can detect this common heart rhythm disorder. But whether this feature can improve your health remains unclear.

In 2018, the FDA granted marketing clearance for the first smart watch capable of capturing the heart's electrical "signature," known as an electrocardiogram or ECG. An app enables the watch to detect atrial fibrillation (afib), the most common heart rhythm disorder (see "What is atrial fibrillation?" on page 272). Today, four additional smart watches with similar capabilities have FDA clearance, and more are expected on the market soon.

Because bouts of afib are often short-lived and sometimes symptomless, diagnosing it can be challenging. An annual ECG at your doctor's office, which lasts less than 10 seconds, may not pick up afib if it is occurring only occasionally. And unless you have symptoms, medical devices that check the heart for longer periods of time don't make sense.

But your smart watch can continuously monitor your pulse for an abnormally rapid or irregular heart rate and tell you to when record an ECG, which involves opening an app and touching the side of the watch for 30 seconds. In theory, this capability could pick up more cases of afib, which is important because afib raises the risk of stroke. Knowing you have the problem means you can take action. For people at higher risk, taking anti-clotting medications may help lower stroke risk.

The current evidence

But what do we actually know about how well these consumer devices work, and who might benefit from using one? If you already have one of these smart watches or are considering getting one, here's what you should know.

Currently, there are no randomized trials using smart watches to screen for afib that show a health benefit associated with their use. However, an analysis using simulated data based on average Americans suggests the strategy would be cost-effective in people ages 65 and older, says cardiologist Dr. Shaan Khurshid, a research fellow at Massachusetts General Hospital and one of the lead authors of the study, which was published in 2022 in *JAMA Health Forum*. "In older adults, consumer wearable devices have the potential

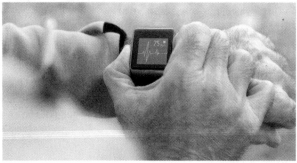

© Nastasic | Getty Images

Many smart watches can continuously monitor your pulse for abnormalities and tell you when to record an electrocardiogram.

to improve outcomes and lower costs by decreasing strokes," he says.

How reliable are the readings? According to a study published in 2023 in *JACC: Clinical Electrophysiology*, about a quarter of the ECG readings from five smart devices were deemed "inconclusive." But setting those cases aside, the devices were all highly accurate in finding afib. The tested devices were the Apple Watch 6, the Samsung Galaxy Watch 3, the Withings ScanWatch, the Fitbit Sense, and the AliveCor KardiaMobile (a credit-card-sized device you touch with your fingers and use with a smartphone).

There are some drawbacks. The devices are not cheap: most ECG-enabled smart watches start at around $250. People should also be aware of the potential emotional cost of a false-positive result (when the ECG incorrectly reports afib), which could cause anxiety. In addition, processing the sheer volume of patient data available is already a challenge for many doctors, and the need to review multiple smart watch ECG tracings could further strain our health care system. Finally, the people who would likely benefit most from afib screening may be the least able to afford or know how to use a consumer device, an issue that could further exacerbate existing health disparities.

The bottom line

For people considering buying a smart watch, the ECG recording capability is a potential added benefit, says Dr. Khurshid. "But if you don't want to spend the ▸▸

money, there are many other ways to screen for afib," he adds. These strategies, which include simply checking your own pulse or wearing a heart monitor for a couple weeks, depend on your afib risk and symptoms.

If you already have afib, however, a smart watch may help you monitor the condition over the long term, which could help inform your doctor's treatment advice.

What is atrial fibrillation?

Atrial fibrillation (afib) is a heart rhythm disorder that causes a rapid, irregular heartbeat. These bouts may occur for occasional, brief periods or much longer—even permanently in some people. About one in 11 people ages 65 and older has the condition, which is more common in those with high blood pressure, obesity, and sleep apnea.

Possible symptoms include shortness of breath, fatigue, and dizziness, but sometimes afib goes unnoticed. Recognized or not, this erratic heart rhythm can cause blood to pool in the heart's upper chambers. This increases the likelihood of clots, which can travel to the brain and block blood flow, causing a stroke.

Want to age in place? Tap technology

Aging in place remains a vaunted ideal for older adults, with more than three-quarters wishing to remain in their homes and communities. In pursuit of this goal, more than half of older adults use assistive technologies such as health apps and fitness trackers, according to a recent poll.

Published in 2023, the *U.S. News and World Report* survey questioned 2,000 Americans 55 and older (57% women), 53% of whom reported using assistive tech. Top-used types included medical- or health-related mobile apps (25%) and wearable medical alert trackers (17%), as well as smart home devices (which control temperature, lighting, and other features), hearing assistance devices, and grocery or food delivery apps. The vast majority of survey respondents said assistive technologies improve their quality of life, helping them feel more independent (55%), safer (44%), healthier (33%), or mobile (20%).

"These findings don't surprise me—I think these technologies offer huge benefits," says Katherine Lyman, a geriatric nurse practitioner at Beth Israel Deaconess Medical Center.

Some older adults are so committed to the idea of aging in place that they're likely to remain in less-than-ideal surroundings to do so, Lyman says.

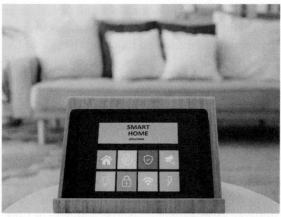

© Westend61 | Getty Images

Smart home devices are among many forms of assistive tech.

Assistive technologies can bridge this gap—but only if they're used to the fullest.

Wearable medical alert trackers offer "all sorts of early warning systems, and if your device is sending you a message that there's some sort of potential danger, you can't ignore it," she says. "It's an opportunity to use that information—to reach out to your family or your doctor—and get help to shore up your defenses."

The latest in medical alert systems

Cell phone and "smart" technology are making the devices more convenient.

Medical alert systems have come a long way since they first became popular in the 1980s. Like most gadgets, they've taken a big leap forward as technology has advanced, especially in the past few years.

One exciting development is the ability to integrate a medical alert monitoring service with an electronic gadget you already have, such as a smartphone, smart watch, or a smart speaker. But the marriage is still young. "While the integration has progressed, there's a long way to go before these tools become mainstream. Use of smart speakers in households is still relatively low, and medical alert companies are very cautious about adopting these new innovations. Still, there is great potential," says Dr. Joseph Kvedar, a Harvard Medical School professor and editor in chief of the journal *npj Digital Medicine*.

What types of systems does that leave us with? Here's a look.

Monitored home systems

Monitored home medical alert systems typically consist of a waterproof alert button (worn as a pendant or watch) that can transmit a signal to a base unit. The base plugs into your landline.

When you press the button, if you're within range of the base (about 1,000 feet), the base calls a monitoring center. Trained operators then talk to you through a speaker in the base and can call your loved ones or paramedics.

One new aspect of these systems is that some now come with built-in cellphone technology, meaning they don't require a landline. And some companies now offer systems that consist only of a voice-activated cellphone (it looks like a speakerphone) that connects you to a monitoring center when you call out to it.

On the horizon: a voice-activated unit that can contact a monitoring center and function as a smart speaker—a small tabletop speaker with a virtual assistant that connects to the Internet, understands your voice commands, and carries out tasks.

Monitored portable systems

Thanks to cellphone technology, you can now get an alert button that can contact a monitoring center

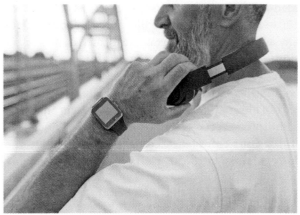

© Eleganza | Getty Images
Have a smart watch you use to track health and communicate? You might be able to connect it to emergency monitoring services.

without a base unit. Most of these devices are waterproof and look like small garage door openers. You can keep the device in your pocket or wear it around your neck or clipped onto your waistband, and it will work anywhere there's cellular service.

These alert buttons have speakers, so you can talk to an operator. They might also have fall detection capability and GPS technology, which enables operators to send help to your exact location. Many portable devices can also be paired with a medical alert company's app that allows your family to communicate with you and see where you are.

A recent development: some devices look like a smart watch, with a button to call for help along with other features typical of smart watches, such as a pedometer, heart rate monitor, weather app, calendar reminders, and even the ability to receive texts.

Monitoring service only

Do you already own a smartphone, smart watch, or smart speaker? You might be able to get medical alert monitoring services for it, without buying any other equipment.

For example, if you have an Amazon Echo device (a smart speaker), you can pair it with Amazon's Alexa Together, a subscription medical alert monitoring service.

And some companies, such as Lively (www.lively. com), now offer a subscription medical alert ▸▸

▶▶ monitoring app, which you can download to a smart speaker or a smart watch.

Costs and alternatives

Medical alert monitoring isn't cheap. Costs range from $20 to $50 per month, depending on the company and any additional services you select (such as fall detection or apps that enable your family to connect to your device). There may also be fees for activation and equipment (up to a few hundred dollars).

The alternative is to get an alert system that isn't monitored. You can get a smart speaker and have it call your emergency contacts (but not 911, due to regulatory hurdles). Your smartphone probably already has an emergency button built into it (these features vary by phone; for instance, you might press and hold the side button). You can also download free "panic button" apps for your smartphone or smart watch that will notify your emergency contacts that you need help.

And many nonmonitored safety button devices are available online for less than $50; you can pair one of these with your smartphone to contact loved ones in an emergency. But will your loved ones see these notifications? Will they be able to reach you? These are all important considerations.

One thing is certain: as technology continues to improve, so will our options. 🛡

Bad bedfellows

Sleep trackers have pros and cons, but the devices may also lead to slumber-sabotaging anxiety.

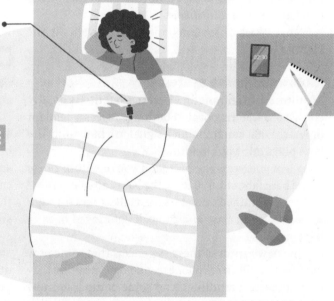

© Kudryavtsev Pavel | Getty Images

They seem like a promising health tool, but sleep trackers aren't yet as accurate as you might expect.

You woke up with a pep in your step, feeling energetic and well rested. But wait: your sleep tracker says otherwise. Does the data change your plans for the day and how you'll approach bedtime that night? Are you now anxious when you'd been feeling calm?

The rise of sleep tracking devices—which monitor physiological factors related to sleep—has made this conundrum increasingly relevant. A 2023 survey by the American Academy of Sleep Medicine shows that more than one-third of Americans have used electronic sleep tracking devices.

Seven hours of sleep each night are generally adequate for an average adult, Harvard experts say. But many folks are fixated on getting a "perfect" eight hours after learning that sleep deprivation can raise the risks of an array of potentially serious health problems, including obesity, diabetes, and cardiovascular disease. The quest for better sleep may backfire, however, leading to anxiety and stress that can thwart restful slumber.

"We do need to lower the emotional temperature a bit and be rational about this," says Dr. John Winkelman, chief of the Sleep Disorders Clinical Research Program at Harvard-affiliated Massachusetts General Hospital.

"Many people still don't respect the importance of sleep, but using sleep trackers feeds into some people's anxieties," he says. "Anxiety and psychological arousal are the opposite of what we need when we sleep."

Influential data

Many types of devices are marketed to track sleep, ranging from watches and rings to smartphone apps and mattress monitors. Some measure whether you're asleep or not by recording aspects such as movement, heart rate, body temperature, and breathing patterns—all of which change at different sleep stages.

The data these devices generate can also hold a lot of sway over how people feel each day. A small 2018 study in the *Journal of Sleep Research* demonstrated this phenomenon. It involved 63 adults with insomnia who were given wrist-worn sleep trackers. In the morning, half of them received information telling them they'd slept poorly, while the others were told they'd slept well—regardless of their actual sleep quality. All reported on their mood and alertness several times over the course of the day.

The 32 participants who were told their sleep was poor reported lower alertness during the day and greater sleepiness in the evening compared to those given positive feedback. And people told they had restful sleep reported a significantly higher level of positive mood and alertness.

"In fact, there was no meaningful difference in sleep quality between the two groups," Dr. Winkelman says. "I'm a little bit addicted to my Fitbit, but I don't use it to inform how I feel during the day. I just like knowing the data and thinking about the relationship of the data to how I think I slept. But understand: those two things are far from synonymous."

Pluses and pitfalls

Using sleep trackers can present distinct pros and cons, Harvard experts say. Among the pros:
- They can make you more aware of your sleep patterns.
- They can offer affirmation if you're trying to form better sleep habits. "Trackers allow people to see if their bedtimes and wake times aren't stable, which they should be," Dr. Winkelman says. "Our sleep is really best when we're on a regular schedule."
- They can identify a potential sleep disorder by spotlighting signs such as awakening many times during the night. "Some trackers offer information about

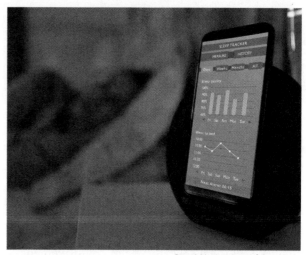

© monkeybusinessimages | Getty Images

Don't let information from sleep trackers overwhelm you.

your oxygen variability," Dr. Winkelman says. "They can be very helpful in identifying sleep-related breathing disorders, such as sleep apnea."

But the devices can also lead to an unhealthy preoccupation with sleep, which can fuel insomnia, Dr. Winkelman says. Here are some other downsides:
- Interpreting and using the data can be confusing. For example, your tracker may tell you that you're apparently not sleeping very deeply, but you might not know how to change that.
- Focusing on sleep data may lead some people to ignore how they actually feel after sleeping. "Can you wake up without an alarm clock? Make it through the day without feeling exhausted or drinking five cups of coffee?" asks Dr. Elizabeth Klerman, a professor of neurology at Massachusetts General Hospital and the Division of Sleep Medicine at Harvard Medical School. "To me, those are probably much more useful metrics."

A lack of accuracy

Sleep trackers are only as useful as the data they produce—which aren't always accurate. A small 2019 study in the journal *Sensors* compared several types of sleep trackers to the gold standard of sleep measurement, a sleep study called polysomnography. After comparing 27 nights of sleep study recordings in 19 participants ages 19 to 64 (66% women) with sleep tracker data from the same nights, researchers found the trackers lacking.

Specifically, the devices had difficulty detecting participants' wake periods, which hindered their ▸▸

▶▶ ability to estimate total sleep time and sleep quality. However, the sleep trackers accurately detected the most basic sleep parameter—the actual amount of time participants spent in bed.

"They're not accurately reflecting how much sleep people are getting, or the depth of sleep or type," Dr. Klerman says. "I think they're more accurate now than they used to be. On the other hand, they haven't been tested on every type of person who wears them."

Sleep-boosting measures

If you've found that anxiety surrounding sleep is keeping you from restful slumber, Harvard experts suggest seeking a special type of cognitive behavioral therapy, called CBTi, that's designed to improve insomnia.

"The cognitive part works on anxious thoughts, while the behavioral part actually decreases the amount of time you spend in bed so you're really sleepy when you get there," Dr. Winkelman says.

Here are some other tactics to improve your sleep:

Set consistent bed and wake times. You can use a tracker to help you do this or merely rely on the clock. But either way, the practice should prod you to wind down calmly before bed.

Don't check sleep data first thing in the morning. Start your day, decide how you feel, and then look at your sleep tracker.

Monitor substance use surrounding sleep. Pay attention to when you last used caffeine, alcohol, and tobacco, which can all affect sleep quality.

Consider your medication use. Ask your doctor if any prescriptions or supplements you take might make it harder to fall or stay asleep. Tweak the use of those medications if possible.

Stay alert for breathing issues. If your bed partner says you snore or gasp frequently while sleeping, tell your doctor. Ditto if you can't sleep lying down and need to sit up, which usually indicates breathing problems. "A tracker may not catch that," Dr. Klerman says. "That's really good evidence you should see a health professional." ▮

What color is your sleep noise?

It may seem paradoxical that a noisy environment could promote sleep. But some people prefer not to slumber in total silence—instead, they add background sound to the bedroom to sleep more soundly.

Recent years have seen a proliferation of sleep machines and apps that emit various audio frequencies that sound similar to static from an untuned radio or TV. Some people profess that listening to these monotonous sounds before or during sleep can help them drop off more easily and stay asleep longer, calming them and drowning out background noise like traffic or creaky pipes.

These sounds have colors assigned to them based on each noise's strength and frequency:

White noise is perhaps the best-known of all noise colors and contains all audio frequencies. It can be intense and high-pitched, resembling a fan, air conditioner, or vacuum.

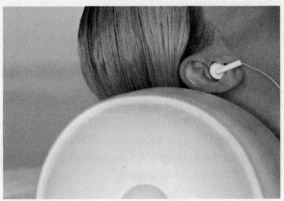

© Image Source | Getty Images

Background sound from white, pink, or brown noise machines or apps may promote sleep.

Pink noise is lower-pitched than white noise. It sounds like steady rain, wind blowing through trees, or waves on a beach.

Brown noise sounds more bass, like a rushing river, pounding surf, or strong winds.

by **ANTHONY L. KOMAROFF, M.D.,** Editor in Chief, *Harvard Health Letter*

Will artificial intelligence replace doctors?

Q *Everyone's talking about artificial intelligence, and how it may replace people in various jobs. Will artificial intelligence replace my doctor?*

A Not in my lifetime, fortunately! And the good news is that artificial intelligence (AI) has the potential to improve your doctor's decisions, and to thereby improve your health—if we are careful about how it is developed and used.

AI is a mathematical process that tries to make sense out of massive amounts of information. So it requires two things: the ability to perform mathematical computations rapidly, and huge amounts of information stored in an electronic form—words, numbers, and pictures.

When computers and AI were first developed in the 1950s, some visionaries described how they could *theoretically* help improve decisions about diagnosis and treatment. But computers then were not nearly fast enough to do the computations required. Even more important, almost none of the information the computers would have to analyze was stored in electronic form. It was all on paper. Doctors' notes about a patient's symptoms and physical examination were written (not always legibly) on paper. Test results were written on paper and pasted in a patient's paper medical record. As computers got better, they started to relieve doctors and other health professionals from some tedious tasks like helping to analyze images—electrocardiograms (ECGs), blood samples, x-rays, and Pap smears.

Today, computers are literally millions of times more powerful than when they were first developed.

© Sergey Dogadin | Getty Images

More important, huge amounts of medical information now are in electronic form: medical records of millions of people, the results of medical research, and the growing knowledge about how the body works. That makes feasible the use of AI in medicine.

Already, computers and AI have made powerful medical research breakthroughs, like predicting the shape of most human proteins. In the future, I predict that computers and AI will listen to conversations between doctor and patient and then suggest tests or treatments the doctor should consider; highlight possible diagnoses based on a patient's symptoms, after comparing that patient's symptoms to those of millions of other people with various diseases; and draft a note for the medical record, so the doctor doesn't have to spend time typing at a computer keyboard—and can spend more time with the patient.

All of this will not happen immediately or without missteps: doctors and computer scientists will need to carefully evaluate and guide the development of new AI tools in medicine. If the suggestions AI provides to doctors prove to be inaccurate or incomplete, that "help" will be rejected. And if AI then does not get better, and fast, it will lose credibility. Powerful technologies can be powerful forces for good, and for mischief.

Is sex hormone therapy safe for your heart?

New evidence provides some clarity on the long-controversial practice of sex hormone use in both men and women.

The two main sex hormones—estrogen and testosterone—have wide-ranging effects in the body, including on the cardiovascular system. Produced primarily by the ovaries (estrogen) and testes (testosterone), these hormones affect not just your sexual function but also blood pressure, cholesterol, and other factors that influence heart health.

As people age, the natural decline in sex hormone levels sometimes causes undesirable symptoms, such as hot flashes or a flagging sex drive. Doctors can prescribe pills, patches, gels, and creams containing estrogen or testosterone to ease those symptoms. But are these products safe for your heart?

Some studies have suggested protective effects, while others have reported dangers to the cardiovascular system. But there's been far more research on estrogen, which is often given in combination with progesterone, another sex hormone. In fact, there were no long-term findings on testosterone therapy in men until 2023. Here's a review of the current evidence on this topic.

Testosterone therapy

When men reach their mid-20s, their testosterone levels start to gradually fall. The term andropause, which refers to this age-related hormone drop, was coined back in the 1930s, but the push to treat the phenomenon is far more recent. In the early 2000s, direct-to-consumer advertisements suggested that low testosterone could make men feel tired, dull, and depressed and that testosterone therapy could restore their energy, alertness, and sexual function. This marketing trend, along with the release of an easy-to-use gel formulation of the drug, led to a sharp rise in testosterone prescriptions.

According to the American Urological Association (AUA), testosterone therapy is recommended only for men with low blood levels of testosterone (defined as less than 300 ng/dL) and associated symptoms, which might include a loss of muscle mass, sleep problems, and a reduced sex drive. Yet up to a quarter of men don't have their testosterone levels checked before starting treatment. And of those who do, nearly half

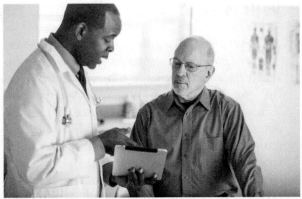

John Fedele | Getty Images

Men with low blood testosterone levels and related symptoms may qualify for the therapy.

don't get rechecked once they do start, according to the AUA, which recommends stopping the therapy if symptoms don't improve.

Several observational studies found a possible increased risk of heart-related problems from testosterone therapy in older men. As a result, in 2014, the FDA issued a warning cautioning against the practice. But the latest research offers some reassurance about testosterone's cardiovascular safety, according to Harvard Medical School professor Dr. Aria Olumi, chief of urologic surgery at Beth Israel Deaconess Medical Center.

Published in 2023 in *The New England Journal of Medicine*, the study included more than 5,200 men who were at high risk for cardiovascular problems and had low testosterone levels. Over a follow-up period averaging nearly two years, men using testosterone were no more likely to have serious heart-related problems than those using a placebo.

Still, it's worth noting that about two-thirds of the men in both groups dropped out of the study. Plus, the report did not include information about whether testosterone therapy improved any symptoms related to low testosterone, Dr. Olumi notes.

"I see men who have been prescribed testosterone by another physician and have continued taking it for years. But they admit that they're not really sure it's doing anything for them," he says. What's more, many men have low testosterone levels and feel perfectly fine, he adds. For men with low testosterone and related symptoms, it's now considered safe to try testosterone. "But if you don't feel better after six months, there's no reason to keep taking it," says Dr. Olumi.

Estrogen therapy

In contrast to the gradual decline in hormone levels men experience, hormone levels drop rather abruptly when women reach their late 40s and early 50s. About 75% of women say they experience symptoms such as hot flashes and night sweats around the time of menopause. Some have only mild, occasional symptoms. But others are so uncomfortable and debilitated that the experience impairs their sleep, mood, and day-to-day function.

Hormone therapy can ease menopausal symptoms, but lingering concern about possible heart-related risks—documented in a major trial published in 2002—has left some doctors reluctant to prescribe the therapy.

"It's a conundrum that comes up fairly often, because all women go through menopause," says Dr. Emily Lau, a cardiologist at Massachusetts General Hospital who specializes in women's cardiovascular health. Research over the past two decades has painted a clearer picture of the cardiovascular risk, which depends on the timing and type of hormone therapy

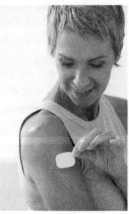
© BSIP | Getty Images
Transdermal estrogen patches are safer than estrogen pills.

a woman takes, as well as her own underlying risk of heart disease, she says. (To assess your 10-year risk, see www.health.harvard.edu/heartrisk).

First, women shouldn't start taking systemic hormone therapy (that is, in pill or patch form) after age 60 or more than 10 years after menopause begins. Second, women should use the lowest possible dose of hormones to ease their bothersome symptoms and ideally re-evaluate the need for the therapy every year, according to Dr. Lau, who co-authored an in-depth article about menopausal hormone therapy published in 2023 in *Circulation*.

For healthy women with a low 10-year heart disease risk (less than 5%), all forms of hormone therapy are acceptable. But for those with a risk of 5% to 10%, experts recommend transdermal patches, which are less likely to trigger blood clots than hormones taken in pill form. Women at high risk (greater than 10%) should avoid systemic hormone therapy if possible.

A new, nonhormonal drug called fezolinetant (Veozah) for treating hot flashes and night sweats could be a good alternative, says Dr. Lau. Finally, it's worth noting that vaginal estrogen products (creams, suppositories, and rings), which can relieve vaginal dryness and discomfort during sex, do not appear to be linked to any increased heart risks. 🛡

Genetic profiling for heart disease: An update

Tests that analyze millions of common DNA variants may help predict heart attacks with more precision. For now, the potential benefits are greatest for people under 50.

As the leading cause of premature death in the United States, cardiovascular disease is to blame for more than $150 billion in lost productivity each year. Thanks to decades of research, we know a great deal about what predisposes people to coronary artery disease, the most prevalent form of heart disease and the root cause of most heart attacks. However, doctors

still can't predict heart attacks very accurately. Some people who appear prone to heart attacks never have one, while others succumb to heart disease despite having no obvious risks.

Can genetic profiling help? Perhaps, according to a 2022 scientific statement from the American Heart Association that looked at the promise and ▸▸

▶▶ challenge of such testing. Using a small sample of blood or saliva, these tests analyze millions of common variants in your DNA to create what's known as a polygenic risk score. You can have zero, one, or two copies of any gene variant, each of which may either raise or lower your risk of coronary artery disease.

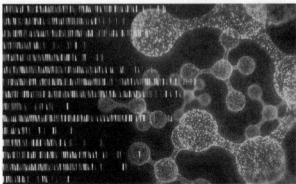

© Yuichiro Chino | Getty Images

A polygenic risk score analyses more than three million variants, each of which contributes a small amount to a person's cardiovascular risk.

Millions of variants

"Ten years ago, there were just 20 or 30 known variants that affect coronary artery disease, but today there are more than three million," says Dr. Nicholas Marston, a preventive cardiologist at Harvard-affiliated Brigham and Women's Hospital. Scientists discover variants by comparing the genetic codes of people without coronary artery disease to those of people with the disease. Many of these variants occur in genes known to affect heart disease, such as those related to cholesterol, blood pressure, and blood clotting. Others aren't well understood and may provide targets for future research, potentially fueling new drug discovery efforts, Dr. Marston says.

The evidence to date

A polygenic risk score reflects the overall impact of all the variants together and is expressed as a percentile. But a high score (for instance, the 95th percentile) doesn't mean you have a 95% chance for developing the disease. Rather, it means that among 100 people, your score is higher than 95 people and the same as or lower than five.

So far, research using polygenic risk scores for coronary artery disease suggests they may offer modest improvements for predicting risk in people who are middle-aged or younger. In some cases, the score can help doctors decide whether to be more or less aggressive in prescribing cholesterol-lowering medications like statins, says Dr. Marston. For example, a 35-year-old man with a father who died of a heart attack at age 45 may wonder what he can do to escape that fate, especially if his cholesterol numbers look fine. Standard risk calculators to guide statin treatment don't apply to people under 40, so a polygenic risk score can help the doctor decide if and when the man should start a statin.

In addition to statins, more powerful cholesterol-lowering drugs like alirocumab (Praluent) and evolocumab (Repatha) are available. These drugs are expensive, and insurance doesn't always cover them. So it doesn't make sense to give them to everyone. A polygenic risk score may help identify which heart attack survivors would benefit most from these medications, says Dr. Marston.

Who offers polygenic risk scores?

Currently, people can find their scores by participating in a research study, such as the Electronic Medical Records and Genomics Network (eMERGE) study. Scientists at some hospitals at Harvard and nine other institutions around the country are investigating the genetic risk of several heart-related conditions, as well as cancer and other diseases (see www.emerge.study).

A handful of direct-to-consumer companies also provide cardiovascular-based scores for $250. Dr. Marston has recommended the test for several of his patients, who must pay out-of-pocket since insurance doesn't cover the tests. Another limitation: the scores are based mainly on people with European ancestry, which means the scores may not be reliable for people of different ethnicities. But efforts to expand the diversity of the data are under way.

For older people, polygenic risk scores for heart disease aren't as helpful. By the time you're 70, decades of lifestyle habits have shaped your risk, and genetic factors are less relevant. "Ultimately, you want the results to be actionable. We won't see a big uptake for using polygenic risk scores until they demonstrate a role in medical decision making," says Dr. Marston. 🛡

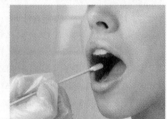

© Peter Dazeley | Getty Images

A cheek swab can collect a DNA sample.

5 trends in cardiology to watch

Known as "the father of modern cardiology," Harvard Medical School professor Dr. Eugene Braunwald shares his perspective on promising future directions in the field.

Longtime readers of the *Heart Letter* know that most of our stories focus on steps you can take right now to improve your heart health. But, once in a while, we look ahead at what's on the horizon in this dynamic field. To that end, we consulted Dr. Eugene Braunwald, Distinguished Hersey Professor of Medicine at Harvard Medical School, where he has worked since 1972. At age 94, he continues to work and publish, adding to the more than 1,100 articles he has authored since the early 1950s. His pioneering research helped elucidate how heart attacks happen, which ushered in new ways to treat and prevent them.

Dr. Braunwald's discoveries also advanced the understanding of hypertrophic cardiomyopathy, valvular heart disease, and heart failure. (His life and research are described in *Eugene Braunwald and the Rise of Modern Medicine*, written by former *Harvard Heart Letter* editor in chief Dr. Thomas H. Lee.) The trends Dr. Braunwald is most excited about, summarized below, may one day affect heart health at every stage of life—from birth to old age.

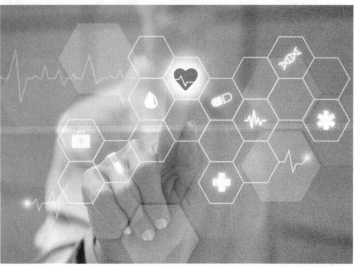

© Westend61 | Getty Images

In coming years, advances in genetics, cell therapy, and transplantation will improve and extend the lives of people affected by cardiovascular disease.

1 Primordial prevention

Dr. Braunwald: The future of cardiology will focus on preventing heart disease very early in life, a concept known as primordial prevention. Instead of waiting until people develop risk factors such as high blood pressure, high cholesterol, or diabetes, and treating them, we will be able to identify and prevent the development of those conditions in the first place. Many of these conditions are caused not by a single gene but by many genes. We now have specialized genetic tests to create polygenic risk scores that help predict cardiovascular risk [see "Genetic profiling for heart disease: An update," page 279]. In the future, these tests will become more accurate and less expensive, so I foresee doing these tests in newborns.

For example, if a baby has genes linked to the development of high blood pressure by age 30, you could modify that child's diet to prevent the problem.

Focusing on prevention very early in life could make a huge difference in reducing cardiovascular disease, which remains the most common cause of death in adults worldwide.

2 Targeting inflammation

Dr. Braunwald: For people who already have heart disease, medications that lower blood pressure and cholesterol are an important part of avoiding future heart problems. Until recently, however, there haven't been any drugs to address inflammation, which ignites the artery-damaging process that leads to a heart attack. But in June 2023, the FDA approved the anti-inflammatory drug colchicine [Lodoco] for people who have or are at high risk for heart disease. The drug, which has been used for many years to treat gout, can lower the risk of heart attack and related problems by about 30%. Investigators and the pharmaceutical industry are now looking very closely at this category of medications. Going forward, I predict there will be a whole battery of new anti-inflammatory drugs. It will be similar to the current situation with high blood pressure, where we have many different drugs that doctors can use to treat this common problem. ▶▶

3 Cardiac cell therapy

Dr. Braunwald: A heart attack cuts off blood flow to part of the heart's muscle, creating damage that scars the heart. Over time, especially in people with repeat heart attacks, this can impair the heart's ability to function normally, leading to heart failure. For more than two decades, scientists have tried to repair damaged hearts using cardiac cell therapy, also known as stem cell therapy. The original concept was to infuse large numbers of stem cells derived from bone marrow into the heart to regenerate heart muscle cells. While the initial results appeared promising, these cells aren't incorporated into the heart muscle, and they quickly

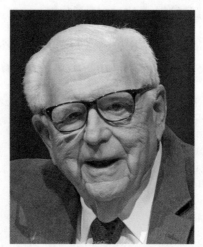

Photo courtesy of Dr. Eugene Braunwald

Dr. Eugene Braunwald, whose career at Harvard Medical School spans more than half a century, is widely considered the most influential cardiologist of our time.

disappear. Now, several other techniques are being explored, including isolating the substances released from transplanted cells that appear to be responsible for their benefits. By making these substances—which include factors that encourage blood vessel growth—in the lab, we might be able to provide "cell therapy without cells." I'm also excited about the promise of pluripotent stem cells, a discovery based on technology that was awarded the 2012 Nobel Prize in Physiology or Medicine. These are cells that have been reprogrammed into their embryonic state and can therefore be directed to generate any type of adult cells, including heart muscle cells.

4 Transplanting pig hearts

Dr. Braunwald: Despite steady progress in heart transplantation, many hundreds of people die each year waiting for a heart transplant. Over the years, there have been a number of successful interspecies transplants—known as xenotransplantation—including in non-human primates. In the past two years, two men with end-stage heart failure received transplants using genetically modified pig hearts. [One survived for six weeks, the other for two months]. Pigs are a logical choice because their hearts are similar in size to a human's. In both cases, several genes in the donor pig were inactivated and human genes were inserted into the pig's genome to stop the recipient from rejecting the new organ. These early studies have paved the way for further advances in xenotransplantation.

5 Improved left ventricular assist devices

Dr. Braunwald: A left ventricular assist device, or LVAD, is a small pump implanted in the chest to help a greatly weakened, failing heart deliver blood to the body. In addition to becoming smaller, more powerful, and less expensive, LVADs will undergo other improvements in the coming years. Current devices use a driveline, a cable that passes through the skin to connect the pump to a battery and control system worn outside the body. In the future, devices will be charged through the skin without requiring a driveline, which is a common place for infections. Another potential advance is the use of biocompatible materials in the pump, which means patients might not need to take anti-clotting drugs. People with advanced heart failure may receive an LVAD temporarily while waiting for a heart transplant, or even instead of a transplant, in what we call "destination therapy." ♥

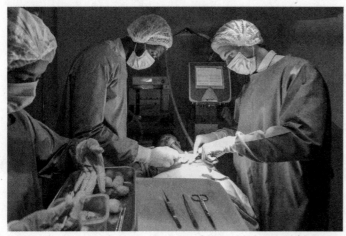

© Akarawut Lohacharoenvanich | Getty Images

A recent advance in heart transplantation involves using genetically modified pig hearts that might one day replace human heart donations, which are in very short supply.

Gene therapy for cardiovascular disease

This trailblazing technique is being tested in people with inherited forms of heart disease, but challenges remain.

Over the past decade, the Nobel-prize-winning technology known as CRISPR has transformed biomedical research, enabling scientists to edit DNA far more easily and precisely than ever before. In late 2023, the first medical use of the gene editing tool was approved to treat sickle cell disease, an inherited blood disorder that causes excruciating pain, organ damage, and strokes.

Investigators are also using gene editing to develop novel therapies for several types of heart disease. Clinical trials are currently under way among people with three genetic conditions: abnormally high cholesterol; a type of heart muscle disease; and a form of heart failure that results from amyloid deposits. Preliminary results in small numbers of people appear promising.

However, there are still some considerable challenges related to developing and delivering gene therapy for heart disease, says Dr. Calum MacRae, vice chair for scientific innovation in the Department of Medicine at Harvard-affiliated Brigham and Women's Hospital. "Sickle cell disease results from a single, specific genetic defect. Most cardiovascular genetic disorders are caused by different genetic defects in each family, and the factors leading to clinical disease are less well known," he says. Gene variants can also have complex effects throughout the entire body, and editing the defect in single tissues may have unpredictable effects, he adds. Delivering the ideal "dose" of gene editing technology to the right types of cells may be an issue. There are also concerns about off-target effects elsewhere in the genome, as well as possible inflammatory reactions to the viruses or lipid particles used deliver the therapies.

Here's a brief summary of current gene therapies for heart disease.

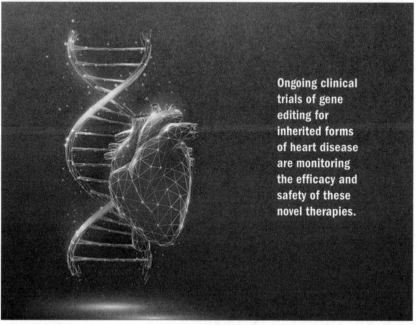

Ongoing clinical trials of gene editing for inherited forms of heart disease are monitoring the efficacy and safety of these novel therapies.

© Alena Butusava | Getty Images

Familial hypercholesterolemia (FH). About one in 250 people has a variant in the PCSK9 gene that causes extremely high levels of harmful LDL cholesterol. FH is one of the leading causes of premature heart attacks (those that occur before age 45 in men and 55 in women). A new gene editing therapy essentially turns off the PCSK9 gene in the liver. Early data found that a single infusion led to drops of 39% to 55% in LDL cholesterol. The nine adults who received the therapy (all of whom had one FH variant) had cardiovascular disease and high LDL, despite taking maximum doses of cholesterol-lowering drugs. The company continues to enroll people for the study, all of whom will be followed for another 14 years, which the FDA requires for all participants in any human genome editing trials.

Hypertrophic cardiomyopathy (HCM). An estimated one in 500 people have HCM, which results from variants in genes that affect the structure of the heart's muscle. More than a dozen genes have been linked to HCM, but the disorder is most often connected to variants in the myosin binding protein 3 (MYBPC3) gene. In people with these variants, the heart's walls may become abnormally thick, restricting blood flow ▸▸

and leaving the heart prone to dangerous, potentially fatal heart rhythms. A gene therapy trial that uses a virus to deliver a working copy of the MYBPC3 gene to the heart muscle began in the fall of 2023.

Transthyretin amyloid cardiomyopathy (ATTR-CM). The exact prevalence of this rare disorder is unclear because it is difficult to diagnose, but an estimated 5,000 to 7,000 new cases are identified in the United States each year. It occurs when a gene variant causes the liver to make an abnormal form of transthyretin (TTR) protein. Clumps of TTR build up, causing the heart's left ventricle to stiffen and weaken, potentially leading to heart failure. A trial using gene editing to stop the production of the abnormal TTR protein showed dramatic drops in the protein among the 60 people who received the therapy.

The big picture

The above conditions can all be treated with existing medications or procedures. The overarching problem is that they're usually discovered only at very advanced stages, after a person has developed severe symptoms. "The biggest unmet need in cardiovascular genetic disorders is identifying people when early, preventive interventions are feasible. Currently, most of these cases go undetected," says Dr. MacRae.

Still, gene therapy trials should radically improve recognition of these inherited heart diseases. "As we expand our detection of disease and the underlying gene defects, we will begin to better understand how these conditions affect patients and how therapies of differing risk and benefit can best be implemented," says Dr. MacRae.

IN THE JOURNALS

RNA-based drug shows promise for lowering blood pressure

A single injection of a new RNA-based drug may lower blood pressure for up to six months, according to a small study published in 2023 in *The New England Journal of Medicine*.

The drug, zilebesiran, is an example of a new class of medications called small interfering RNA (siRNA) drugs. It works by interfering with the liver's production of angiotensinogen, a protein that plays a key role in high blood pressure.

Researchers tested seven different dosages of the drug in 107 people. Higher doses led to drops of at least 10 points in systolic blood pressure (the first number in a reading) and 5 points in diastolic

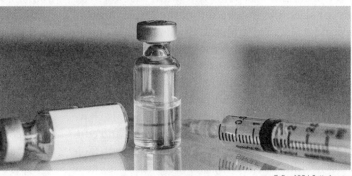

© Pua108 | Getty Images

blood pressure (the second number) after two months, and the effects lasted for six months.

The changes stayed consistent throughout the day, and few side effects were reported. Two larger trials of the drug are currently under way.

ADVANCES IN HEALTH TECHNOLOGY

by **ANTHONY L. KOMAROFF, M.D.,** Editor in Chief, *Harvard Health Letter*

Does your gut affect your risk for Alzheimer's disease?

Q *I know that your genes and lifestyle can influence your risk of getting Alzheimer's disease. Now I read that microbes in our guts also may be involved. Really?*

A Genes and lifestyle both influence our risk of getting Alzheimer's disease. And, as strange as it may seem, so may the microbes in our gut.

We've known for nearly 200 years that microbes live on and in us. We thought they were just living off the warmth and nutrients that our bodies provided to them—invisible freeloaders that had no effect on our health. Beginning about 20 years ago, we began to learn that was wrong. Like humans, microbes have genes. All of the different genes of the microbes that live on us or in us, collectively, are called our "microbiome." To our surprise, we've learned that these microbe genes can make chemicals that can affect human health.

We now know that our microbiome can affect our risk for obesity, diabetes, atherosclerosis, and other important diseases. A study reported in 2023 in the prestigious scientific journal *Brain* finds that our microbiome may even influence our risk of developing Alzheimer's disease.

Previous studies had reported that in people with Alzheimer's disease, some particular species of gut bacteria are more prevalent, while other species are less so, compared to people without the disease. But that did not answer the cart-and-horse question: does the disease affect the difference in the gut bacteria, or does the difference in the gut bacteria affect the disease?

The new study provides provocative evidence that the gut bacteria may actually influence the risk of getting the disease. The research team took a group of healthy young rats and eliminated all bacteria from their guts. Then the team collected bowel movement samples from people with Alzheimer's disease and from people with normal cognition and no signs of the disease. Such samples are full of gut bacteria. Then the samples from humans were squirted into the rats' guts.

The microbiome from people with Alzheimer's disease—but not the microbiome from people without the disease—caused some Alzheimer's-like changes in the rats' brains. Those rats also developed memory impairments. Moreover, the rats that received the microbiomes from the most severely affected Alzheimer's patients developed the greatest brain abnormalities and memory problems.

It will require much more research to confirm that our gut microbiome influences our risk of Alzheimer's disease—and, if so, how it does so. The answer to that last question could someday point to treatments that can treat or even prevent Alzheimer's disease.

© chombosan | Getty Images

Some evidence links gut bacteria and the risk of Alzheimer's disease.

by **ANTHONY L. KOMAROFF, M.D.**, Editor in Chief, *Harvard Health Letter*

Can we fix Alzheimer's genes?

Q *Alzheimer's disease runs in my family. Could scientists fix the genes that cause the disease?*

A Your question highlights something important. Even just 30 years ago, we didn't know for sure if any genes increased the risk for Alzheimer's disease, and we surely had no tools for fixing such defective genes. Today, we do know of several important genes, and we have gene editing tools, like CRISPR. But we're not yet able to prevent the disease in someone like you. Here's why.

A few cases of Alzheimer's occur in younger adults and are predominantly caused by defects in a handful of genes. It's possible that someday CRISPR could work for this type of Alzheimer's. However, it won't be easy. While CRISPR can easily edit genes in cells in a laboratory dish, using CRISPR to edit the genes of cells deep inside the body of a living person is much harder: attempts to edit genes inside the cells of living animals are just in their infancy.

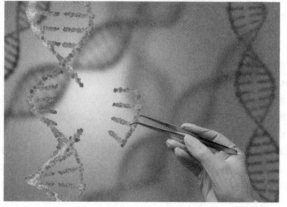
© rommma | Getty Images

Gene editing probably won't prevent Alzheimer's anytime soon.

Most cases of Alzheimer's, however, occur in older adults and do not appear to be caused just by a few defective genes. Indeed, lifestyle—particularly exercise, diet, and amount of high-quality sleep—affects the risk of developing Alzheimer's at least as much as genes.

Also, there is growing evidence that smoldering, chronic, low-grade infections of the brain acquired earlier in life—infections that produce no symptoms—may provoke the development of some cases of Alzheimer's. Some infectious agents, particularly viruses, can quietly infect the brain and can't be eradicated; they remain for the rest of a person's life.

How might this increase the risk of Alzheimer's? One characteristic of Alzheimer's is accumulations (plaques) in the brain of a molecule called amyloid-beta. Everyone's brain has the ability to make amyloid-beta. Unfortunately, amyloid-beta is a "good news–bad news" molecule. It helps fight infections of the brain; that's the good news. The bad news is that amyloid-beta cannot eradicate some infections. When the brain is infected with an agent that cannot be eradicated, amyloid-beta keeps being produced, and keeps trying and failing to eliminate the infection. Over the long term, the buildup of amyloid-beta damages the cells that do the thinking (the neurons).

So, I doubt that gene editing techniques like CRISPR are going to prevent Alzheimer's—at least, not for a long time. But I'm more optimistic about medicines that reduce the levels of amyloid-beta and another molecule, tau, that appears important in causing Alzheimer's, based on very recent research. And I'm also optimistic that as we learn more about the role of infections that may increase the risk of Alzheimer's, we may develop treatments and vaccines that target those infections and reduce that risk.

Be cautious with new Alzheimer's disease test

You don't need your doctor's okay to get it, but some experts say it's not ready for prime time.

The idea of getting Alzheimer's disease is troubling for anyone. And if you have a family history of the condition or if you've been experiencing persistent memory loss, you might wonder if it's time to seek testing. Traditionally, the process starts with a doctor visit and evaluation. However, you can now order an Alzheimer's blood screening on your own. The question is—should you?

Ordering without a doctor visit

The screening is called AD-Detect. It's available through Quest Diagnostics for $399, plus a $13 fee for physician services. Anyone 18 or older can go online and order AD-Direct, without a doctor visit, and a Quest-affiliated doctor will review the order to determine if it's medically necessary.

Eligibility is based on risk factors such as a family history of Alzheimer's, a decline in thinking skills (memory problems and getting lost, for example), previous head trauma or brain injuries, or excessive alcohol use.

If the test is prescribed, you go to the nearest Quest lab to have your blood drawn. Quest analyzes the sample, looking for two types of proteins: amyloid-beta 40, which is naturally present in the brain and considered normal; and amyloid-beta 42, which is involved in forming Alzheimer's brain plaques.

To see your results (a comparison of the protein levels), you log on at the Quest portal. You can also chat with a Quest-affiliated doctor about your results and next steps (it's covered in your fees).

Concerns to consider

Ordering the new Alzheimer's screening comes with risks.

It's not FDA-approved. The screening doesn't need the FDA's okay to be marketed to consumers.

It's only a screening tool. A positive result means that your risk of getting Alzheimer's is increased, but it does not mean that you definitely have Alzheimer's.

We don't know how accurate it is. Very little information about AD-Detect is available to the public. No peer-reviewed research on the screening has been published. So we don't know the risk of false results. A

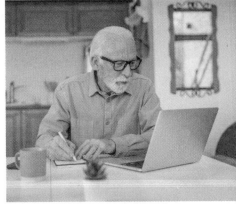
© Miljan Živkovic | Getty Images
Be thoughtful before self-ordering an online screening test for Alzheimer's disease.

false-negative result (one that says your risk is low or normal when, in fact, it's increased) might give you a false sense of security and cause you to delay pursuing diagnosis and treatment, even if you're having symptoms. A false-positive result (one that says your risk is increased when, in fact, it's normal or low) might cause you undue stress and anxiety, plus time and expense in seeking further testing.

"There are few diagnoses I can think of that would be worse to hear. It might cause anxiety, depression, and even an alteration of life plans for the entire family," says Dr. Andrew Budson, a lecturer in neurology at Harvard Medical School and chief of Cognitive and Behavioral Neurology at the VA Boston Healthcare System.

There's a delay to speak with a doctor. It can take a few days to speak with a Quest-affiliated doctor about your results, which might be stressful.

You might need further testing. If the results suggest you need additional testing, you'll have to turn to a specialist. Would you have access to a neurologist who specializes in Alzheimer's care, and facilities offering tests you might need? Would it be hard to get an appointment to discuss your next steps? "The wait to see dementia specialists can be six months or longer," Dr. Budson says.

Getting a diagnosis

An Alzheimer's diagnosis requires much more than a blood screening. It involves a comprehensive evaluation of your current and past health problems, physical and neurological exams, family history, blood tests to rule out hidden conditions that might be causing memory problems (such as vitamin B_{12} deficiency), and imaging tests.

"I would start with a brain MRI or a CT scan to look for structural problems like strokes or brain tumors. If we've ruled out everything and I still suspect Alzheimer's disease, I might also order an amyloid PET scan or a test of spinal fluid that could contain Alzheimer's markers," Dr. Budson says.

Doctors can also order blood tests designed to help diagnose Alzheimer's. Like the AD-Detect screening, these tests look for amyloid proteins, but they go further by looking for other markers of Alzheimer's. "But these tests aren't yet as accurate as a spinal fluid test or a PET scan," Dr. Budson says.

What you should do

Self-ordered screening blood tests may someday have a role in investigating a possible Alzheimer's diagnosis, but Dr. Budson thinks they're not a good idea today. "If you have concerns about Alzheimer's disease, talk to your primary care doctor. Investigate your risks together. If necessary, get recommendations for an Alzheimer's specialist," he says. "This could be one of the most important decisions of your life. Approach it as carefully as possible." ▌

IN THE JOURNALS

Nasal spray slows rapid heart rhythm

A nasal spray containing the experimental drug etripamil can quickly and effectively treat an abnormally fast heart rhythm called supraventricular tachycardia (SVT), according to a new study.

Caused by an electrical misfire that overrides the heart's natural pacemaker, SVT occurs sporadically and can lead to heart rates as high as 180 to 200 beats per minute. While it may resolve on its own, SVT may persist and make people dizzy or lightheaded. Coughing or gagging sometimes helps, but people usually need to go to an emergency room for an injection of a drug to slow the heart.

Published in 2023 in *The Lancet*, the study included 184 people who were followed for nearly two years. When people used etripamil spray at home, it was twice as effective as a placebo spray in restoring SVT back to a normal heart rhythm (and helped them avoid emergency department visits). The company that makes etripamil has submitted the drug for FDA approval and expects a decision in spring 2025.

IN THE JOURNALS

Two-dose shingles vaccine is still highly effective after four years

The CDC recommends adults ages 50 and older get two doses of the recombinant zoster vaccine (Shingrix), with the doses separated by two to six months, to prevent shingles. But how long can it offer protection? According to a 2024 study involving almost two million people published by the *Annals of Internal Medicine,* the two-dose vaccine was still 73% effective four years later. However, in those adults who received only one dose instead of the recommended two, the effectiveness dropped rapidly after the first year and only offered 52% protection against shingles after three years.

These results reinforced the importance of getting the second dose. But even if you miss the usual two-to-six-month window for the booster, it may not be too late. The researchers also found that the vaccine's effectiveness did not suffer if the second dose was delayed beyond six months.

The vaccine also was slightly more effective in people who got the shots before age 65 compared with those who were vaccinated later in life.

ADVANCES IN HEALTH TECHNOLOGY

Chapter 12

Savvy Patient

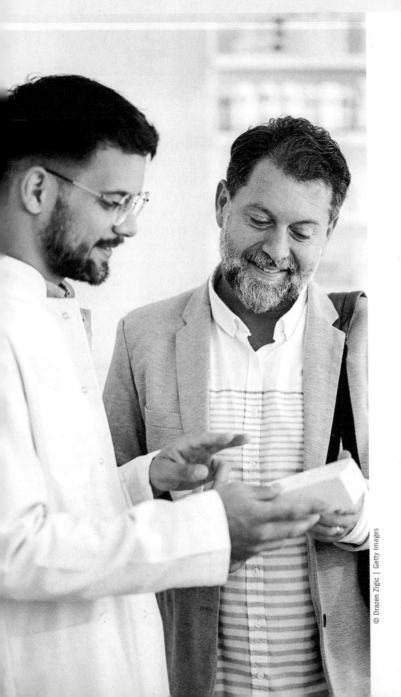

© Drazen Zigic | Getty Images

Healthy Habits!
5 Things You Can Do Now

1 **Conduct a health review.** An annual review of your health data is a wise way to keep on top of goals. (page 290)

2 **Tackle medical anxiety.** What your doctors want you to know to feel comfortable. (page 293)

3 **Heading for the hospital?** Our tips for preparing will set you up for success. (page 298)

4 **Consider a plus-one at your next appointment.** Bringing someone along can help you track details and ensure important information is communicated. (page 303)

5 **Take medication as prescribed.** Learn how to make doing so easier. (page 311)

Time for your annual health review

Begin the new year by looking at where you've been and where you want to go.

The start of a new year is always a great opportunity to re-engage with your health. And one of the first steps is to conduct a personal health review. "It's a way to measure where your health stands now, outline what goals you hope to accomplish, and devise a strategy in partnership with your physician, mapping out how to reach them," says Dr. Jeremy Whyman, a geriatrician and specialist in internal medicine and palliative medicine at Harvard-affiliated Beth Israel Deaconess Medical Center.

A personal health review follows a three-step process: gathering all your current health information, listing your goals, and sharing everything with your doctor during a scheduled wellness visit.

Gather the information

First, make a list of key health points from the past year. "Include everything from routine check-ins with other specialists to urgent care visits to diagnostic tests," says Dr. Whyman. "Be as detailed and concise as possible. Nothing is not relevant when looking at your overall health." Here are some examples of information you should collect (your patient portal can help):

- Have you seen a new doctor or specialist for any reason?
- What tests did you have and what were the results and conclusions reached?
- What medications do you currently take and do you take them regularly? Did you begin taking any new medications? Did you stop taking any, or was your dose adjusted?
- What routine check-ups did you have (dental, eye, skin, hearing, foot)? What were the results? Were any recommendations given?
- Did you have any surgery or treatment?
- Did you suffer from an injury? Even a minor one?

Another component of important health information you need to record: lifestyle habits or issues, such

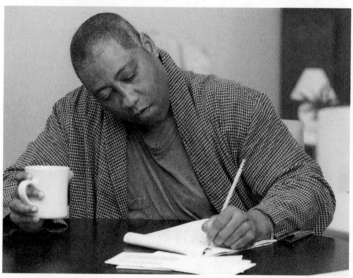

© Hill Street Studios I Getty Images

Listing your current health information and future goals can help create a strategy for success.

as exercise routine, weight pattern, diet, and emotional health. Here's a look at what points you should include and how each can fit into your future health goals.

Exercise. Outline your regular exercise activities—what you do daily and weekly, and for how long (for example, strength training, aerobic exercise, flexibility, or some combination). Also, highlight if these are new endeavors or continuous ones and how motivated you feel about your overall exercise efforts. "You might be ready to increase your efforts in certain areas or be open to adapt your usual workouts with something new to increase motivation," says Dr. Whyman. "Be explicit with your physician about what you are and are not ready to pursue. This helps focus the conversation during the visit." Also, note any injuries or recurring aches that may have hindered your workouts, like a sore knee or back. "If you have had physical therapy for an issue, make sure you include that, too," says Dr. Whyman.

Weight. Has your weight gone up or down over the past year? Did it fluctuate? Do you feel you are at a comfortable weight? "If weight loss is a goal, define a reasonable idea of how much you should aim to lose," says Dr. Whyman.

Diet. Do you follow a specific diet or eating plan, like a Mediterranean diet? If not, what do your daily meals look like? "It's difficult to provide detailed accounts of every daily meal, but try to paint a picture of your usual eating habits and be as honest as you can. It's so important for your physician to know the good and the bad," says Dr. Whyman. What area(s) do you think are your strengths (for example, eating whole grains for breakfast and fruit for snacks) and weaknesses (for instance, skipping meals or eating too much red meat or snack foods)?

Mental health. How has your mood been over the past year? Have you experienced any periods of time where you've felt depressed or anxious? Did you suffer a personal loss or setback? "Everyone has the occasional down day, but note any specific times where you felt low or anxious for an extended period, or if it interfered with your life, preventing you from being with friends or family, doing important work or even completing routine tasks that usually come easy to you," says Dr. Whyman. "A lot of men often don't like talking about their mental health, but it could be an underlying barrier that needs to be addressed."

Outline your goals

Next, choose three health goals and rank them. "You don't want to take on too much, but selecting three goals is manageable, and prioritizing them helps you and your doctor determine what changes need to be made first," says Dr. Whyman.

Some examples: increase strength and endurance to interact with grandchildren, improve your functional fitness so you can do daily chores, and continue to live independently. "Think in terms of what you would like to achieve in the short term and the long term," says Dr. Whyman.

Schedule a wellness visit

When you schedule your annual get-together with your primary care physician, make sure the office staff indicates it is an "Annual Wellness Visit." Then it will be fully covered by Medicare, as well as by most other health insurance plans.

This consultation can help your doctor identify areas that need improvement or adjustments and devise a strategy to follow. "Your physician is like a quarterback overseeing the entire offense," says Dr. Whyman.

For instance, knowing what other health care you have received, including drug prescriptions, can help your doctor determine if any changes in doses should be addressed with your specialists to match your health goals.

Regarding exercise, your doctor may advise strategies to overcome obstacles and address your goals—for example, adopting a step counter to help you walk more, switching to a treadmill or elliptical trainer, or hiring a personal trainer to increase strength training. "He or she also can help identify problems or barriers that may hinder your exercise, like arthritis or tendinitis," says Dr. Whyman.

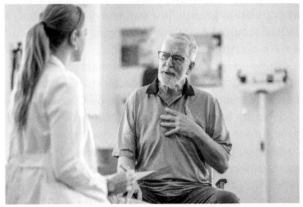

© FatCamera | Getty Images

Health care professionals can work with you to track key health data and provide support to reach your goals.

Your doctor can also suggest changes to your eating habits, like increasing protein to combat natural muscle loss and offering healthy alternatives to satisfy cravings. Seeing a nutritionist may be recommended if you have trouble making healthy choices. If you have weight issues (significant losses or gains), the conversation might reveal other undiagnosed issues such as depression or a thyroid problem.

Your doctor will also want to ensure you are up to date on cancer screenings based on your age and family history. For men, this may include colon cancer screening and possibly PSA blood testing for prostate cancer. Your doctor will also review your immunization history and recommend vaccines or boosters for which you are due. 🛡

The secret to finding a primary care provider: Be flexible

Be open to seeing a physician, nurse practitioner, or physician assistant for primary care.

Forget being finicky if you're looking for a new primary care physician: it's hard enough just finding one who's taking new patients. That's due to a doctor shortage in the United States, fueled by such factors as population growth, low pay, physician burnout, a lack of required postgraduate training programs, and a wave of retirements.

The shortage is becoming so serious that some states are trying to make it easier for doctors to practice there, or they're creating new medical schools. And Congress is debating how to increase the number of training programs in the country. Those measures aren't going to help you get a new primary care physician anytime soon, however, so you need to be flexible about the type of health professional you seek. Fortunately, you have options.

Primary care physicians

This category includes several kinds of primary care doctors. They've all earned a bachelor's degree (which takes three or four years), graduated from medical school (which takes four years), completed a training

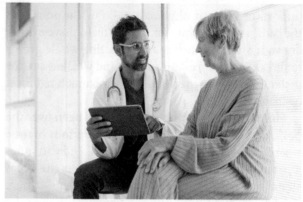

© Solskin | Getty Images

It's important to have a primary care provider in place before serious health problems develop.

program (which takes at least three years), and passed licensing exams. They all promote wellness and preventive care and treat a wide range of conditions. But each doctor's focus is a little different.

Internal medicine specialist. An internist treats adults only and has completed training in a hospital and subspecialty clinics (such as cardiology or gastroenterology) for every organ system in the body.

Internal medicine-pediatrics. A "med-peds" physician treats adults and children and has trained in both internal medicine and pediatrics.

Family practitioner. This doctor can treat children and adults and has a broader scope than an internist or med-peds physician. For example, some family practitioners can perform minor surgery and even deliver babies.

Geriatrician. A geriatrician deals with the medical complexities of older patients with many chronic conditions. Geriatricians also consider the many issues that affect older adults, such as social or functional limitations.

Other primary care providers

You can also turn to an advanced practitioner for primary care: a nurse practitioner (NP) or a physician assistant (PA). Both are licensed and can diagnose and treat patients, order medical tests, and prescribe medication. But there are differences in their training and autonomy.

The NP becomes a registered nurse first (with a two- or four-year degree), and then earns a master's or doctorate degree in advanced practice nursing (which takes two to three years). NPs can practice

---

Resources to find providers

Tap into these resources when looking for a primary care provider:

Referral lines. Hospitals often have referral lines that can direct you to primary care providers taking new patients.

Your family, friends, and doctors. They may have recommendations for providers they trust.

Online reviews. Look at physician review sites, but take reviews with a grain of salt unless there's a large number of comments pointing one way or the other.

---

medicine independently in about half of the United States. In many states, however, they must collaborate with a doctor.

The PA has a health- or science-related bachelor's degree and a master's degree from an accredited physician assistant program (which takes two to three years). Unlike NPs, PAs are not permitted to practice independently. They must work in collaboration with a doctor.

Doctors vs. advanced practitioners

Is there a difference in the quality of care you'll receive if you go to a doctor versus an advanced practitioner? "It's difficult to say. Studies comparing the quality of care between the two groups are inconclusive. But if you spend four years in medical school and three-plus years in a training program, it's probably true that you'll perform better than advanced practitioners in some regards, since you have more training," says Dr. Anupam Jena, the Joseph P. Newhouse Professor of Health Care Policy at Harvard Medical School and co-author of the book *Random Acts of Medicine.*

Still, Dr. Jena notes that NPs and PAs are skilled clinicians who can spot medical problems and, if they can't treat them, connect you to the care you need. So don't fret about the type of primary care provider you see.

"The priority is establishing the relationship. Otherwise, if you're sick, and you don't have someone you can call, you'll have to go to an emergency department or a walk-in clinic. That's not optimal," Dr. Jena says. "You want a relationship with someone who knows you and can make recommendations you'll listen to. And ideally it's important to have that in place before a serious problem develops."

Afraid to visit the doctor?

You're not alone if medical anxiety is endangering your health.

Even after many years of seeing Dr. Daniel Sands, a primary care doctor at Harvard-affiliated Beth Israel Deaconess Medical Center, Maggie could best be described as a reluctant patient. "She was deathly afraid of doctors and hospitals and very anxious every time she came in, but knew she had to sometimes," Dr. Sands recalls.

But Maggie's hesitancy cost her dearly, preventing her from getting care that might have kept her healthier and stronger. She skipped vaccinations against illnesses that could worsen her chronic lung disease. And although she had terrible arthritis in her knees, she refused to even consider joint replacement surgery to make her more comfortable and mobile.

Maggie (whose name has been changed to protect her privacy) is a prime example of medical anxiety, a sometimes crippling fear of doctors and medical settings. It's a pervasive issue: in 2023, nearly half of American adults reported feeling anxious before a doctor's appointment, an increase from 39% the previous year, according to a nationally

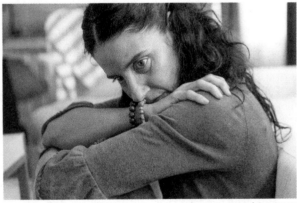

© valentinrussanov | Getty Images

Anxiety that causes people to avoid getting health care is a common problem.

representative survey of 2,000 people by market research company OnePoll.

Dr. Sands sees patients with medical anxiety once or twice a month and encounters a severe case like Maggie's a few times a year. But four in 10 adults polled in 2023 said their anxiety compels them to ▸▸

▸▸ put off seeing a doctor—a decision with potentially wide-ranging health implications.

Serious consequences

Why is health care hesitancy dangerous? It can dissuade people from seeking ongoing monitoring (such as cholesterol and blood pressure checks) or cancer screenings (such as mammograms and colorectal exams). Such anxiety can even stop some people from taking care of serious issues that might shorten their lives.

"So much of what we do depends on follow-up," Dr. Sands says. "If you miss a cancer screening, you have a higher risk of developing cancer. With uncontrolled high blood pressure, you could have a stroke or heart attack or develop kidney or heart failure. Poorly controlled diabetes greatly increases the risk

for heart attacks, kidney failure, blindness, and even amputations."

"Depending on what the problem is, all those things are at play," he says. "At worst," he adds, "you could die before your time."

List of triggers

Medical anxiety differs from health anxiety or hypochondria, which involves an extreme preoccupation with developing serious illnesses such as cancer, heart problems, or neurological illnesses. But it may overlap with "white-coat hypertension," a surge in blood pressure experienced by as many as 30% of people when measured during a doctor's visit, according to American Heart Association research.

For these folks, white-coat hypertension is essentially a fight-or-flight response marked by an increase

---

Be comfortable asking your doctor about a second opinion

If your home needed a new roof, you might get quotes from several companies before making such a weighty financial decision. So why wouldn't you seek advice from more than one doctor if you're facing a weighty medical matter?

Seeking a second opinion is fairly common. But some people are concerned their doctor would be insulted by the request—though they shouldn't be, says Dr. Daniel Sands, a primary care doctor at Beth Israel Deaconess Medical Center.

"Patients should feel comfortable asking for a second opinion," Dr. Sands says. "It shouldn't be a personal affront or a matter of ego to a doctor—it should be a matter of being open to hearing what another health professional says."

Most situations don't call for a second opinion. You don't need one for a minor health problem. And, if you're pleased with your care, you don't need to ask if another doctor would approach it differently.

But wanting a second opinion doesn't necessarily mean you don't trust your doctor. In certain situations, it's just wise to do so—especially if you need major surgery or cancer treatment, Dr. Sands says.

"For any life-changing diagnosis or potentially fatal condition, a second opinion is called for," he says. "Cancer is a good example, since there may be more than one way to treat it, so it might be worthwhile to get information from two or three separate places."

If you feel trepidation about asking for a second opinion, Dr. Sands offers this approach. "Ideally, I'd say, 'I appreciate the time you spent with me and the thought you've put into this. I think you'll understand why I'd like to get a second opinion. Is there someone you recommend I consult with?' A lot of times, they'll point you toward someone specific," he says.

If you're uncomfortable with that tactic, Dr. Sands suggests speaking with your primary care doctor and asking for her guidance. "She can help set up a second opinion," he says.

If your doctor does seem insulted by your request, you don't need to confront her—but you should still follow your instincts. "End your appointment in a normal way and seek a second opinion elsewhere," Dr. Sands says.

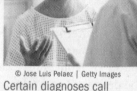
© Jose Luis Pelaez | Getty Images
Certain diagnoses call for a second opinion.

in stress hormones. The trigger might be the stress of getting to the doctor's, or just the sight of a doctor. (The reaction is named for the traditional white lab coat many clinicians wear.) "It might be the antiseptic smell of the doctor's office," Dr. Sands says. "And for some people, it might just be being touched."

People who have undergone trauma or abuse may be especially prone to medical anxiety, Dr. Sands says. What else can provoke fear? Needles or shots are on the list, along with the prospect of a painful test or procedure or receiving bad news or a serious diagnosis. Those latter two reasons were cited by about 40% of the 2023 poll respondents who reported medical anxiety.

Ways to cope

Anxiety about medical care doesn't usually exist in a vacuum, Dr. Sands says. People with it often have generalized anxiety that also crops up outside of health care settings. "In my experience, going to the doctor only makes it worse," he says.

Dr. Sands recommends that people with medical anxiety seek treatment, which may include psychotherapy, medication, or both. "These kinds of situations often call for professional help," he says.

He offers these additional coping strategies if doctors or medical settings make you anxious:

Identify what worries you. Doing so may take its power away or prod ideas about how to respond. "If you can identify your triggers, you can try to talk yourself through them," he says. "But you should also share them with your doctor. If your doctor doesn't ask, say, 'These are things that make me concerned or anxious.'"

Do a cost-benefit analysis. Weigh the long-term health benefits of getting needed health care against your short-term discomfort. This is perhaps easier said than done when you're anxious, Dr. Sands acknowledges.

Bring someone along. Having a trusted companion at your side during your appointment can calm frayed nerves.

Request sedatives. Short-acting medications may help you stay more relaxed during anxiety-provoking procedures, but they can also involve drawbacks, such as being unable to drive afterward. For more involved, longer procedures, your doctor may have the option to perform them under anesthesia. Using either sedatives or anesthetics involves carefully weighing the risks and benefits. Ask your doctor about the pros and cons.

Try relaxation techniques. Meditation or deep breathing can help allay anxiety while you're in the waiting room. "It's a great way to relax and bring your blood pressure down," Dr. Sands says. 🛡

The colonoscopy diet

What you eat before, right after, and in the days following a colonoscopy can make a difference for the procedure and your gut health.

A colonoscopy reigns as the gold standard screening test to look for colorectal cancer and other bowel problems. It's an outpatient procedure that allows your doctor to peek inside your colon using a thin, flexible tube with an attached camera, inspect the colon lining, and even remove potentially cancerous growths.

But the doctor's expertise isn't all that's needed to make the procedure a success. Your preparation—what you eat, and the way you clean out your gut beforehand—is essential to give your doctor the best view of the colon lining. The post-procedure diet is also important for your comfort and gut health. Here's what you need to know about a "colonoscopy diet."

Three days beforehand

The mission to prepare your colon for a colonoscopy starts a few days before the procedure. "During this time, we advise that you eat a low-fiber diet. These foods are easy to digest and move through the colon faster than high-fiber foods. This will make colon prep easier," says Dr. Andrew T. Chan, a gastroenterologist and director of epidemiology at Harvard-affiliated Massachusetts General Hospital Cancer Center. ▸▸

▶▶ Eating a low-fiber diet doesn't mean you can ditch all healthy food and reach for chips and soda instead. It means eating foods such as animal protein (eggs, cheese, fish, poultry); certain cooked vegetables (carrots, green beans, potatoes, pumpkin, yams, or zucchini and other squash); low-fiber fruits (bananas, peaches, pears); and (if your doctor says it's okay) low-fiber breads such as white, sourdough, or refined wheat breads.

A low-fiber diet also nixes foods such as legumes (beans, lentils, peas), whole grains (whole-wheat crackers, cereals, breads, popcorn, granola), nuts, seeds, dried fruit, and high-fiber raw fruits or vegetables (especially asparagus, broccoli, Brussels sprouts, cabbage, cauliflower, and celery).

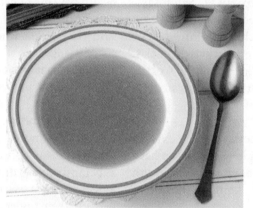

© Madeleine_Steinbach | Getty Images

Switch to low-fiber foods, such as plain chicken soup, two to three days before colonoscopy.

The day before the colonoscopy

Unless your doctor has prescribed the type of colonoscopy prep that's done only on the day of the procedure, the day before a colonoscopy is when you should have only clear liquids. Examples include clear broth or bouillon, black coffee, plain tea, clear juice (apple, white grape), clear soft drinks or sports drinks, Jell-O, and popsicles. Then, in the late afternoon, you take laxative pills and solutions and drink lots of fluids to clean out your colon.

Note: Avoid foods or drinks that are red, blue, or purple. Just like they can temporarily stain your tongue, they can also stain the lining of your colon, which might make it hard for your doctor to examine it properly. So stay away from grape, raspberry, or cherry Jell-O or popsicles; go for the lighter-colored flavors instead, such as banana.

The day of the colonoscopy

A colonoscopy requires you to receive a powerful sedative: most people remain conscious, but are very relaxed and less likely to feel any discomfort. You also may have little memory of the procedure. Because of the sedative, you probably won't be allowed to eat or drink anything on the day of your procedure, unless your doctor has advised you to continue taking your usual prescription medications (such as drugs that treat high blood pressure) with a sip of water, or has directed you to begin the colon prep on this day.

After the procedure, you'll be allowed to resume your normal diet. But should you? A sudden injection of fiber—such as a bowl of black bean soup with whole-wheat crackers on the side, or chickpea pasta tossed with olive oil with grilled asparagus—might cause gas, bloating, and discomfort.

"Some people are able to start eating a full diet right away without discomfort, while others may require a slower introduction of their usual foods. So it might be wisest to restart your normal diet gradually over the next day or so," Dr. Chan says.

Gut health reset?

With your colon cleaned out, you might wonder if you'll now have an opportunity to create a healthier population of gut microbes than you had before the procedure. Is it possible? The jury is still out. "There is no clear evidence that you can more favorably repopulate your gut bacteria over the long term after a colonoscopy with any particular dietary changes," Dr. Chan says.

What we do know is that your gut is home to trillions of mostly beneficial microbes—bacteria, viruses, fungi—that help digest your food and keep you healthy. These bugs fight harmful pathogens; make vitamin K and other important chemicals; affect the way medications work; influence your immune system, heart health, and cancer risk; and possibly play a role in healthy aging and longevity.

We also know that what you eat can help gut microbes thrive. For the best results, feed them a fiber-rich diet that includes fruits, vegetables (especially dark, leafy greens), legumes (beans, peas), and whole grains (quinoa, oats, whole wheat, brown rice). These are the kinds of foods found in a Mediterranean-style diet, which also includes lean proteins (poultry and fish), olive oil, nuts and seeds, dairy foods (milk and cheese), and limited amounts of red wine.

It's a diet that will keep your gut microbes happy and help you maintain many other aspects of good health. 🍷

by **HOWARD LeWINE, M.D.,** Editor in Chief, *Harvard Men's Health Watch*

Why do medical guidelines change frequently?

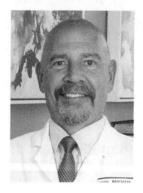

Q*I find it disconcerting that medical recommendations and guidelines seem to change so often. For example, I recently read there may be another change in colon cancer screening recommendations. How does a person decide what's right?*

AThere are several reasons why these changes happen. One reason is that ongoing research provides new information that leads to new guidelines. Another issue is different expert opinions. As you pointed out, a good example of this is the controversy this year regarding when people at average risk for colon cancer should begin screening.

Many clinicians, such as myself, use guidelines from the U.S. Preventive Services Task Force (USPSTF) as the go-to standard. For each guideline, the USPSTF recruits 16 experts from different specialties to research and discuss the potential benefits and harms of screening and other methods aimed to promote health and prevent disease. The summary recommendation is then released for public comment.

However, other professional organizations can evaluate the same medical evidence, and their experts may arrive at recommendations that are different from the USPSTF's. Unlike medical decisions that are straightforward—for example, taking an antibiotic for strep throat—almost all screening recommendations are developed for medical questions that have no obvious right answer.

Your concern about differences in colon cancer screening is a timely example. In response to the rising number of colon cancer cases in adults younger than age 50, the USPSTF lowered the age to begin screening to 45. However, the highly respected American College of Physicians (ACP) looked at the same data and concluded that the benefits did not outweigh the potential harms from screening until age 50.

What all the experts agree on: screening for colon cancer saves lives. My preferred strategy encourages all people at average risk of colon cancer to get at least one colonoscopy between ages 45 and 50. If the initial colonoscopy is normal, then you and your doctor can decide on your future screening strategy, which may be colonoscopy once every 10 years, stool testing every two years, or sigmoidoscopy every five years in addition to stool testing.

I personally will continue to have periodic screening colonoscopies as my choice. There are two main advantages of colonoscopy. The presence or absence of polyps helps determine my future colon cancer risk. And removing a polyp or early cancer improves the likelihood that it won't become a serious problem.

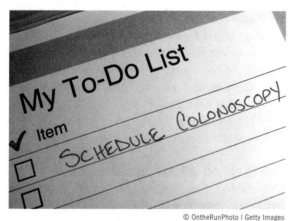

© OntheRunPhoto | Getty Images

Recent colon cancer screening guidelines are an example of how new information can change recommendations.

6 things to do when heading for the hospital

Thorough planning will help you avoid hassles and confusion.

You don't always get to prepare for a prolonged hospital stay. But when you know you'll be hospitalized for a few days—such as for an elective procedure—do more than just pack a small bag before you go. Here are six tasks for your to-do list.

1 Print important documents

Your hospital might not have current information in your file, even if you've been there before and your doctor is affiliated with the facility. To be proactive, pack a few documents (print them out in case hospital staffers don't have the time to upload the information in electronic form).

One document should be a list of your emergency contacts, chronic conditions, and medications (including supplements) and their doses. This is essential information that doctors use to make decisions about your care.

Another document should be a copy of your advance directive, which might include

- a living will detailing the kind of medical care you'd like if you're unable to make your own decisions
- a health care proxy form designating who'll make health care decisions if you can't (it's especially helpful when decisions aren't black and white)
- a POLST (physician orders for life-sustaining treatment) form signed by your clinician; this option for people with serious medical conditions turns your health care preferences into a medical order that must be followed.

If you need an advance directive, download the forms for free from your state. The AARP offers handy links (www.health.harvard.edu/freepad). Some forms must be witnessed or notarized, preferably before a hospital stay.

2 Alert your health care proxy

Tell your health care proxy when and why you're going to the hospital, and what should or shouldn't be done if you can't make decisions. Your proxy can only help you if he or she knows what you want.

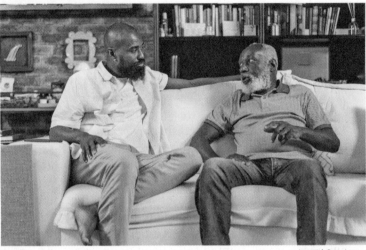

andreswd | Getty Images

Tell your health care proxy what should or shouldn't be done if you can't make decisions.

"Often, when we have to call the proxy, the person says, 'I don't know, I've never talked to my friend or family member about it.' Those situations can be tough for health care proxies, because sometimes we're asking them to make decisions about high-risk treatments," says Dr. Jose F. Figueroa, a hospitalist at Harvard-affiliated Brigham and Women's Hospital, and a health policy and management researcher at the Harvard T.H. Chan School of Public Health.

3 Pack a little extra

Planned short hospital stays sometimes turn into longer ones or lead to a stay in a rehabilitation facility. That could leave you without enough clothes, electronic devices, or device chargers. Dr. Figueroa recommends either packing for such an event, or packing an extra bag to leave at home and arranging for a friend to deliver it if necessary.

4 Establish a toothbrushing plan

Ask a friend, family member, or your nurse to help ensure that your teeth are brushed daily. "Bacteria in the mouth sometimes get into the lungs and cause pneumonia. Good oral hygiene, including toothbrushing, can lower the risk of pneumonia by decreasing the amount of bacteria on the teeth and in the mouth. We have evidence about this in patients in the intensive care unit, and it's reasonable to think it applies to all patients," says Dr. Michael Klompas, a researcher and infectious disease specialist at Brigham and Women's Hospital (see "Toothbrushing can be a literal lifesaver in the hospital" below).

5 Get a discharge buddy

When it's time to leave the hospital, your nurse will provide you with instructions about your care. "But it's a vulnerable time to be getting a lot of information, such as details about new medications, old medications, and when you're supposed to see a doctor again. Being confused about what to do next can lead to medication mistakes and hospital readmissions," Dr. Figueroa says.

Before your stay, ask a friend to be there at discharge time—in person or on the phone—to jot down details and ask questions. "Have the friend ask about medication changes you should be aware of, signs to be worried about, when to call the doctor, and whether you have any new appointments set up or need to make them," Dr. Figueroa advises.

6 Arrange a ride home

You may have a way to get to the hospital, but many people forget about the ride home. "We never advise driving yourself home. You might be on medications that affect your ability to concentrate, or you might be confused or weak after a hospital stay," Dr. Figueroa says. If you don't have a friend who can take you home, ask your doctor's office, religious organization, or senior center about ride opportunities. If you can afford it, hire a health aide to drive you. Just make sure there's someone to help get you inside your home and settled. A little advance planning will go a long way. 🛡

IN THE JOURNALS

Toothbrushing can be a literal lifesaver in the hospital

Regular toothbrushing can help save hospital patients' lives during their stays in intensive care units (ICUs), according to a Harvard study published in 2023 by *JAMA Internal Medicine*. Researchers combined the results of 15 randomized clinical trials that included about 2,800 ICU patients and found that twice-a-day toothbrushing was associated with lower rates of death compared with not regularly brushing.

Patients who had their teeth brushed daily also had shorter ICU stays and spent less time on a mechanical ventilator. (Since ICU patients are often unable to brush on their own, toothbrushing was done by the hospital care team.) The reason? Regular toothbrushing appears to protect ICU patients from getting pneumonia, the most common ICU-acquired infection, according to

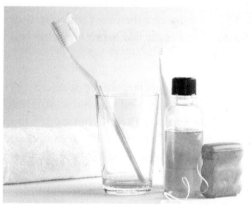
© simarik | Getty Images
Twice-daily tooth brushing in the hospital helps avoid lung infections.

the researchers. While the trials did not focus on non-ICU patients, the researchers added that regular toothbrushing might offer similar protection from pneumonia during regular hospital stays, but more research is needed.

Staying safe while getting well

Adverse events—many of them potentially preventable—can leave hospital patients vulnerable. How can you protect yourself?

You're ensconced in a hospital bed, surrounded by dedicated doctors and nurses and relieved to be recovering in a place whose mission is to get you well.

But are you safe? That may seem like a strange question when you're in a facility intended to restore your health or even save your life.

More than 33 million people were admitted to the nation's 6,000 hospitals in 2022, according to the American Hospital Association. About 13 million of them were 65 or older. All of them showed up there at a vulnerable moment, trusting they'd be cared for safely.

But sometimes things go wrong. Despite the best efforts of your medical team, adverse events and medical errors can happen.

"Hospitals are not as safe as they could be," says Dr. David Bates, chief of the Division of Medicine at Harvard-affiliated Brigham and Women's Hospital and director of its Center for Patient Safety Research and Practice.

"It's certainly unsettling," adds Dr. Bates, who led a 2023 study looking at adverse medical events during hospitalizations published by *The New England Journal of Medicine*. "That being said, there are certain strategies patients and their families can take to protect themselves."

What can go awry?

Dr. Bates's efforts—which largely replicated a 1991 Harvard analysis—also showed that hospital-related adverse events happen up to 10 times more often than they did 30 years ago, though the study design and some definitions of harm differed. "I was surprised there is as much harm as there is," he says.

He and colleagues analyzed a random sample of 2,809 patient admissions at 11 Massachusetts hospitals in 2018. Preventable medical events occurred in nearly 7% of all admissions, while serious and potentially life-threatening preventable events arose in 1%.

What constitutes a medical adverse event? Examples include patients receiving the wrong medication or dose, getting a new infection while in the hospital, developing bed sores, or falling.

"Preventable adverse events typically happen because someone makes a mistake, or more than one,

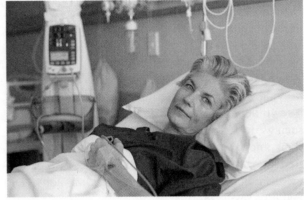
© Ridofranz | Getty Images

Patients and family members can take proactive steps to lower the odds of adverse events.

in the process of care," Dr. Bates says. "I think a lot of it is just the pressures of giving care today."

Various hospital protocols are often able to identify these problems before a patient is harmed. "At the same time, while we have better equipment now, sometimes the risk of what we do has simply gone up," Dr. Bates says. "We now do surgery for more serious problems and have more powerful medications, so it is not surprising to see some adverse events."

Protection strategies

The fallout from an adverse hospital event can affect a patient's physical, mental, and financial health. You may end up staying in the hospital longer or facing a prolonged recovery at home. Depression is often part of the aftermath, Dr. Bates notes, "and the older you are, the more likely you'll experience an adverse event and that it will affect you psychologically."

While adverse events often aren't preventable—and they're rarely the fault of the patient—Dr. Bates offers ways your own vigilance might reduce the odds of you suffering from a mishap.

Get a care partner. Ask your spouse, adult child, or another loved one to remain close at hand while you're hospitalized. This trusted person can serve as a second set of eyes and ears and is particularly valuable if you're too sick to keep tabs on the care you're getting. "Ideally they'd always be there, but the more they can be, the better," Dr. Bates says.

Track your medications. It's crucial to know which drugs you usually take and what they're for. It's also especially valuable if a family member can help sort out any questions about new or unfamiliar medications—or the discontinuation of something you've been taking. "Your medication list will likely change quite a bit during your hospitalization, so you want to keep a list you came in with and a list you leave with," he says.

Understand your fall risk. Your care team should review which situations may increase your risk of falling and let you know when you should push a call button for help. "Often, what happens in the hospital can make you weak to an extent you don't expect," Dr. Bates says. "You may get up when you shouldn't, or get up without help, and go down unnecessarily."

Move around if you can. There's a reason hospital staff gets you out of bed quickly after surgery, whenever possible. Moving your body within 24 hours of surgery—transferring from bed to chair, rising from a chair, exercising in or out of bed, sitting in a chair rather than bed to eat your meals, or walking the hallways—helps maintain muscle strength, lowers the risk of postoperative complications, and reduces

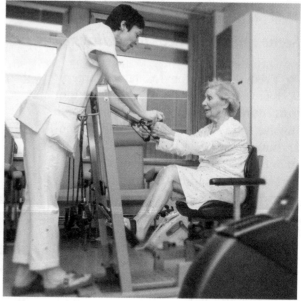

© Thierry Dosogne | Getty Images

Moving around soon after surgery can lead to faster and stronger recovery.

the length of patients' hospital stays, according to a 2022 study in the *Journal of Comparative Effectiveness Research.* ♥

IN THE JOURNALS

Are you missing out on this crucial cardiovascular therapy?

New evidence suggests that most people with heart failure aren't getting cardiac rehabilitation, a recommended treatment that can help lengthen life and is covered by Medicare. An analysis of almost 70,000 people in the United States hospitalized for heart failure in 2010 to 2020 found that only 25% were referred for cardiac rehab. The referral rate was similar for 8,300 people with Medicare who were fit enough for rehab six weeks after leaving the hospital, but only 4% of those who got referrals took part in such programs. People who weren't referred were more likely to be older, Black, have a lot of health problems, or live in a rural area. The findings were published in 2023 by *Circulation: Heart Failure.* Cardiac rehab is a medically supervised three-month program for people who have heart failure or chronic chest pain (angina) as well as people who've had a heart attack, heart bypass surgery, a heart transplant, stenting to open arteries, or valve surgery. But people often miss out on cardiac rehab because of bias in referrals, transportation issues, or fear of being too unfit to take part. (Tai chi also provides benefits similar to cardiac rehab; see "For mellow movement that helps your heart, try tai chi," page 97.)

Do you need a medical escort?

Some minor medical procedures can't happen unless you bring someone along.

Need a colonoscopy? Cataract surgery? Extensive dental work? These minor procedures and others like them, which involve intravenous (IV) sedation or general anesthesia, aren't trivial when you factor in one thing: all require a medical escort—someone who can usher you home safely afterward.

This seemingly small detail is becoming increasingly significant as more older adults lead solo lives. About 27% of the more than 54 million Americans who are 65 and older live alone—and most of them are women, according to the U.S. Administration for Community Living.

Outpatient surgery centers, doctors' offices, and clinics usually require you to submit the name and contact information of the person who'll take you home after a screening test or same-day surgery. Many of these facilities won't allow you to leave unescorted, for fear your safety might be compromised.

If you don't have an escort, the stakes quickly climb. "Many people will forgo the procedure because it's too complicated to get it done," says Dr. Suzanne Salamon, clinical chief of gerontology at Harvard-affiliated Beth Israel Deaconess Medical Center.

"I've seen people go without needed screening or treatment," agrees Katherine Lyman, a geriatric nurse practitioner at Beth Israel Deaconess Medical Center. "It's heartbreaking that we have these barriers."

Transportation pitfalls

Overcoming this hurdle is becoming an issue for many older adults as the population ages. If you're single, your grown kids or other family members don't live nearby, and friends can't fill in, you may find yourself in a predicament.

Calling a cab or taking the bus won't suffice, compounding the problem. The same is true for rideshare services such as Uber or Lyft. Why? The drivers, however friendly, don't have a stake in your safety and typically won't accompany customers into their home.

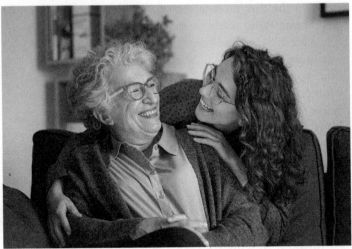

© Ridofranz | Getty Images

A medical escort ensures that you get settled safely in your home after you've had a minor procedure.

"Uber or taxi drivers are not going to walk you out of the car and help you get into bed," Dr. Salamon says. "It's not in their job description, and if the patient falls, that could be trouble."

The concern is indeed warranted, Harvard experts say. Anesthesia and sedatives tend to remain in your system for many hours after a procedure, even if you feel otherwise fine. You might go home and happily sink into the sofa, but you might also be nauseated, vomiting, in pain, or unable to make cogent decisions.

"The anesthesia may be brief, but it can still knock you out to the point where you're not able to get home on your own without support," Lyman says.

And "anything involving general anesthesia raises the risk of you falling or being confused afterward," Dr. Salamon says.

Try these workarounds

If you don't have a medical escort handy, Harvard experts encourage you to think out of the box. Try one of these strategies:

Ask your doctor for guidance. Some medical offices employ a social worker or resource specialist to help coordinate this type of service.

Rely on community. "If you're tapped into a church, temple, or another house of worship, very often they have a cadre of volunteers that do just this," Lyman says.

Contact local organizations. Your area's Office on Aging might point toward volunteer or paid medical escort services. "They're not only sympathetic, but have a wealth of resources they can hook you up with," Dr. Salamon says.

Check with home health aide agencies. While these organizations typically hire out professionals who spend a certain number of hours with clients every week, some also offer medical escort services.

Brainstorm alternatives. Sometimes clinicians can use local anesthesia in place of IV sedation or general anesthesia, so you can drive yourself home or take public transportation afterward. Alternatively, they may be able to help by monitoring you in the office for a few hours after your procedure before you drive home. 🛡

Why you might want to bring a plus-one to your next doctor's appointment

Going to a routine doctor's visit on your own seems pretty straightforward. But for some people, it's anything but. Nearly four in 10 adults have felt anxious before such appointments, while almost half have left a visit feeling confused, according to a nationally representative 2022 survey of more than 2,000 Americans conducted by market research company OnePoll.

"It's a big problem," says Katherine Lyman, a geriatric nurse practitioner at Beth Israel Deaconess Medical Center. "They're worried about what the doctor will find and what they'll hear. Are they going to uncover a dreaded disease?"

One way to smooth your concerns is by bringing someone with you. Ideally, this person would be a family member or good friend who's aware of your home life, what medical issues you face, and your medication use. Alternatively, try looping in a family member over speakerphone during the appointment.

When should you ask for such assistance? Harvard experts point to these solid reasons:

You're upset. Your symptoms may be distressing, or you worry your clinician won't take them seriously. The person who goes with you can help you convey fraught or embarrassing information in a clear, organized way.

You're overwhelmed. If you expect a difficult diagnosis or exhaustive information about treatment options, your plus-one may be better equipped to focus on what your doctor says. She can also write down important details and help you follow through.

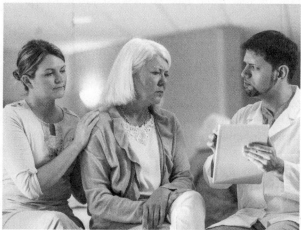

© kali9 | Getty Images

A family member or friend can ease your anxiety and track important details during a doctor's appointment.

You're forgetting things. Your companion can remind you what you planned to discuss with the doctor and help you recall what she said. "Many times people with memory issues will report problems they've had for years or forget to tell me problems that are really concerning," says Dr. Suzanne Salamon, clinical chief of gerontology at Beth Israel Deaconess. "The visit can really be fruitless."

You've been falling. As hard as it is to admit, divulging this information to your doctor is crucial to prevent a future calamity. A family member or friend who knows what's happening can provide useful context.

You're considering a major medical procedure. Your loved one can ask pivotal questions you might overlook and take notes on what to expect during the procedure and your recovery.

What to do about medical gaslighting

If you feel like your doctor is dismissing your health concerns, you may be experiencing medical gaslighting.

The term "gaslighting" is usually applied to personal relationships, when a partner's manipulation causes you to doubt your mental capacity, ideas, and feelings. But in recent years, gaslighting has been recognized in medical settings, too.

Medical gaslighting describes when health care professionals seem to invalidate or ignore your concerns. It can be linked to missed diagnoses, delayed treatment, and poor health outcomes. It might damage your trust in the health care system and make you less likely to seek care.

Potential causes

Why does gaslighting occur? It can be unintentional. "The health care provider might have poor communication skills, or have limited time to speak with a patient, or not be medically knowledgeable enough to know what to do," says Dr. Jonathan M. Marron, a physician and director of clinical ethics at the Harvard Medical School Center for Bioethics.

Medical gaslighting might also stem from having an illness that isn't well understood, such as long COVID. "Gaslighting might also occur when someone has a disorder that doesn't have a straightforward test for diagnosis," Dr. Marron says. And it is possible that, if the doctor is puzzled by a person's symptoms and bothered by that, the doctor might react by saying the person's symptoms are unimportant, reflecting their own uncertainty or insecurity.

And unfortunately, medical gaslighting also can result from conscious or unconscious bias. "We know there is a significant amount of unconscious bias in the practice of medicine. Studies show that those from marginalized groups, especially women and people of color, are more likely to have their concerns or questions not taken seriously, which can be associated with worse health outcomes," Dr. Marron says.

Avoiding medical gaslighting

To avoid medical gaslighting, Dr. Marron advises going to an appointment as prepared as possible. Consider bringing
- a journal tracking the symptoms you've been having
- a brief and precise expression of your medical concerns

- a short list of questions for the clinician
- a buddy who can support you, take notes, and observe your interaction with the clinician.

At the start of the appointment, tell the clinician you have a short list of questions you'd like to ask at the end of the appointment. "If you don't know what to ask," Dr. Marron says, "you could try, 'If you were in my shoes, what should I be asking right now?' Don't leave without understanding the big-picture plan and next steps."

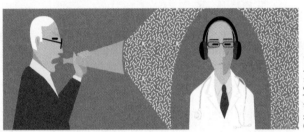

Confronting gaslighting

Dr. Marron says one challenge of medical gaslighting is that most clinicians probably don't feel they do it. That makes for tricky ground if you perceive that you're being gaslighted. How can you cope in the moment?

Take a step back. "Maybe there's a misunderstanding between you and the clinician. It's okay to say that and then reframe your question or request and see if it garners a different response," Dr. Marron advises.

Ask your buddy for support. Perhaps your friend can advocate for you and lend credibility to what you're saying or asking the clinician.

Prepare for some discord. If the appointment seems to be going south, it's okay to note your concerns. "Calling out gaslighting is reasonable. But understand that it may not be the most comfortable conversation. Some clinicians might feel they're being attacked. Be clear that it's not your intent," Dr. Marron says.

Get a different clinician. If you and the clinician can't reach a resolution, it might be a good idea to move on. You deserve compassionate treatment. "Everyone has the right to change clinicians or get a second opinion," Dr. Marron says. "The more you and your family members are aware of it and feel empowered, the less likely it will have a negative impact on you." ▮

Reframing hospice and palliative care

Sometimes viewed as "giving up," these crucial services instead offer life-affirming benefits during difficult times.

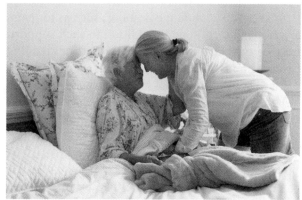

© manonallard | Getty Images

Prioritizing comfort is central to hospice care.

When Jimmy Carter decided earlier this year to opt for hospice care at his Georgia ranch after a series of hospital stays, the 99-year-old former president made a deliberate choice: no more trips to the ER, and no more aggressive, time-consuming treatments.

Instead, the revered statesman reached for more of the good stuff: time with his cherished wife of 77 years, Rosalynn. Moments relishing their large extended family. And more peanut butter ice cream, his favorite treat.

After a life well lived, Carter clearly saw himself at a crossroads. And his decision epitomized a shift in understanding of the aim of hospice itself—not as an act of "giving up," but instead a choice to prioritize comfort and make the most of everyday moments. But many people are still missing this key insight into hospice—and the related practice of palliative care— that could improve their ability to live the way they want when they're seriously ill, Harvard experts say.

"Choosing hospice doesn't mean you're giving up getting medical care; it's focusing on comfort with the medical care you do receive," says Dr. Carine Davila, a palliative care physician at Harvard-affiliated Massachusetts General Hospital.

"Maybe we can't control a disease, but we can control where we are and who we're with," agrees Sarah Byrne-Martelli, a board-certified chaplain and bereavement coordinator in the Division of Palliative Care and Geriatric Medicine at Massachusetts General Hospital. "When people are offered the choice of being stuck in a hospital or being home with their family and dog, watching their favorite shows and eating their favorite meals, they often choose the latter. We can help them paint a picture of what they want the end of life to look like, and for most, it's not being stuck in an ICU."

Differences in approach

Fundamental to understanding your choices is knowing the difference between palliative care and hospice. The two overlap, but aren't the same.

Palliative care focuses on symptom relief and management for people who are seriously ill at any stage, not just the end of life. It can also be offered alongside potentially curative treatments. "Palliative care offers an extra layer of support to patients, families, and the teams taking care of them," Dr. Davila says.

Hospice, on the other hand, makes the dying process more comfortable for people with serious illnesses. While this approach is often offered to those expected to survive six months or less, many people opt for hospice care even when the end of life may be further off. This can include people with terminal conditions such as late-stage cancer, but also those with several chronic illnesses such as kidney disease, diabetes, or heart failure that together can shorten life. Like President Carter, some people who enter hospice have also endured multiple hospitalizations, becoming weaker with each.

"Palliative care is a bigger umbrella, where we help people at all stages of illness, while hospice is focused on the end stage of life," Dr. Davila says.

Layers of support

Hospice care occurs at two main levels. "Routine" hospice care, which applies to the vast majority of hospice patients, involves a broad team supporting them in their home with medication, medical equipment, nurse visits, and social and spiritual support. Meanwhile, patients who need round-the-clock nursing care to stay comfortable can be cared for in either a hospital-based hospice unit, dedicated hospice facility, or nursing home.

The hospice team equips patients' homes with items such as a hospital bed, shower chair, and assistive devices like canes, walkers, or wheelchairs. It also ▸▸

makes sure certain medications, such as for pain, are ready and waiting. In addition to such support, hospice typically also offers a 24/7 hotline enabling patients and families to ask questions at any hour.

"It's a holistic way of looking at total pain. You might be having physical, spiritual, emotional, or social pain," Byrne-Martelli says. "We see you as a whole person."

Tough decisions

Long-established research shows that palliative care can extend life. A seminal 2010 study in *The New England Journal of Medicine* suggested that patients newly diagnosed with terminal lung cancer who began receiving palliative care along with their cancer treatment lived nearly three months longer than others who received standard cancer care alone. Patients receiving palliative care were less likely to need aggressive cancer treatments at the end of life, although that option remained available.

The palliative care patients were also happier, more mobile, and in less pain as their time shortened. "With better symptom management, people may tolerate their treatments better and may be able to continue on them longer," Dr. Davila notes.

For now, aggressive medical care remains common at the end of life, according to a 2023 study published in *JAMA Network Open*. Researchers analyzed five years of cancer registry data, nursing home assessments, and Medicare claims to evaluate "aggressive end-of-life care" such as repeated emergency room visits or ICU care among 146,000 older adults with advanced cancer (average age 78, 48% women). Most received aggressive treatment in their final 30 days of life, and one-quarter

How to approach hospice care for yourself or a loved one

If someone you know has been told they have six months or less to live, it's wise to consider hospice sooner rather than later—as grueling as that decision may be, Harvard experts say.

"That type of prognosis should be an automatic trigger to think about it," says Dr. Carine Davila, a palliative care doctor at Massachusetts General Hospital.

Considering hospice care doesn't mean you have to follow through, says Sarah Byrne-Martelli, a chaplain and bereavement coordinator at Massachusetts General Hospital. "You can always meet with a hospice admission nurse to get more information—it doesn't mean you have to sign up. You don't have to commit to anything, but they can share what services they offer."

Harvard experts offer these tips to smooth the decision:

Talk to the care team. Ask for their honest appraisal of the situation and if hospice is appropriate.

Ask about enrollment. A doctor may have to initiate the hospice process with a referral. Often, a specific hospice agency serves a particular geographic area.

Ask family and friends about their experiences. Has someone you know had a good or bad experience with a family member in hospice? Ask for suggestions.

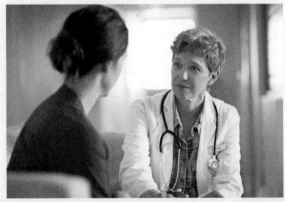

© kupicoo | Getty Images

It's wise to learn about hospice care sooner rather than later.

Call a hospice agency. Ask questions, or schedule an informational visit to get more details.

Assess your home's layout. Hospice programs will send medical equipment such as a hospital bed, commode, and wheelchair to the patient's home. Consider which equipment might be needed and where it will placed.

Don't think of it as a failure. "Do your best to embrace this as the next chapter of life," Byrne-Martelli says. "And know that even though it's scary, there are people who've been supporting this process for a long time and can help."

underwent cancer treatment such as surgery, radiation, or chemotherapy.

"Part of it is that people opt for aggressive treatment because they're hoping for a miracle and wrestling with grief, fear, and uncertainty. The tricky thing, of course, is that healing can occur in different ways and not always on our timeline," Byrne-Martelli says. "When we can talk about what it means to live well and what their spiritual values are, sometimes people can say, 'I don't need to try this fifth surgery because it might actually cause more suffering. Maybe it makes more sense to put my energy toward comfort and quality of life.'"

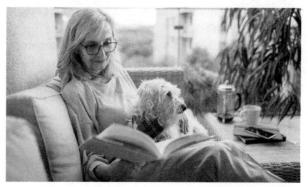

© Halfpoint Images | Getty Images

Most hospice patients would rather enjoy the comforts of home than be in the hospital.

Healing actions

One of the biggest under-recognized benefits of hospice care is the ability to carry out your own priorities. Team members ask patients what they want and support them toward reaching those goals—whether that's to attend a grandchild's graduation or wedding, take a trip, or just walk their favorite path in the woods each day.

"Sometimes parents want to spend time creating a memory book, or writing letters to their children to mark important future milestones, knowing they won't be there for some of those life events," Dr. Davila says. "Those are examples of really powerful meaning-making for patients and families that also create things these families will be able to hold on to."

Byrne-Martelli took weekly walks with a man in hospice care whom she visited for many months. He spent that time telling her about "his life, his kids, his regrets, and his joys," she recalls. "It was almost like he was taking the time to very intentionally wrap up his life. Having the space to share that with someone can be really healing in and of itself." ♥

Time for a new knee? Ask these questions first

Gather as much information as possible to make an informed decision about a total knee replacement.

When a worn knee starts to give you trouble, non-surgical treatments are the first line of defense. Weight loss, physical therapy, or injections may help reduce your pain. If your knee doesn't respond to those approaches, it's time to consider a joint replacement. And you'll need information to make a decision about the surgery, which is a big commitment.

Here are some questions to ask and a sneak peek at what your doctor might say, courtesy of Dr. Antonia Chen, an orthopedic surgeon and director of research for the Division of Adult Reconstruction and Total Joint Arthroplasty at Harvard-affiliated Brigham and Women's Hospital. ▶▶

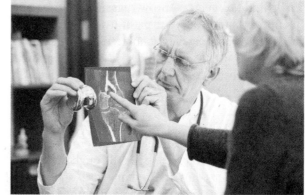

© Jan-Otto | Getty Images

Ask your doctor about the surgical steps and new parts used in knee replacement surgery.

Q: What should I look for in a knee replacement surgeon?

Dr. Chen: Ideally your surgeon would be someone who is board-certified in orthopedic surgery, fellowship-trained, and a specialist in knee replacement. But that type of expert might not be available in your community. If not, look for an orthopedic surgeon who's been performing knee replacements for at least two years, and make sure the surgeon you choose performs at least two knee replacements a month.

Q: What type of prosthetic is best?

Dr. Chen: The gold standard knee replacement is made of cobalt chromium with polyethylene (plastic) in between the metal pieces. Sometimes, the bone behind the kneecap will be replaced with polyethylene (see "Anatomy of a knee replacement," page 309). There are additional materials, such as titanium or zirconium, that can be used in knee replacements. The best prosthetic will be the one your surgeon is comfortable implanting, unless you have a metal allergy, which you should discuss with your doctor.

Q: How should I prepare physically for a knee replacement?

Dr. Chen: Pre-surgery physical ability predicts your post-surgery physical ability. So work on bending, straightening, and strengthening the knee as much as possible before surgery. Physical therapy can help, and so can exercises that you can do at home.

Q: How should I prepare my home for recovery?

Dr. Chen: Remove anything that might cause you to slip and fall, such as throw rugs, floor clutter, and furniture that blocks your path. It will help to have certain types of equipment at home, including a walker and a cane. You can also consider getting a raised toilet seat and a bedside commode, but not every patient will need these.

Q: Which surgical approach will you take?

Dr. Chen: There are three main approaches. One goes around the kneecap, one goes through the middle of the quadriceps muscles, and one goes underneath the quads. There are pluses and minuses for each one, and it mostly depends on the approach your surgeon is most experienced with.

Q: Will you use robotic tools?

Dr. Chen: Some studies have shown that robotic surgery is more precise than traditional surgery. I personally use robotic tools, but robotics are not available at every hospital.

Q: What are potential surgery complications, and what will you do to reduce them?

Dr. Chen: Knee replacement risks include bleeding, blood clots, and infection. We use devices to stop bleeding at the time of surgery, and we may apply a tourniquet. You will likely get an antibiotic before surgery to prevent infection and a blood thinner after surgery to prevent clots.

Q: Will I have to stay overnight in the hospital?

Dr. Chen: Most people go home on the day of their surgery or stay overnight in the hospital for one night. Home health services can provide visiting nurses or physical therapists who go to a patient's home after surgery.

Q: How much pain will I have, and how will you treat it?

Dr. Chen: The first two to six weeks after surgery will be very painful, and we have an extensive plan to treat it. We start right before surgery, giving the patient painkillers such as acetaminophen (Tylenol) and celecoxib (Celebrex), as well as spinal anesthesia. During surgery, I'll inject a number of different analgesics and anti-inflammatory medicines into the knee. After surgery, we use narcotics such as oxycodone (OxyContin) only sparingly. If necessary, we can prescribe low-level narcotics such as tramadol (Ultram). But we prefer that you use acetaminophen around the clock. It may not work well on its own, but adding a nonsteroidal anti-inflammatory drug such as naproxen (Aleve) or a nerve medication called gabapentin (Neurontin) can improve pain relief.

Q: What do you do to ward off stiffness and swelling?

Dr. Chen: These side effects can happen right after knee surgery. It's important to get right into physical rehabilitation to prevent stiffness. To reduce inflammation, I like my patients to use ice or an ice machine that circulates cold fluid around the leg.

Q What will rehab look like?

Dr. Chen: If you are deconditioned or undergo surgery in both knees at the same time, you might need to go to an in-house rehab facility after surgery and stay for a week or two. If you're stronger, you can go home and have a physical therapist visit the home, or go to an outpatient facility for physical therapy. The rehab process can last up to three months. And it's a year for a full recovery.

Q When will I be active again?

Dr. Chen: You might have to walk with a walker or crutches for one or two weeks, and then walk with a cane or one crutch for another two to four weeks. It can take three to six months to get you back to brisk walking, six to nine months for activities such as tennis or golf, and nine months to one year for skiing.

Q How long will the prosthetic last?

Dr. Chen: The plastic part of the prosthetic knee will wear out in about 15 to 20 years, and you might need surgery to replace it.

Q What if I want to wait before considering surgery?

Dr. Chen: It's your choice: you'll be limited by your pain, and the pain is unlikely to improve. The good news is that waiting won't make your knee much worse. So if you don't want to go through a major surgery and a long recovery, don't do it. Wait until you're ready. 🌢

Anatomy of a knee replacement

The knee is a hinge formed by the bottom of the thighbone (femur) and the top of the shin bone (tibia). In front of them is the kneecap (patella). The ends of the bones are cushioned by cartilage. As cartilage wears out over time, the bones rub against each other, causing pain.

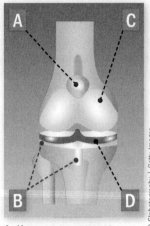

© SIphotography | Getty Images

A: Kneecap component

B: Tibial component

C: Femoral component

D: Plastic spacer

In a knee replacement, the surgeon removes the damaged ends of the thigh and shin bones and replaces them with artificial parts. The prosthetic on the thighbone is made of metal (typically cobalt chromium). The prosthetic on the shin bone is made of metal (typically cobalt chromium or titanium) and has a plastic piece on top. The plastic is polyethylene, a strong, slippery material that acts as cartilage.

The kneecap may also need to be lined with plastic to glide over the other two bones.

Decoding medication instructions

Here's a little insight about the generic directions that often accompany prescriptions.

The doctor prescribed your new medication, and you picked it up promptly. Now comes the job of taking the drug, which can be tough if directions are vague or confusing. Here are some common instructions that can trip people up, along with what they really mean.

Take as needed

"Take as needed" allows you the flexibility to determine when you need the medicine for symptom relief. But the instructions require additional guidance.

"It's not safe to take a medication anytime you feel you need it, whether it's a pill, a topical lotion, or ▸▸

▶▶ a cough syrup. You need to know the intent of the drug, what it does, and the maximum amount you can have in a day. Is it one dose or three? And you need to know how far apart doses should be spaced," says Joanne Doyle Petrongolo, a pharmacist at Harvard-affiliated Massachusetts General Hospital.

Take once daily
When exactly is the "once" in "once daily"? It depends. Some drugs are best taken in the morning, such as thyroid pills that you need to take on an empty stomach. Some are better taken at night. "For example, cholesterol-lowering medications are generally taken once a day at bedtime, since your body produces more cholesterol overnight," Doyle Petrongolo says. "And sometimes it is wiser to take certain antidepressants or antihistamines close to bedtime, since they can make you drowsy in the day."

Take one tablet, twice a day
This is another instruction with vague timing. "You might interpret this in different ways. I was just working with a gentleman whose interpretation was to take pills at 9 a.m. and 1 p.m., which was too close together," Doyle Petrongolo says. "If the label says 'twice daily,' it usually means once in the morning and once at night, about 12 hours apart."

Take with food
This direction is intended to help you absorb certain drugs or to avoid the stomach irritation they can cause. But does "take with food" require a snack or a meal? At what point in the process do you take the pill? And does the type of food matter?

"You need to prepare your stomach by putting food in it first. Typically, that means you can take the medication after a few bites or a whole meal," Doyle Petrongolo says. "But some medications, such as nonsteroidal anti-inflammatory drugs, might require an ample meal beforehand to prevent stomach irritation."

Does the type of food matter? "That depends on the prescription," Doyle Petrongolo says. "For example, certain antivirals or antifungals are absorbed best after

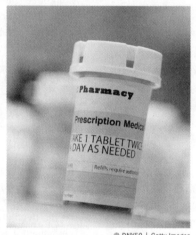

© DNY59 | Getty Images

Don't guess what vague drug instructions mean. Ask your doctor or pharmacist for clarification.

a fatty meal. In other cases, a few crackers will suffice." Pharmacy websites often provide specific advice. You can also ask your doctor or pharmacist.

Take with water
If the label says "take with water," it might be to ensure that the drug is properly eliminated through the kidneys. But often it's simply to prevent a pill from sticking to sensitive tissues while going down.

"With certain osteoporosis drugs, for example, we recommend taking them with eight ounces of water and not lying down for 30 minutes afterward. You want an adequate amount of fluid and time to avoid having them irritate the lining of your throat or esophagus," Doyle Petrongolo says.

Limit sun exposure
Some medications can make you more sensitive to sunlight while you're using them, leading to a bad rash or sunburn after sun exposure. This can happen with certain prescription drugs, such as some diuretics, antibiotics, antihistamines, antiseizure medicines, and antidepressants, as well as some over-the-counter products, such as topical treatments for acne that include the ingredient benzoyl peroxide.

How much should you limit sun exposure? "Avoid being in direct sunlight for long periods. And when you're outside, always wear a sunscreen with a sun protection factor [SPF] of 30 or more. Wearing sun-protective clothing like shirts and hats will also be helpful," Doyle Petrongolo says.

When directions are unclear
If you're unsure exactly how to take a medication, even if it was already explained to you, ask for clarification. Ideally this will happen when your doctor gives you the prescription, but it's okay to call and ask later. You also can talk to your pharmacist about the best way to take a drug, either when you pick up your prescription or sometime later. "Don't feel embarrassed. We understand that it can be confusing," Doyle Petrongolo says. "We want you take the medication correctly so it has the best chance of working." ▮

Medication-taking made easier

Shocking numbers of people don't take their prescriptions at the right dose or frequency—or even at all. Learn ways to make the task less onerous.

Six decades ago, a crooning Mary Poppins told us it takes just a spoonful of sugar to help the medicine go down. But reality is a bit more nuanced: a sour taste isn't the only thing that can turn us off from taking medication—and there's far more than one strategy to make the task easier.

About half the time, people on their own choose to alter how much, how often, or how long they take a medication—or whether to take it at all. In fact, 20% to 30% of new prescriptions are never filled, according to the CDC.

Such medication nonadherence (as it's called) can gravely threaten your health, says Dr. Suzanne Salamon, clinical chief of gerontology at Harvard-affiliated Beth Israel Deaconess Medical Center. It's linked to about 125,000 deaths in the United States every year, according to the CDC.

"A huge number of people don't take their medications as directed," Dr. Salamon says. "It's no joke, and unfortunately it can very easily happen without anyone noticing. Most people don't want to admit to anyone they're not taking their pills."

Reasons for nonadherence

About three-quarters of Americans ages 50 to 64 take prescription drugs, a proportion that climbs to nine in 10 people ages 65 and older. This translates into many occasions and reasons to do it wrong. Dr. Salamon highlights common explanations patients offer for not taking their medications:

Too many. It can seem overwhelming if you've been prescribed multiple drugs, especially if you need to take each one at various intervals during the day. "Sometimes the burden of pills gets so high that people stop taking everything," she says.

Burdensome side effects. From leg cramps to nausea to weight gain and more, there's a huge range of unwelcome offshoots from prescription drug regimens. "Every medication we take has some sort of side effect, and some people are really sensitive to them," she says.

Lack of symptoms. If you feel well over all, you may not think a prescription is necessary. "If someone

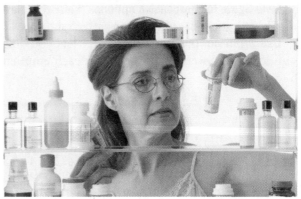

© Jose Luis Pelaez Inc | Getty Images

Every year, about 125,000 Americans die because they don't adhere to their prescribed drug regimen.

hasn't explained why they need to take the medication, many people won't do it," Dr. Salamon says.

Expense. Some people can't afford to fill prescriptions or are forced to take less to make their supply last longer. "Cost is a huge factor," she says.

Forgetfulness. This can happen to anyone, but it's more common among people with memory problems. "If there's no family member watching closely, or patients haven't spoken to their clinician, it can be hard to find out they're forgetting to take their pills," she says.

Depression. "When people get depressed, sometimes they throw their hands up and say, 'What's the point?' It's very important to address this feeling of hopelessness," Dr. Salamon says.

Easing the task

It's crucial to let your doctor know if you're not taking your prescription drugs—and why. Start by asking her to review your medication list, since "deprescribing" drugs can be just as important to your health as starting a new, necessary prescription.

"Some people were put on medications years ago and don't need them anymore," Dr. Salamon says. "Discuss with your doctor which medications you could really live without."

Also try these additional ways to keep up more easily with your medication regimen: ▶▶

▸▸ **Find flexibility.** Doctors can often streamline dosing schedules by reducing the number of times per day a drug is taken or prescribing long-acting or combination versions. "Moving all medications to once-a-day dosing isn't necessarily ideal, but it's often possible," she says.

Investigate less-expensive options. "Your clinician may be able to find a cheaper alternative," she says.

Use a pill container. An organizer lets you dole out doses for a week at a time. Then, each emptied compartment confirms that you remembered to take your pills. Readily available in stores and online, some pill containers include sections for multiple doses at various times of the day.

Track doses with tech. Replace standard drug bottle caps with timer caps. Found in pharmacies and online, these incorporate built-in timers that track when you last took your medication and alert you when the next dose is due. ◆

Stopping a medication? Check first, quit safer

Talk to your doctor before quitting prescription and over-the-counter drugs that you take regularly.

You may have many reasons why you'd like to stop taking a certain medication. Maybe it's causing unwanted side effects, you don't think it's working, you feel that you've healed and no longer need it, or you can't afford it. That doesn't mean it's safe to quit a drug cold turkey. Abruptly stopping a medication can be risky and even life-threatening.

Rebound effects
Many medications work by blocking or activating certain body chemicals or processes. When you stop taking a drug suddenly, symptoms or problems that were controlled can return with a vengeance—meaning they might be worse than they were before treatment. That's called a rebound effect.

"Two prime examples are medications used to treat high blood pressure. If you decide to stop taking the alpha blocker clonidine [Catapres], your blood pressure might increase considerably. Abruptly stopping a beta blocker might cause your heart rate to rise rapidly, which might result in chest pain or even a heart attack," says Joanne Doyle Petrongolo, a pharmacist at Harvard-affiliated Massachusetts General Hospital.

Other drugs with potential rebound effects include proton-pump inhibitors, such as omeprazole (Prilosec), used to treat heartburn; the sleep medication zolpidem (Ambien), if it's stopped abruptly after long-term use; and the over-the-counter nasal decongestant spray oxymetazoline (Afrin), if it's been taken for more than three days.

Withdrawal symptoms
Sometimes quitting a drug is a shock to your body. As it adjusts, you might experience symptoms that are mild or moderate—such as mood changes, insomnia, nausea, diarrhea, muscle pain, or changes in appetite. In some cases, symptoms can be severe: hallucinations, delirium, seizures, or suicidal thoughts. "Symptoms tend to be more severe and last longer—more than a few days—if you've been taking higher doses for a long period of time," Doyle Petrongolo says.

Medications that can cause withdrawal symptoms are often those that affect the brain and nervous system: prescription painkillers such as oxycodone (OxyContin) or hydromorphone (Dilaudid); antidepressants such as selective serotonin reuptake inhibitors (SSRIs), serotonin-norepinephrine reuptake inhibitors (SNRIs), or tricyclics; anti-anxiety medications such as benzodiazepines; nerve pain medications such as gabapentin (Neurontin); and antipsychotic medications.

Talk to your doctor
Consult with your doctor before quitting a drug. "If you feel you no longer need it, ask if the doctor agrees. You could have a false sense that you've healed, while in reality you're better only because you've been taking

Tapering off a drug

The way to stop taking a medication safely is to gradually reduce its dose and frequency. But there isn't a one-size-fits-all approach. It depends on the particular drug, the current dose and frequency, the length of time you've been on it, and your particular health needs. So you need your doctor's guidance on how to taper down.

What might an example of tapering look like? "If you take a 40-mg proton-pump inhibitor for heartburn twice a day, your doctor might recommend going to a 40-mg pill in the morning and a 20-mg pill at night for a few days, then a 20-mg pill twice a day for another few days, then a 20-mg pill once a day for a little while, and then a 20-mg pill every other day for a few days," says Joanne Doyle Petrongolo, a pharmacist at Harvard-affiliated Massachusetts General Hospital. "But please don't attempt it yourself. There are many variables and risks, and you need a doctor to evaluate what's best for you."

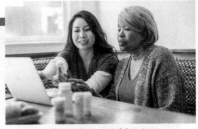

© MoMo Productions | Getty Images

Your doctor will take your health and symptoms into account to help you taper off a drug.

your pills," Doyle Petrongolo says. "If you're experiencing side effects from a medication, or you don't feel it's effective, there might be something else you can take."

If you're having difficulty paying for your medication, Doyle Petrongolo recommends asking your doctor if it's possible to prescribe a more affordable alternative. Or ask your pharmacist about ways to reduce drug costs, such as using drug discount cards or applying for a manufacturer's patient assistance program. "We have a number of strategies we can share with clients and programs we can direct them to," Doyle Petrongolo says.

If you'd still like to quit a medication, do so only with your doctor's guidance (see "Tapering off a drug" above). Until you get that information, don't stop taking any prescribed drug. 🛡

IN THE JOURNALS

Potency of these Alzheimer's pills might not match the label

Here's an example of why you must be especially careful when selecting supplements: Harvard Medical School researchers say that galantamine, a plant extract used in prescription medications to treat Alzheimer's, is often mislabeled and sometimes contaminated with bacteria when it's sold as a dietary supplement. Scientists compared 11 brands of prescription generic galantamine and 10 brands of over-the-counter galantamine dietary supplements. "In the generic drug, the amount of galantamine listed on the label accurately represented the amount of galantamine in the pills and, importantly, no bacterial contamination was found," says Dr. Pieter Cohen, the study's lead author and an associate professor of medicine at Harvard Medical School. "But 90% of galantamine dietary supplements contained an inaccurate amount of galantamine, ranging from less than 2% to 110% of the labeled quantity. Disturbingly, 30% were also contaminated with bacteria that could, if consumed at higher levels, cause diarrheal illnesses." The results were published in a research letter in 2024 by *JAMA*. To ensure that you're getting safe supplements, Dr. Cohen urges you to look for certification seals from vetted independent third parties, such as the U.S. Pharmacopeia (www.quality-supplements.org) and NSF International's Certified for Sport program (www.health.harvard.edu/nsf/cps). And talk to your doctor before taking any dietary supplement.

by **HOWARD LeWINE, M.D.,** Editor in Chief, *Harvard Men's Health Watch*

How can I reduce my number of daily medications?

Q *I now take nine pills every day. My doctors have added new medicines over the years, but not once have they suggested stopping one of them. How do I know that I really need all of these medications indefinitely?*

A We are fortunate today to have many excellent medications to better treat chronic conditions and help ward off serious complications. But when a person is seeing multiple specialists or has been in the hospital (a time when prescriptions are often adjusted), it's common to end up with one or more new drugs without a clear indication about how long to continue taking them.

In general, each doctor you are seeing is not likely to alter your current therapy unless you are having symptoms that could be related to side effects. If you are feeling okay, the tendency for the doctor is to not make any changes.

But perhaps you didn't mention that you're feeling less energetic, attributing it to age, when it might be related to one of your drugs. Still, even if you feel perfectly fine, it's good to consider whether less is more.

Here's my suggestion on how to approach this question. First, make sure you understand the reason you regularly take each of your prescribed drugs. If you are not completely sure, ask the prescribing doctor for an explanation.

Then, on your next visit to your primary care physician, you can review your medications and discuss how you might safely reduce the dosage(s)

or perhaps even do a trial period of not taking one or two. It could even be possible that you are taking two of the same drugs because one pill may be a generic and the other is a brand name, adding to the confusion. At least once a year, take all your pills and bottles with their prescription labels to your doctor to ensure you are getting it right. Or don't wait, and take them to your pharmacist sooner.

© MirageC I Getty Images

Speak with your doctor about reducing the number or dosage of your medications.

A typical example is taking a daily baby aspirin, which one of your doctors may have recommended years ago to prevent a heart attack or stroke. But new guidelines suggest that people without cardiovascular disease have a risk of bleeding from daily aspirin that outweighs any benefit in heart attack or stroke prevention, and it may be best to stop taking it.

Most older people today take at least one drug for a common chronic condition like high blood pressure, high cholesterol, or type 2 diabetes. If your numbers for any of these conditions are within your health goals, then perhaps you can reduce your medication load. Lifestyle changes can also help reduce your need for some drugs. For instance, losing weight, improving your diet, or getting more exercise could keep you close to your goal numbers for blood pressure, cholesterol, or blood sugar with less medication.

Don't get duped: Here's how to avoid online pharmacy risks

Medication deals on the internet often come with a steep price.

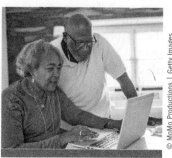

Type the words "best online pharmacy" into a search engine, and you'll find countless options promising prescription drugs delivered right to your door at discount prices. Just be careful if you plan to place an order. Many online pharmacies are unscrupulous purveyors of potentially harmful products. It takes some know-how to identify legitimate pharmacies selling approved medications.

Online pharmacy dangers

The vast majority of online pharmacies are rife with risks, according to the FDA and the National Association of Boards of Pharmacy (NABP), an independent nonprofit group.

The NABP has found that at least 40,000 online pharmacies aren't complying with patient safety standards or laws; about 95% of websites offering prescription-only drugs operate illegally; and 89% of illegal online pharmacies don't require prescriptions for prescription-only drugs. Yes, it really is that bad.

What does that mean for consumers?

You don't know who you're dealing with. "It could be a pharmacy in another country that doesn't have the same level of quality control that we do, or it could be a fake pharmacy with a legitimate-looking storefront," says Joanne Doyle Petrongolo, a pharmacist at Harvard-affiliated Massachusetts General Hospital.

You don't know what you're getting. "You can't tell if the pill you get has been stored properly, if it's expired, if it's the correct strength, or even if it's the right medication. Also, you don't know what else is in the product," Doyle Petrongolo says. The NABP found that some pills contain dangerous substances along with the medicine.

You're risking more than your health. The NABP reports that some online pharmacies are out to steal your personal information (putting you at risk of identity theft) or install malware on your computer.

Don't be scared off

Despite the risks, there are plenty of licensed, legitimate online pharmacies. Using them has many benefits. The main one is cheaper prices for certain drugs. "You can sometimes save hundreds of dollars, so it's worth considering," Doyle Petrongolo says.

Other reasons to use online pharmacies include the convenience of having medications delivered directly to your home, and privacy if you're too embarrassed to pick up certain drugs at the corner drugstore.

Ordering safely

To order prescriptions with the confidence that you're getting legitimate products, learn the signs of safe online pharmacies. These companies

- are licensed with a state board of pharmacy
- have a physical address and phone number, preferably in the United States
- require a doctor's prescription
- have a licensed pharmacist available to answer your questions
- have prices that aren't too good to be true
- clearly state that they don't sell your personal information.

How can you tell all that by looking a website? Doyle Petrongolo recommends using the NABP's Buy Safely tool (https://safe.pharmacy/buy-safely), which allows you to type in an online pharmacy website (the website address, not the name of the pharmacy) to see if it's been verified by the NABP.

You can also look for a symbol on the pharmacy website indicating that it's NABP-accredited. The ▸▸

Warning signs of bogus online pharmacies

Avoid online pharmacies that

- ▸ don't require a doctor's prescription
- ▸ aren't certified by the National Association of Boards of Pharmacy
- ▸ don't have a licensed pharmacist on staff to answer your questions
- ▸ offer discounts that seem too good to be true
- ▸ don't protect your personal and financial information.

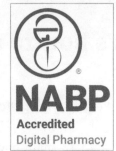

NABP symbol: Courtesy National
Association of Boards of Pharmacy

symbol is a vertical infinity sign (like the number 8) inside a circle and has the words "NABP Accredited Digital Pharmacy." Examples of online pharmacies with this symbol are Amazon's pharmacy service (https://pharmacy.amazon.com) and HealthWarehouse.com (www.healthwarehouse.com).

And before you order anything online, remember you can sometimes find prices

Look for this symbol on a pharmacy website.

that are just as good—or better—at a local pharmacy. "You don't have to look for deals on medications that have been around for a long time, like hydrochlorothiazide or atenolol to treat blood pressure, or simvastatin to treat high cholesterol," Doyle Petrongolo says. "You think they'll be more affordable somewhere else, but they're actually often cheaper—just a few dollars—at a local drugstore or big-box store."

Medication disposal: How—and why—to do it safely

Read this before tossing out or keeping old or unneeded drugs.

If you're doing any spring cleaning this year, remember to look in your medicine cabinets to weed out expired or unneeded medications. Hanging on to them is risky, since outdated medicines can lose their effectiveness or even harm you. And having used medication equipment (such as needles) around can hurt you and others. Fortunately, it's simple to dispose of these items safely.

What needs to go

Candidates for disposal include any expired or unneeded prescription or over-the-counter medications (including vitamins, herbs, and other supplements) and used medication equipment. Beyond pills, hunt for liquids, ointments, lotions, patches, aerosol cans (such as inhalers), spray bottles, droppers, and needles.

"It could be an expired cold remedy, an antibiotic you didn't finish, pain pills left over from surgery, or a blood pressure medication that wasn't strong enough and was discontinued. Don't keep it. You might think you'll need it one day, but you shouldn't take it if it's expired. It might not work effectively," says Joanne Doyle Petrongolo, a pharmacist at Harvard-affiliated Massachusetts General Hospital.

Disposal options

Once you've gathered your expired or unneeded medications, use one of the following options to dispose of them.

Take-back sites. You might hear a lot about take-back initiatives during April and October, when local law enforcement agencies team up with the Drug Enforcement Agency for National Prescription Drug Take Back Day. The option allows you to bring medications to particular drug take-back sites and drop them off (for free). But pharmacies, hospitals, health departments, and law enforcement agencies often provide medication disposal kiosks that are accessible year-round.

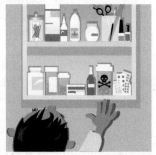

© Aleutie | Getty Images

Having old or unneeded drugs around the house poses a danger to you and others.

When going this route, keep at least a portion of the prescription labels on the drugs so you can tell what they are, but remove or scratch out personal information. Note: Needles are never accepted, and liquid or aerosol medications might not be. Call ahead for details.

Medical waste collection sites. Your city or county may allow medication disposal at the local landfill or health department. This is helpful for safely getting rid of liquid drugs, inhalers, or needles. Keep needles in a sealed plastic container (many drugstores and local health departments offer these containers for free). "If you don't have one, put the needles in an empty laundry detergent bottle or another plastic container,"

Doyle Petrongolo suggests. "Call your sanitation or health department to find what will be accepted."

Disposal at home. As a last resort, it's okay to toss medications into the trash with careful preparation. Some drugstores provide free packets of a powder you mix with water in the medication container, making the drug unusable and safe to throw away.

Another option: The FDA recommends that you mix medicines with unappealing substances such as dirt, cat litter, or used coffee grounds; place the mixture in a sealable plastic bag or container; and throw the bag or container in your trash. This practice may not be allowed for needles or aerosol cans, so be sure to ask your sanitation department for rules first.

With any prescription bottles or boxes, remember to remove and shred the labels and recycle the containers when possible. 🛡️

Improper disposal

You definitely do not want to dispose of medications by pouring them down the drain, flushing them down the toilet, or tossing them into the trash without special preparation. That's how chemicals wind up in soil, waterways, and groundwater. Used needles that are thrown out can also poke holes in garbage bags, potentially hurting sanitation workers. Needles flushed down the toilet can also get stuck in plumbing or equipment at a local water treatment plant.

The FDA notes that some medications are so sought-after for misuse, and so potentially deadly, that if none of the methods of disposal in the accompanying article is possible for you, you should flush the drugs. Drugs on the FDA Flush List include those with opioids, such as any drug whose label contains the words "hydrocodone," "buprenorphine," "fentanyl," or "oxycodone," as well as certain non-opioids such as diazepam rectal gel, methylphenidate patches, and drugs with the words "sodium oxybate." However, some communities don't allow this practice. Contact your local health or sanitation department for more on medication disposal that meets all regulations.

Is that dental pain an emergency?

Use this guide to understand what's behind your pain and how quickly you need to seek help.

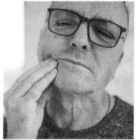
© vitapix | Getty Images
Call your dentist as soon as possible if you suspect infection in your teeth, jaw, or gums.

Agonizing tooth pain, sharp jaw discomfort, a dull ache in your gums—each one is a sign of dental trouble or something more serious. Unfortunately, many people put off a call to the dentist—a potentially risky move.

"As we age, we can feel less pain in our teeth because the nerves inside them shrink, and dentin—a porous material beneath enamel—builds up. So something can fester for a long time and turn into a bigger, more complex problem," says Dr. Lisa Thompson, a geriatric dentistry specialist at the Harvard School of Dental Medicine.

Here's what causes dental pain, how to identify it, and when you should call your dentist or even 911.

Tooth pain

Tooth pain can stem from several problems. Perhaps the most common is a cavity, a tiny hole in the tooth.

Plaque—a sticky mix of food particles and bacteria covering the outer layer of a tooth, the enamel—creates chemicals that break down the enamel. The deeper the cavity, the more likely the nerve in the tooth will be exposed, resulting in sharp pain and sensitivity to hot or cold foods. Those symptoms can also come from a cracked tooth or a cracked or loose filling, which can expose the nerve.

Tooth pain might also be due to trauma, such as accidentally biting down on a fork. That can bruise the ligament holding your tooth in the jaw, generating an initially sharp and then dull ache in the tooth.

If you experience tooth pressure when you bite down on food, have sinus pressure without nasal congestion, or a have a bad (acidic) taste in your mouth, it could ▸▸

▶▶ be that a cavity or cracked tooth has led to a painful infection at the root of the tooth, creating a small pocket of pus called an abscess.

Gum pain

Gum pain tends to be an achy soreness rather than a sharp pain. It has many potential causes. It might be as simple as having sensitive gums, brushing your teeth too vigorously, or having irritation from a bit of food (such as a piece of popcorn) stuck in your teeth or in the space between your gum and teeth.

Gum pain can also come from a cut if something poked you (such as a corn chip), irritation from toothpaste that contains sodium laurel sulfate, or canker sores (aphthous ulcers).

Pain in the gums can also be due to dentures that don't fit well or aren't cleaned regularly. "You might see red bumps on the irritated area or have a burning sensation from a fungal infection," Dr. Thompson says.

Another possibility: plaque buildup at the bottom of teeth is irritating the gums and causing gingivitis, an early stage of gum disease marked by swollen, bleeding gums. Untreated gingivitis can progress below the gum line and eventually become periodontal disease, which wears away the ligament and bone holding the tooth in place, leading to gum pain, abscesses, and tooth loss. Signs of an abscess caused by gum disease include a pimple of pus on the gum or facial swelling.

Jaw pain

Jaw pain can be sudden and sharp, or a chronic tenderness that gradually increases over time. Dull, chronic jaw pain usually comes from a problem with the temporomandibular joint, where the jaw bone meets the skull on either side of your head. Trouble related to this joint is called a temporomandibular disorder, or TMD.

"You can get TMD from injury such as joint dislocation or from problems related to muscles, stress, arthritis, and even behaviors you aren't even aware of. Maybe you grind your teeth at night, chew gum, or bite on a pen," Dr. Thompson says.

Be especially vigilant about a pain that suddenly affects your neck and lower jaw. That can be a form of the pain called angina caused by narrowed heart arteries—or it could even be a symptom of a heart attack. Heart-related jaw pain can occur without the more common heart attack symptoms such as chest pain and shortness of breath.

What you should do

Sudden neck and lower jaw pain can signal an emergency. Call 911, especially if you have known heart problems. All other tooth, gum, and jaw pain should trigger a call to your dentist—as soon as possible if you suspect a cracked filling or tooth, gum disease, or an abscess.

"Bacteria from the abscess can get into the bloodstream and travel to other spaces in your body, such as your brain or heart. It can be life-threatening. If your dentist can't see you immediately, go to an emergency department, although there's not much they can do but give you antibiotics until you can get to a dentist," Dr. Thompson says. "If you suspect that your diet, behavior, or brushing habits might be causing pain, go ahead and experiment: get a soft toothbrush, use a Waterpik, switch toothpastes. And keep brushing and flossing your teeth every day." 🛡

How well do you worry about your health?

Many of us worry, yet a lot of what we focus on poses little risk.

Don't worry. It's good advice if you can take it. Of course that's not always easy, especially for health concerns. The truth is: it's impossible (and ill-advised) to never worry about your health.

But are you worrying about the right things? Let's compare a sampling of worries to the most common conditions that actually shorten lives. Then we can think about preventing the biggest health threats.

Dangerous but rare health threats

The comedian John Mulaney says the cartoons he watched as a child gave him the impression that quicksand, anvils falling from the sky, and lit sticks of dynamite represented major health risks. For him (as is true for most of us), none of these turned out to be worth worrying about.

While harm can befall us in many ways, some of our worries are not very likely to occur:

▸ **Harm by lightning:** In the United States, lightning strikes kill about 25 people each year. Annually, the risk for the average person less than one in a million. There are also several hundred injuries due to nonfatal lightning strikes. Even though lightning strikes the earth millions of times each year, the chances you'll be struck are quite low.

▸ **Dying in a plane crash:** The yearly risk of being killed in a plane crash for the average American is about one in 11 million. Of course, the risk is even lower if you never fly, and higher if you regularly fly on small planes in bad weather with inexperienced pilots. By comparison, the average yearly risk of dying in a car accident is approximately 1 in 5,000.

▸ **Snakebite injuries and deaths:** According to the Centers for Disease Control and Prevention, an estimated 7,000 to 8,000 people are bit by poisonous snakes each year in the United States. Lasting injuries are uncommon, and deaths are quite rare (about five per year). In parts of the country without poisonous snakes, the risk is essentially zero.

▸ **Shark attacks:** As long as people aren't initiating contact with sharks, attacks are fairly uncommon. Worldwide, about 70 unprovoked shark attacks occur in an average year, six of which are fatal. In 2022, 41 attacks occurred in the United States, two of which were fatal.

▸ **Public toilet seats:** They may appear unclean (or even filthy), but they pose little or no health risk to the average person. While it's reasonable to clean off the seat and line it with paper before touching down, health fears should not discourage you from using a public toilet.

I'm not suggesting that these pose no danger, especially if you're in situations of increased risk. If you're

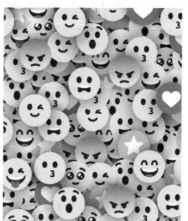

© Ihor Biliavskyi | Getty Images

The most common health risks are far more preventable than many realize.

on a beach where sharks have been sighted and seals are nearby, it's best not to swim there. When in doubt, it's a good idea to apply common sense and err on the side of safety.

What do Google and TikTok tell us about health concerns?

Analyzing online search topics can tell us a lot about our health worries.

The top Google health searches in 2023 were:
▸ How long is strep throat contagious?
▸ How contagious is strep throat?
▸ How to lower cholesterol?
▸ What helps with bloating?
▸ What causes low blood pressure?

Really? Cancer, heart disease and stroke, or COVID didn't reach the top five? High blood pressure didn't make the list, but low blood pressure did?

Meanwhile, on TikTok the most common topics searched were exercise, diet, and sexual health, according to one study. Again, no top-of-the-list searches on the most common and deadly diseases.

How do our worries compare with the top causes of death?

In the United States, these five conditions took the greatest number of lives in 2022:
▸ heart disease
▸ cancer
▸ unintentional injury (including motor vehicle accidents, drug overdoses, and falls)
▸ COVID-19
▸ stroke.

This list varies by age. For example, guns are the leading cause of death among children and teenagers (ages 1 to 19). For older teens (ages 15 to 19), the top three causes of death were accidents, homicide, and suicide.

Perhaps the lack of overlap between leading causes of death and most common online health-related searches isn't surprising. Younger folks drive more searches and may not have heart disease, cancer, or stroke at top of mind. In addition, online searches might reflect day-to-day concerns (how soon can my child return to school after having strep throat?) ▸▸

▸▸ rather than long-term conditions, such as heart disease or cancer. And death may not be the most immediate health outcome of interest.

But the disconnect suggests to me that we may be worrying about the wrong things—and focusing too little on the biggest health threats.

Transforming worry into action

Most of us can safely worry less about catching something from a toilet seat or shark attacks. Instead, take steps to reduce the risks you face from our biggest health threats. Chipping away at these five goals could help you live longer and better while easing unnecessary worry:

▸ Choose a heart-healthy diet.
▸ Get routinely recommended health care, including blood pressure checks and cancer screens, such as screening for colorectal cancer.

▸ Drive more safely. Obey the speed limit, drive defensively, always wear a seatbelt, and don't drive if you've been drinking.
▸ Don't smoke. If you need to quit, find help.
▸ Get regular exercise.

The bottom line

Try not to focus too much on health risks that are unlikely to affect you. Instead, think about common causes of poor health. Then take measures to reduce your risk. Moving more and adding healthy foods to your meals is a great start.

And in case you're curious, the average number of annual deaths due to quicksand is zero in the United States. Still a bit worried? Fine. Here's a video that shows you how to save yourself from quicksand, even though you'll almost certainly never need it: https://www.youtube.com/watch?v=7CIOWh1JNTs. ♥

---

5 great tips for sustainable summer living

Stay cool and find joy with planet-friendly ideas to enhance summer life.

Sustainable living treads lightly on natural resources and follows a "rethink, reuse, repurpose" mantra to minimize waste.

Big and small wallet-friendly tips can help you save money and befriend our planet this summer, says Dr. Wynne Armand, a primary care physician at Harvard-affiliated Massachusetts General Hospital and associate director of the Mass General Center for the Environment and Health. Here are five great tips to get you started.

1 Embrace the 5 Rs
Refuse, reduce, reuse, repurpose, and only then recycle is a well-laid out sustainability strategy promoted online by the Cincinnati Recycling and Reuse Hub. Do you really want or need a shiny new object? Where can

you share tasks or tools? What could you swap, give away, or buy used? How could you slim down your recycling stream?

Give yourself permission to start here: Nobody is perfect. We all have preferences and sustainability blind spots, fumbles, and "sorry, just no" feelings. Start where you are and add on when you can.

2 Cut down on cooling energy
Summer heat can endanger your health, and paring back on energy use isn't always possible or wise. Still, it may be possible to:

Stay cooler naturally. Pull down shades during daytime hours to block out hot sun. Open windows at night if the temperature cools down, and

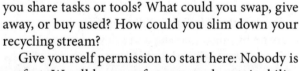
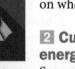
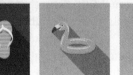

© bortonia | Getty Images

to capture cross breezes if possible. Dress in loose cotton clothes and wear a shading hat when outdoors. Remember that sun bounces off lighter colors and is soaked up by black or darker colors. Make your own shade by carrying an umbrella on sunny—not just rainy—days. "Prepare meals that don't require cooking or baking, since that saves resources and keeps your home cooler," advises Dr. Armand.

Seek shade and cool spots. If you don't have air conditioning or you worry about the bills, green, leafy spaces like parks can help cool you down. Cities and towns often open cooling centers, splash pads, and public pools. Public buildings like libraries and malls are available during daytime hours for anyone trying to beat the heat.

Turn up the temperature. On air conditioning, that is. If you're fortunate enough to have air conditioning at home, follow natural cues. When you're shivering, sweater-seeking, or tucked up under blankets, push the temperature up to save energy and money.

3 Save resources

A sharp eye for energy savings may help pare down bills, too.

Electrify. Shrink your carbon footprint and help cut air pollution by using electric grills, mowers, and other landscaping tools. When tools or appliances need to be replaced, consider electric options.

Conserve energy. Turn off electrical equipment that is not in use in the office and at home, such as lights, TVs, computers, copiers, and printers.

Go low when demand is high. "During peak electricity demand, ensuring stability of the grid is essential to public health," says Dr. Armand. "Avoid using appliances like dishwashers, washers, or dryers during periods of high demand. Instead, do these chores—and charge your electric car, if you have one—late at night." Some energy-hogging appliances have timers to help with this.

Sign up for Shave the Peak alerts. Know when to curb your electricity use to avoid times when your local electric grid is relying on nonrenewable, expensive, polluting fossil fuels.

4 Stay heat-aware and hydrated

Saving resources is a worthy goal, but not at the expense of staying safe and healthy when summer temperatures spike.

Make plans to stay cool. When summer swelters, having an affordable, personal plan to cool down—especially during heat waves—can be lifesaving.

Watch out for signs of dehydration. Drinking plenty of water and eating water-rich foods like lettuce, cucumbers, melon, and citrus fruits can help you stay well hydrated. Water-filling stations for reusable bottles cut down on single-use plastic bottles and help save money at the grocery store.

Know how to treat heat rash and more serious heat-related illnesses. The small, itchy red or darkened bumps of heat rash (prickly heat) occur when sweat ducts become blocked or inflamed. This makes it harder for children and adults to cool their bodies down. Generally, too much heat can harm our bodies, particularly if we work outdoors, take certain medicines, or have certain illnesses.

5 Kickstart sharing circles

Sharing circles can help you expand a wardrobe or tool shed or your taste in foods—all while building community.

Start local, then consider expanding. Brainstorm with a few friends on what you all might like to share or swap. Think seasonal: gardening tools, outside décor, summer sports (because not everyone needs to own a paddleboard). Local clubs, block associations, or public spaces like libraries and schools may be willing to host community swaps and shares. Some communities have swap sheds, and some libraries loan gadgets and even appliances like a portable induction cooktop burner, tech and home-improvement tools, games, and much more.

Summer supper club. Perfect for those overloaded with summer harvests from window boxes, community gardens, or a CSA share. Build a theme around what's fresh, local, and low-cost. Plant-forward menus are good for health and for the planet. Cultural inspiration always helps. And having one person cook—or stressing no-cook recipes—saves resources.

Cut your clothing allowance. Tired of your wardrobe? Gather friends for a summer clothes and accessories swap. Be sure to agree on rules: gently-used, carefully washed, no stains, and so on.

Hot spots. "Gathering at a friend's or neighbor's home for fun games and festivities on hot days is a great way to build community while saving on energy costs for cooling. And rotate for that next hot day!" says Dr. Armand. 🛡

Index

ABCDE guide, 164
abdominal bloating, 126, 233, 265, 296, 319
abdominal exercises, 7, 27, 78, 199, 213–14
abdominal (belly) fat, 178, 216, 243, 246–47, 249
abdominal pain, 82, 156
abdominal pull-in, 27
accountability partners, 15, 187, 207
ACE (angiotensin-converting enzyme) inhibitors, 72, 74
acetaminophen (Tylenol), 147, 154, 308
acid reflux, 32, 148–49
actinic keratoses (AKs), 165, 167
activity trackers, 187, 191, 193
acts of kindness, 47
acupuncture, 140, 143, 147
    electroacupuncture, 144–45
adaptive servo ventilation (ASV), 150
added sugars, 127–28
AD-Detect, 287–88
addictions
    alcohol use disorder, 43, 236, 267
    opioid use disorder, 145–47
    weight-loss drugs for, 267–68
adenosine triphosphate (ATP), 19
advance directives, 298
adverse hospital events, 300–301
Advil. See ibuprofen
aerobic exercise. See exercise
ageism, 10
age-related macular degeneration, 35
age spots, 165, 167, 221
aging (aging well), 3–30
    5 healthy habits, 3
    boosting energy and, 19
    group housing trends, 22–23
    hearing aids and, 23
    house hunting and, 29–30
    reversing, 12
    role of positive attitude, 3, 9–10
    role of social connections, 24–25
aging in place
    house hunting, 29–30
    technology, 272, 273–74
airplane crashes, 319
air pollution, 321
alcohol (alcohol use), 58, 120–21, 250–51
    aging and, 10
    amount of, 250–51
    binge drinking, 21, 43, 251

Dry January challenge, 101, 120–21, 235
    fatigue and, 138
    heartburn and, 149
    heart health and, 121
    hypertension and, 75
    men and, 250–51
    women and, 217, 234, 235–36
alcohol use disorder, 43, 236, 267
aldosterone, 71–72, 75
alendronate (Fosamax), 261
Aleve. See naproxen
alfuzosin (Uroxatral), 76
alirocumab (Praluent), 280
allergies, 129, 158–60
allergy shots, 159–60
almond milk, 91, 123
alpha-hydroxy acids, 221
alpha-linolenic acid (ALA), 110–11
alternate-nostril breathing, 8
Alzheimer's disease, 33–37, 285–88.
    See also dementia
    erectile dysfunction drugs and, 254
    exercise for, 32
    genetics and, 285, 286
    gut and, 285
    lifestyle changes for, 34–35
    medications for, 36–37, 313
    multivitamins for, 31, 37
    tests, 263, 287–88
ambulatory blood pressure monitoring (ABPM), 62
amino acids, 224, 248
amitriptyline (Elavil), 76, 156
amphetamines, 141
amyloid-beta, 32, 35, 36–37, 286, 287–88
androgen deprivation therapy, 260
anemia, 18, 137, 193
angina. See chest pain
angiotensin-receptor blockers (ARBs), 72, 74
annual wellness visits, 291
anosmia, 133–34
antacids, 90, 148
antibiotics, 173, 229, 297, 310, 316
    for Lyme disease, 139–40
antidepressants, 19, 119, 147, 156, 219, 232, 310, 312
anti-germ habits, 5–6
antihistamines, 19, 155, 159, 310
anti-inflammatory medications, 281, 308, 310. See also NSAIDs
anti-obesity medications, 112–13, 263, 264–68

antioxidants, 65, 102, 106, 126, 154, 180
anxiety
    forgiveness and, 49
    gardening for, 3, 12
    herbal remedies for, 53
    medical, 289, 293–95
    positive attitude for, 9
    resilience plan for, 57–58
aortic stenosis, 67
apathy, 42
appetite
    apple cider vinegar and, 126
    intuitive eating and, 122
    protein intake and, 113
    weight-loss drugs for suppressing, 267–68
apple cider vinegar, 126
appointments, plus-ones for, 289, 303
apps
    afib, 263, 271–72
    alcohol use, 121
    breathing, 63
    for chronic pain, 142
    fitness, 97, 187, 191, 193, 206, 291
    heart health, 263, 269, 271–72
    medical alert systems, 273–74
    sleep trackers, 274–76
aquatic exercise, 201–4
arm-across-chest stretch, 27
arm curls, 197
arterial plaque. See atherosclerosis
arthritis. See also osteoarthritis; rheumatoid arthritis
    electroceutical therapies for, 145
    exercise for, 157–58
    prevention tips, 21
artificial intelligence (AI) and doctors, 277
artificial sweeteners, 91, 115, 162
artificial tears, 155–56
ashtanga yoga, 212
aspartame, 162
aspirin, 39, 89, 314
assistive technologies, 272, 273–74
asthma, 15, 193
    exercise and the cold, 160
atherosclerosis, 70, 135, 285
Atkins diet, 103
atorvastatin (Lipitor), 70
atrial fibrillation (afib), 84, 271–72
    coffee and, 93
    COVID and, 131
    exercise and, 189
    omega-3s and, 111

cardiovascular-kidney-metabolic (CKM) syndrome, 268, 269
cardiovascular surgeons, 85
caregiving crisis, 217, 238–40
carvedilol, 193
cataracts, 35, 155, 302
cavities, 317
celiac disease, 118
ceramides, 221
cervical polyps, 229
chamomile, 53
chemical peels, 165
chemotherapy, 133, 171, 172, 175, 255, 260, 307
cherry angiomas, 170
chest pain (angina)
    cardiac rehab for, 301
    GERD and, 225
    heartburn, 148–49
    jaw pain and, 318
    warning sign, 82, 83, 312, 318
chest press, 199
chili peppers, 91, 107–8, 109
Chinese diets, 107–8
chiropractic treatments, 140
chlamydia, 229
cholesterol, 80–81
    5 healthy habits, 59
    coffee and, 94
    diet and, 65, 67, 68–69, 105, 106, 111, 112, 123, 127
    exercise and, 200
    medications for, 66–67
    metabolic syndrome and, 87
    RNA-targeted drugs for, 66–67, 284
    statins for, 39, 70–71, 136
cholinesterase inhibitors, 36
chronic conditions, 129–60. *See also specific conditions*
    5 healthy habits, 129
chronic coronary disease, 83
cigarette smoking. *See* smoking
circular thinking, 51–52
"clean beauty," 222
cleaning products, 163
cleanses, 241–42
climate change, 13, 57, 99
clonidine, 312
Clostridium difficile (C. diff), 139–40
clothing, sun-protective, 168–68
coal tar dyes, 163
coffee (caffeine), 93–94, 119, 138, 276
cognition. *See* brain health
cognitive behavioral therapy, 152
cognitive behavioral therapy (CBT), 52
    for hot flashes, 219
    for Lyme disease, 141

for pain, 231
cognitive behavioral therapy for insomnia (CBT-i), 276
cognitive decline. *See also* Alzheimer's disease; dementia
    multivitamins for, 31, 37
    pets for, 31, 55–56, 99
    social interactions for, 8
cognitive rehabilitation, 141
cognitive reserve, 43
cognitive stimulation, 8, 35, 38, 45
colchicine (Lodoco), 281
cold therapy, 153
colon (colorectal) cancer, 184, 320
    screening, 291, 295–96, 297
colonoscopies, 297
    preparation and diet, 295–96
compression stockings, 77
concentration, 42, 130, 140, 141, 175, 255
constipation, 69, 119, 266
continuous positive-airway pressure (CPAP), 150–51
cookware, nonstick, 162
cooling energy, 320–21
core exercises, 213–14
corticosteroids, 209, 260
counting breaths, 63–64
couples and high blood pressure, 66
COVID-19, 129, 130–34, 319
    anti-germ habits, 5–6
    diabetes and high blood pressure, 134
    lessons learned from, 4–5
    long, 129, 130, 131–32
    Lyme disease and, 139
    sense of smell and, 133–34
    vaccinations, 6, 130, 131–32, 270
crawling, 259
CRISPR, 283, 286
Crohn's disease, 118
cross-contamination, 125
curcumin, 126, 154

dairy, 68, 69, 91, 103, 104, 112, 123
DANCERS and dementia, 38
dancing, 11, 32
dapagliflozin (Farxiga), 269
DASH (Dietary Approaches to Stop Hypertension), 32, 102, 103, 104, 106, 111, 118, 177, 179
dating, 252
deadbugs, 214
deadlifts, 199
decongestants, 155, 159, 312
deep breathing, 53, 54, 59, 63–64, 142, 143, 195, 295

dehydration, 119–20, 125, 193, 321
dementia. *See also* Alzheimer's disease
    exercise for, 32
    gum disease and, 28
    hearing and vision problems, 35
    high blood pressure and, 75
    internet use and, 31, 41, 43
    multivitamins for, 31, 37
    sitting and, 39
    TV watching and, 31, 41
dental care, 28–29
    brushing teeth, 28–29, 298–99, 318
    flossing, 7, 29, 318
dental exams, 29
dental pain, 317–18
deodorants, 163
depression
    forgiveness and, 49
    gardening for, 12
    heart disease and, 100
    medication nonadherence and, 311
    pets for, 31, 56
    postpartum, 226
    social interactions for, 8
    symptoms of, 42
    TV watching and, 31, 41
dermatofibromas, 170
detoxes, 241–42
device-guided breathing, 64
dextroamphetamine (Adderall), 141
diabetes, 81, 82. *See also* prediabetes
    aging and, 9
    blood pressure, 76
    COVID and, 134
    diet for, 65, 105–6, 108, 114, 115, 127, 179
    exercise for, 14, 18, 186–87, 188, 202, 209
    gum disease and, 28
    medications, 70, 71, 104, 264–69
    metabolic syndrome and, 87–88
    pregnancy complications and, 227
    race, racism, and, 86–87
    sugar and, 105–6
diabetic neuropathy, 145, 146, 211, 232
diagonal chops, 213–14
diclofenac (Voltaren), 154, 209
diet, 101–28
    4 nutrition myths, 123
    5 healthy habits, 101
    10 popular diets, 102, 103
    80/20 rule, 105
    for Alzheimer's disease, 34, 35
    for arthritis, 21
    for autoimmune diseases, 136
    before bedtime, 242
    for blood pressure, 59, 65, 67

for brain health, 32, 34, 35, 38
for cancer, 161, 177, 179–80
for cholesterol, 65, 67, 68–69, 105, 106, 111, 112, 123, 127
colonoscopies, 295–96
for COVID, 131
DANCERS and dementia, 38
for diabetes, 105–6, 108, 114, 115, 127
for fatigue, 137–38
gardening and, 3, 11
for heartburn, 149
for heart health, 79, 91–92, 102–11
hydration and, 119–20
intuitive eating, 101, 121–23
for Lyme disease, 141
magnesium in, 217, 230
maximizing energy and, 19
Mediterranean. *See* Mediterranean diet
for men, 245, 247, 248–49
for metabolic syndrome, 88
portfolio, 68–69
portion size, 245
post-COVID, 4
protein, 112–13
reviewing goals, 290–91
shopping tips, 127–28
for tinnitus, 152
for women, 217, 223–25, 230, 242
Dietary Approaches to Stop Hypertension diet. *See* DASH
dietary fiber. *See* fiber
dietitians, 143
digestion, 7, 11, 77, 127
discharge buddies, 299, 300
diuretics, 21, 72, 74, 76, 155, 310
dizziness, 36, 42, 73, 76, 82, 125, 140, 145, 232, 233, 253, 272, 288
DNA methylation clocks, 12
docosahexaenoic acid (DHA), 90–91, 110–11
doctors
appointments, plus-ones, 289, 303
approval before exercise, 186–87, 196
artificial intelligence and, 277
fear of visits, 289, 293–95
finding primary care providers, 292–93
medical gaslighting, 304
medications and, 312–13
physician-led walks, 25–26
resources, 292
second opinions, 294
vs. advanced practitioners, 293
wellness visits, 291

dogs
adoption considerations, 55
benefits of, 31, 55–56, 99
donepezil, 36
dopamine, 36, 46, 190
double kickbacks, 204
drinking water. *See* hydration
drugs. *See* medications; *and specific drugs*
dry eye, 155–56
Dry January challenge, 101, 120–21, 235
dry mouth and throat, 125
dulaglutide (Trulicity), 266, 268
duloxetine (Cymbalta), 147

eating. *See* diet
echocardiograms, 82, 83
effort-reward imbalance, 251
eicosapentaenoic acid (EPA), 90–91, 110–11
ejaculation frequency and prostate cancer, 177
electroacupuncture, 144–45
electrocardiograms (ECGs), 82, 277
smart watches, 263, 269, 271–72
electroceuticals, 144–45
electrophysiologists, 85
empagliflozin (Jardiance), 269
endometriosis, 231
endorphins, 45, 63, 138
energy, maximizing, 19–20
energy savings, 321
epidermal cysts, 169–70
erectile dysfunction (ED), 252–53, 254, 259
exercise for, 257
medications, 76
PSA testing and, 181
ER-positive breast cancer, 172
estimated glomerular filtration rate (eGFR), 268–70
estrogen, 172, 218, 221, 229, 231, 233, 278
estrogen therapy, 219, 225, 226, 234, 279
etripamil, 288
evolocumab (Repatha), 280
exercise, 185–216. *See also* strength training; stretches; walking
5 healthy habits, 185
150-minute target, 187–88, 191
activity trackers, 187, 191, 193
for aging, 9–10
for Alzheimer's disease, 34
amount of, 187–88, 191, 197, 200
for arthritis, 21, 157–58

asthma and the cold, 160
for autoimmune diseases, 136
for blood pressure, 18, 59, 63, 77–78, 195
for blood sugar, 199, 201, 209
for bone health, 157, 201, 205, 261
boosting energy, 19–20
for brain health, 32, 34, 38, 45, 54
for cancer prevention, 165, 177, 180
coffee and, 93
DANCERS and dementia, 38
doctor approval before, 186–87, 196
for fatigue, 137, 138
footwear, 185, 210–11
gardening, 3, 11
for heart health, 79, 93, 95–98, 138, 186–91, 198–200, 202–3
heart rate and, 192–93
home workouts, 196–97
hospital stays and, 18, 301
intensity of, 191
for men, 243, 244, 246, 247, 257, 258–59, 261, 262
for mood, 31, 45, 54
for pain relief, 143
for Parkinson's disease, 230
personal trainers, 194–95, 200
post-COVID, 4
recommended goals, 187, 189–90
reviewing goals, 290, 291
for sciatica, 153
short bursts of, 7, 165, 190, 191, 205–6
strong core, 213–14
support for, 15, 187, 207
time of day for, 185, 190, 191
for tinnitus, 152
"use it or lose it," 185, 186–87
water workouts, 185, 201–4
for women, 230, 232–33, 238, 241
exercise mats, 196
exercise stress tests, 83, 92, 192, 227
exhaustion, 136–37
expiration dates, 125
eye exams, 233
eyes and vision
dementia and, 35
dry eye, 155–56
protection tips, 156

face masks, 6, 150–51
falls (falling)
after standing up, 76–77
doctors and, 303
hiking and, 16
in hospitals, 301
men and, 258–59

pacing and, 20
soft landing, 259
tai chi for, 98
women and, 232–33
familial hypercholesterolemia (FH), 283
family history. *See also* genetics
of cancer, 167, 177, 178
of dementia, 32, 33, 34, 287
of melanomas, 166
of osteoarthritis, 157
of pregnancy risk, 228
family practitioners, 292
fasting blood sugar, 87, 269
fatigue, 129, 136–38
causes of, 137
vitality-enhancing tactics, 137–38
fats, dietary. *See* omega-3 fatty acids;
saturated fats; unsaturated fats
fatty liver disease, 105
fermented foods, 91, 92
fezolinetant (Veozah), 218, 279
fiber, 67, 68–69, 108, 296
on food labels, 127
fibroids, 233–34
FINER, 142
finerenone (Kerendia), 269
fish and seafood, 109, 110–11, 180
fish oil, 79, 90–91, 110–11, 177
fit and active. *See* exercise
flat feet, 208
flavonoids, 108
flexitarian diet, 131
flossing, 7, 29, 318
flu shots, 6, 263, 270
food. *See* diet
food labels, 127–28
food poisoning, 101, 124–25
food shopping, 127–28
foot ailments, 208–9
foot care, 208
foot check, 209
foot swelling, 209
footwear, 185, 196, 210–11
foreplay, 252
forest bathing, 16–17
forgetfulness, 38, 74, 303, 311
forgiveness, 48–50
formaldehyde, 163
freckles, 164, 167
fridge, spring cleaning, 124–25
friends (friendships), 5, 8, 9, 12, 33,
98–99
aging well, 24–25
walking with, 3, 14–15
fruits, 102, 103, 104, 106, 108, 110.
See also specific fruits
for cancer, 161, 178, 179–80

eating the rainbow, 127
frozen vs. fresh myth, 123

gabapentin (Neurontin), 140, 147, 220,
308, 312
galantamine, 36, 313
gallstones, 71
gardening, 3, 11–12
gastric bypass surgery, 118
gastroesophageal reflux disease
(GERD), 148–49, 225
gastroparesis, 266
gender differences
alcohol and, 121
pain and, 231
gene editing, 283–84, 286
genetics. *See also* family history
Alzheimer's disease and, 285, 286
biomarker tests, 12, 37, 167, 176
caffeine metabolism, 94
cancer risk and, 172, 184
heart disease, 71–72, 85, 279–80
past lifestyle habits and, 10
RNA-targeted drugs, 66–67, 284
salt sensitivity and, 71–72
stress and, 35
geriatric care managers, 240
geriatricians, 292
gingivitis, 21, 28–29, 318
glaucoma, 35, 155, 159
GLP1 (glucagon-like peptide 1) receptor
agonists, 199, 264–68, 269
glucose. *See* blood sugar
glutamate, 36
goals (goal setting), 291
exercise, 187, 189–90
gonorrhea, 229
good deeds, 31, 46–47
Google health searches, 319
gout, 21, 71, 144, 281
gratitude, 9, 45–46, 100
green leafy vegetables, 34, 35, 104, 120,
127, 217, 230, 296
green tea, 108
group dynamics, 33
group housing trends, 22–23
guilt, 42, 50, 123
survivor's, 161, 174–76
gum bleeding, 29, 318
gum inflammation (gingivitis), 21,
28–29, 318
gum pain, 318
gut microbiome, 91–92, 115, 285, 296
gym classes, 17
gym memberships, 142
gyms, personal trainers, 194–95, 200
gynecological cancers, 229

hair dyes, 163
hair relaxers, 163
hand washing, 3, 6
happiness
good deeds for, 31, 46–47
hobbies for, 3, 8
hatha yoga, 212
hats, 168–69
HDL (good) cholesterol. *See* cholesterol
headaches
alcohol withdrawal and, 43
arthritis treatment, 145
caregivers and, 239
fatigue and, 137
gender differences, 231
mind-body techniques for, 143
phobias and, 42
health care proxies, 298
health club memberships, 142
health reviews, 289, 290–91
health technology, 263–88. *See also* apps
5 healthy habits, 263
Alzheimer's test, 263, 287–88
artificial intelligence and doctors,
277
cardiology trends, 281–82
flu shots, 263, 270
gene therapy for heart disease, 283–
84
genetic profiling for heart disease,
279–80
medical alert systems, 273–74
PREVENT calculator, 263, 268–69
sex hormone therapy, 278–79
sleep trackers, 274–76
wearable trackers, 263, 269, 271–72
weight loss medications, 263, 264–68
healthy fats, 105
hearing aids, 23
hearing loss
dementia and, 35
tinnitus and, 151–52
hearing tests, 23, 233
heart attacks
aspirin for, 89, 314
genetic profiling, 279–80
GLP-1 medications and, 267
inflammation and, 135
lipoprotein(a), 67
loneliness and, 99
metabolic syndrome and, 87–88
pets and, 55
silent, 81–82
stress and, 13
symptoms, 82
testosterone therapy and, 256
heartburn, 32, 148–49

late-night eating, 149
Latin America diet, 109–10
LDL ("bad") cholesterol, 81, 283. *See also* cholesterol
   coffee and, 94
   diet for, 67, 68–69, 104, 105, 112, 123, 127
   RNA-targeted drugs for, 66–67, 284
   statins for, 70, 71
lecanemab, 36–37
left-sided heart disease, 73
left ventricular assist device (LVAD), 282
lightheadedness. *See* dizziness
lightning strikes, 319
lipomas, 169–70
lipoprotein(a) (Lp(a)), 67
loneliness, 8, 33, 46, 98–99. *See also* social isolation
   vs. isolation, 58
long COVID, 129, 130, 131–32
lottery winners, 14
lung cancer, 10, 163, 175, 306
lunges, 199, 207, 214, 215
lungs and pulmonary hypertension, 73–74
lupus, 135, 231
lycopene, 65
Lyme disease, 129, 139–41
   pain management, 140–41
   treatment, 139–40

magnesium, 217, 230
magnetic resonance imaging (MRIs), 183–84
mammograms, 173, 176, 294
massages (massage therapy), 143, 252
mattresses, 162
meat. *See* processed meats; red meat
medical alert systems, 273–74
medical anxiety, 289, 293–95
medical check-ups, 4–5
medical escorts, 300, 302–3
medical gaslighting, 304
medical guidelines, 297
medical records, 277, 298
medical waste collection sites, 316–17
medical worries, 318–20
Medicare, 28, 36, 142, 143, 144, 266, 291, 301, 306
medications, 309–17. *See also specific medications*
   5 healthy habits, 289
   decoding instructions, 309–10
   disposal, 316–17
   men and, 244
   nonadherence, 289, 311–12

online pharmacy risks, 315–16
   rebound effects, 312
   reducing daily number of, 314
   reviewing, 290
   side effects, 19, 311, 312, 313, 314
   stopping, 312–13
   tapering off, 313
   therapy and, 44
   tracking, 301
   withdrawal symptoms, 312
meditation, 9, 46, 54, 141, 143, 153
   DANCERS and dementia, 38
Mediterranean diet, 102, 103, 104, 106, 109, 111, 246, 290, 296
   for brain health, 32, 34, 58
   for cancer, 177, 179
   for gout, 21
melanoma, 164–65, 166–67
memantine, 36
memory loss, 38–39. *See also* Alzheimer's disease; dementia
   DANCERS and, 38
   warning signs, 38
men (men's health). *See also* prostate cancer
   5 healthy habits, 243–62
   alcohol and, 250–51
   diet for, 245, 247, 248–49
   exercise for, 243, 244, 246, 247, 257, 258–59, 261, 262
   falls and falling, 258–59
   heart health and, 244–45, 251
   osteoporosis and, 260–61
   pain gap, 231
   sex life and, 252–54
   testosterone replacement therapy, 243, 255–56, 278–79
   weight gain and, 245–47
menarche, 231
menopause, 220–22, 229
   hot flashes, 217, 218–20
   ovary removal, 226
   skin care products and, 220–22
   uterine fibroids and, 233–34
men's health clinics services, 259
menstruation, 219, 231
mental health. *See also* anxiety; depression; stress
   caregiving crisis and, 239–40
   forgiveness and, 49
   misperceptions, 40–41
   recognizing signs of, 42–43
   reviewing, 291
   rumination and, 51–54
mental lapses, 38–39
mentors (mentorships), 13, 47
metabolic syndrome, 87–88

metabolism, 216, 242, 246
methylphenidate (Ritalin), 141
metoprolol, 193
middle-age weight gain, 18
migraines. *See* headaches
mind. *See* brain health
MIND (Mediterranean-DASH Intervention for Neurodegenerative Delay), 32, 34, 179
mindfulness, 48, 54, 56, 152
   for high blood pressure, 118
   for pain, 141, 142, 143, 153
minimalist shoes, 211
miso, 91
mitochondria, 19
moisturizers, 7, 221–22
moles, 164, 166–67
monitored home medical alert systems, 273–74
monkey mind, 97
monosodium glutamate (MSG), 107
monounsaturated fats, 69, 105
mood
   boosting, 12, 45–46, 48, 54
   exercise for, 31, 45, 54
morning exercise, 190, 191
morning stretches, 7
multitasking, 38, 232
multivitamins, 31, 37, 116
"muscle memory," 186
muscle strengthening. *See* strength training
muscle-strengthening activity, 198
myocarditis, 132

naltrexone (Vivitrol), 147, 264
naproxen (Aleve), 75, 140, 147, 157, 208, 238, 308
naps (napping), 7, 254
nasal rinses, 159
nasal steroid sprays, 159
natural toothpastes, 28–29
nature, 31, 45
   forest bathing, 16–17
neck pain, 82, 145, 203, 228, 318
negative thoughts, 9, 45, 51–54
   four steps for changing, 53
neuropathy, 145, 146, 211, 232
night creams, 220–22
night sweats, 218–19, 279
nonstick cookware, 162
NSAIDs (nonsteroidal anti-inflammatory drugs), 75, 119, 140, 153–54, 157, 208, 308, 310
nurse practitioners (NPs), 292–93
nutrition. *See* diet

nuts and seeds, 7, 68–69, 104, 110–11, 131, 230

oatmeal, 67, 68, 114, 249
oats, 67, 69, 92
obesity
    anti-obesity medications, 112–13, 263, 264–68
    cancer and, 177, 178
    diet and, 108, 114, 128
    exercise for, 191, 201
    gut microbiome and, 92, 285
    heart disease and, 86, 87
    metabolic syndrome and, 87
obituaries, 14
obsessive-compulsive disorder (OCD), 51
obstructive sleep apnea, 150, 226
occupational therapy, 141
olive oil, 69, 103, 105, 106, 110, 123, 179, 296
omega-3 fatty acids, 90–91, 105, 110–11, 177, 180
omeprazole (Prilosec), 126, 312
omnivore diet, 69
online lectures or classes, 142
online pharmacy risks, 315–16
opioids (opioid use disorder), 145–47, 317
oral care. *See* dental care
organ transplantation, 167, 260
orthostatic hypotension, 76–77
osteoarthritis, 157–58, 208–9
    back pain and, 238
    prevention tips, 21, 157–58, 261
    treatment, 208–9
osteoporosis, 260–61
    men and, 260–61
    shrinking height and, 26
    women and, 223, 226, 232, 233
ovary removal, 226
overweight. *See* obesity
oxybutynin (Oxytrol), 220
oxycodone (OxyContin), 146, 308, 312
Ozempic, 264, 265–66, 267, 269

pace (pacing), 15, 20, 205, 209
    for Lyme disease, 129, 141
pacemakers, 85, 145
pain (pain management), 142–45. *See also specific pain*
    5 healthy habits, 129
    alternative therapies, 129, 142–43
    electroceuticals, 144–45
    gender differences, 231
    for Lyme disease, 140–41
    mindfulness for, 141, 142, 143, 153

    for osteoarthritis, 157
    sciatica, 153–54
painful sex, 229, 233
pain medications. *See specific medications*
paleo diet, 103
palliative care, 305–7
pamidronate (Aredia), 261
pancreatitis, 266
pantry, spring cleaning, 124–25
Pap smears, 277
parabens, 163
Parkinson's disease
    blood pressure and, 76
    TV watching and, 41
    women and, 230
paroxetine (Paxil), 76, 219
passionflower, 53
pasta, 18, 122, 224
patient information, 289–321
    5 healthy habits, 289
    changing medical guidelines, 297
    colonoscopy diet, 295–96
    dental pain, 317–18
    finding primary care providers, 292–93
    health reviews, 289, 290–91
    health worries, 318–20
    hospice and palliative care, 305–7
    hospital tips, 289, 298–301
    knee replacements, 146, 307–9
    medical anxiety, 289, 293–95
    medical escorts, 300, 302–3
    medical gaslighting, 304
    medication tips, 309–17
    plus-ones for appointments, 289, 303
    sustainable summer living, 320–21
PCSK9, 66–67, 283
peanut butter, 68, 113, 114, 134
pelvic girdle syndrome, 231
pendulum (exercise), 204
penile shock wave therapy, 259
perimenopause, 221, 223, 233
personal care products, 163
personal health reviews, 289, 290–91
personal trainers, 194–95, 200
pessimism, 42
pets
    adoption considerations, 55
    benefits of, 31, 55–56, 99
PFAS (perfluoroalkyl and polyfluoroalkyl substances), 162
phentermine (Adipex-P), 264
phobias, 42–43
physical activity. *See* exercise
physical therapy, 140, 143, 233
physicians. *See* doctors

physician assistants (PAs), 292–93
physician-led walks, 25–26
phytosterols, 69
pickleball, 214–15
pig heart transplants, 282
pill containers, 312
pink noise, 276
placebo effect, 37, 71, 90, 115, 116, 156, 256
plane crashes, 319
planks, 59, 77–78, 213–14
plantains, 110
plantar fasciitis, 208, 210
plant-based diet, 103, 104, 106, 109
    for brain health, 32, 34, 35, 38
    for cancer, 179–80, 184
    for COVID, 131
    for heart health, 59, 68–69, 88, 90, 91, 92
    milks, 91, 123
    prebiotics, 115
    protein in, 112, 113, 224
plant sterols, 69
plaque. *See* atherosclerosis
platelet-rich plasma (PRP) injections, 259
pneumonia, 298, 299
POLST (physician orders for life-sustaining treatment), 298
polygenic risk scores, 85, 280, 281
polyunsaturated fats, 105, 106
portfolio diet, 68–69
portion sizes, 245
positive airway pressure (PAP), 150–51
positive attitude, 3, 9–10, 100
post-COVID conditions (PCC). *See* long COVID
post-Lyme disease syndrome (PLDS), 139–41
postpartum depression, 226
post-traumatic stress disorder (PTSD), 147
posture, 20, 26–27, 213
potassium, 71, 107, 193
pranayama, 64
prebiotics, 115
prediabetes, 81, 269
pre-eclampsia, 227–28
prefrontal cortex, 38, 45, 48, 56
pregabalin (Lyrica), 140, 147
pregnancy, 233
    complications, 124, 227–28
    diet for, 108, 223
prescription medications. *See* medications; *and specific medications*
preventative care, 243, 244–45

PREVENT calculator, 263, 268–69
primary care providers, 292–93
primordial prevention, 281
probiotics, 92, 115
processed foods, 114–15, 122
processed meats, 108
progesterone, 172, 225, 278
prostate cancer, 177–84
    diet for, 161, 178, 179–80
    exercise for, 177, 180
    PSA testing, 161, 181–82, 183, 184, 291
    weight loss for, 161, 178–79
Prostate Health Index (PHI), 183
protein, 112–13, 223–25, 248–49
    for fatigue, 137
    food sources, 113, 224, 249
    men and, 248–49
    recommended amount of, 24
    women and, 217, 223–25
protein shakes, 225, 249
proton-pump inhibitors, 118, 312, 313
PSA (prostate-specific antigen) testing, 161, 181–82, 183, 184, 291
psoriasis, 135
psychodynamic therapy, 52
pulmonary hypertension, 73–74
purpose in life, 9, 13–14, 46–47
push-ups, 7, 188, 199, 206, 207

quicksand, 319, 320

race (racism) and heart disease, 86–87
random acts of kindness, 47
rectus abdominis, 213
red meat, 90, 92, 103, 106, 108, 112, 115, 123, 179, 180, 250, 291
refined carbohydrates, 18, 123
refined sugar, 105–6, 127–28
religion, 17, 24, 240
residential care homes, 23
resilience plan, 57–58
resistance bands, 200
resistance training. *See* strength training
resistant hypertension, 74–75
respiratory syncytial virus (RSV), 5, 6
respiratory viruses, 5–6
respite care, 240
retinols, 221
rheumatoid arthritis, 135, 136
    fatigue and, 19
    prevention tips, 21
rice, 18, 109–10
rinsing mouth, 28, 29
risedronate (Actonel), 261
rivastigmine, 36
RNA interference, 66–67

RNA-targeted drugs, 66, 284
role models, 13
rosacea, 221
rumination, 12, 51–54
running clubs, 33, 207
running shoes, 185, 210–11

St. John's wort, 53
saline nasal rinse, 159
salmon, 90, 105, 110, 111, 112, 113, 224, 249
salt. *See* sodium
sarcopenia, 188, 248
sardines, 90, 102, 105, 110, 111
SARS-CoV-2, 131
saturated fats, 68, 69, 102, 105, 112, 115, 123
savvy patient. *See* patient information
sciatica, 153–54
scrambler therapy, 144–45
seafood. *See* fish and seafood
seasonal allergies, 158–60
second opinions, 294
    heart disease, 84–85
sedatives, 295, 296
sedentary life, 187–88, 197, 201, 241
    aging well and, 25, 26
    brain and, 39, 45, 54
    core muscle strength and, 213
    dementia risk and, 39
    heart and, 95–97, 98
self-talk, 52
semaglutide, 112–13, 199, 264–68
"senior moments," 38
sense of purpose, 9, 13–14, 46–47
sensory quiet time, 141
serotonin, 46, 190
serotonin-norepinephrine reuptake inhibitors (SNRIs), 312
serotonin reuptake inhibitors (SSRIs), 219–20, 312
sex and sex life
    overcoming barriers, 252–53
    sleeping apart, 243, 253–54
    women bleeding after, 229
sex hormone therapy, 278–79
sexually transmitted infections (STIs), 229
SGLT-2 (sodium-glucose cotransporter-2) inhibitors, 104, 268–69
sharing circles, 321
shark attacks, 319
shingles vaccines, 288
Shingrix, 288
shinrin-yoku, 16–17
shoulder blade squeeze, 27

shoulder pain, 82, 203, 214
sildenafil (Viagra), 76, 253, 254, 257
silent heart attacks, 81–82
simvastatin (Zocor), 70
sitting, 79, 95–97, 197. *See also* sedentary life
    core muscle strength and, 213
    dementia risk and, 39
sit-to-stand, 258
skin canscers, 164–69
    screenings, 166–67, 170–71
    self-exams, 161, 164–65
skin care
    cosmetic treatments, 165
    products and cancer risks, 163
    products and menopause, 220–22
skin lumps and bumps, 169–71
skin self-exam, 161, 164–65
sleep, 274–76
    boosting measures, 276
    for brain health, 32, 38
    coffee and, 93
    DANCERS and dementia, 38
    heart health and, 93, 96
    noise, 276
    partners and, 243, 253
    sex life and, 243, 253–54
    for tinnitus, 152
sleep apnea, 150
    CPAP for, 150–51
    hypertension and, 75
sleep problems (insomnia)
    CBT-i for, 276
    depression and, 41
    fatigue and, 137
    high blood pressure and, 237
    rumination and, 51
    women and, 218, 220
    yoga for, 147
sleep trackers, 274–76
small-interfering RNA (siRNA) drugs, 66–67, 284
smartphones, sanitizing, 6
smart watches
    apps, 263, 271–72
    breathing, 63
    fitness trackers, 97, 193, 263, 269, 272
    medical alert systems, 273–74
smell, 133–34
smoking, 58, 267
    aging and, 6, 10
    heartburn and, 149
    heart health and, 86, 256
    high blood pressure and, 65
    lung cancer and, 10, 163, 175, 306
snacks (snacking), 7, 68, 96, 113, 180, 224, 242

snakebite injuries and deaths, 319
sneakers, 185, 196, 210–11
snuggle time, 254
social isolation, 14, 19, 22, 23, 31, 33, 38, 40, 45, 52, 56, 58
socializing (social connections), 5, 8, 9, 12
    for aging well, 24–25
    for brain health, 33
    for heart health, 79, 98–99
    for stress relief, 17
    walking with friends, 3, 14–15
socks, 210, 233
sodium (salt), 71–72, 115
    blood pressure and, 59, 71–72, 74
    on food labels, 127
sodium-glucose cotransporter-2 (SGLT-2) inhibitors, 104, 268–69
soluble fiber, 69, 127
sotatercept, 73
soybean oil, 69, 90, 105, 110
soy protein, 107–8
soy sauce, 107
specialized communities, 22
spirituality, 17, 24, 240
spring cleaning, 124–25
squamous cell carcinoma (SCC), 165, 170
squats, 7, 59, 77–78, 195, 198, 199, 215
    proper form for, 194
standard American diet (SAD), 91–92
statins, 39, 70–71, 136, 244
    alternatives, 71
step counters, 187, 206, 291
stereotypes
    ageism, 10
    mental health, 40–41
stoicism, 9
strength training, 198–200
    5 healthy habits, 185
    amount of, 187–88, 200
    benefits of, 198–200
    for blood pressure, 77–78
    for brain health, 58
    for fatigue, 137
    for heart health, 96
    injury prevention, 194–95
    for knees, 261
    major muscle groups, 199
    for muscle mass, 19
    for posture, 26
    protein for, 248–49
    "use it or lose it," 185, 186–87
stress (stress reduction)
    for autoimmune diseases, 136
    brain health and, 35
    gardening for, 12

heart and, 86, 97, 251
hiking for, 16–17
pets for, 31, 56
resilience plan for, 57–58
social connections for, 17
for tinnitus, 152
yoga for, 147, 152
stress tests, 83, 227
stretches (stretching)
    morning, 7
    for plantar fasciitis, 208
    post-exercise, 197
    for posture, 27
    for sciatica, 153
    warm ups, 196–97, 215
stretchy bands, 200
strokes, 80–81
    afib and, 271–72
    aging and, 9
    aspirin for, 89, 314
    COVID and, 131
    diet for, 68, 104, 105, 108, 110, 111
    exercise for, 18, 77, 189, 191, 201
    GLP-1 medications and, 267
    gum disease and, 28
    inflammation and, 135
    lipoprotein(a), 67
    loneliness and, 99
    metabolic syndrome and, 87–88
    NSAIDs and, 140
    pets and, 55
    sleep apnea and, 150
    stress and, 13
    testosterone therapy and, 256
    women and, 219, 227
structural racism, 86–87
subcutaneous fat, 246
sugar, 105–6, 127–28
sugary drinks, 18, 102, 106, 108, 162
summer living, 320–21
sunburns, 167, 169, 310
sun exposure, 164–65, 167
    medications and, 310
    UPF-clothing for, 168–69
    vitamin D, 118
sun-protective clothing, 168–68
sunscreen, 7, 168, 169, 221, 260–61, 310
sun spots, 165, 167
supplements, 117–18. *See also specific supplements*
    multivitamins, 31, 37, 116
    safety warning, 117–18
support groups, 142, 176, 207, 231
supraventricular tachycardia (SVT), 288
survivor's guilt, 161, 174–76
sustainable summer living, 320–21
swimming, 32, 136, 158, 185, 201–4

tadalafil (Cialis), 253, 254, 257
tai chi, 27, 79, 97–98, 142, 152, 153, 195, 232, 301
talk test, 192–93
talk therapy, 141, 143
tamsulosin (Flomax), 76
tanning beds, 167
tea, 108, 119
teeth care. *See* dental care
telemedicine, 4–5, 240
    blood pressure and, 64
tempeh, 91, 113
temporomandibular disorder (TMD), 318
tendinitis, 210, 291
testosterone, 253, 255–57, 278–79
testosterone replacement therapy (TRT), 243, 255–56, 259, 278–79
therapists, choosing, 44
therapy. *See also* cognitive behavioral therapy
    for negative thoughts, 52
    tips for getting most out, 44
thyroid problems, 74, 119, 137, 226, 291
TikTok health searches, 319
timer caps, 312
tinnitus, 151–52
tiredness vs. fatigue, 136
tirzepatide (Zepbound), 112–13, 199, 265–66
tobacco. *See* smoking
toenails, 164, 209
tofu, 68, 107, 113, 260
toilet seats, public, 319
tomatoes and blood pressure, 65
tongue scraping, 29
toothbrushing, 28–29, 298–99, 318
tooth pain, 317–18
toothpastes, 28–29, 318
topical painkillers, 154
total knee replacements, 307–9
traditional Chinese diets, 107–8
tramadol, 146, 308
transcutaneous electrical nerve stimulation (TENS) therapy, 144–45
transthyretin amyloid cardiomyopathy (ATTR-CM), 284
treadmills, 197, 262, 291
trekking poles, 16, 205, 207
trichomoniasis, 229
triglycerides, 81, 87, 104, 105, 111, 256, 269
triple-negative breast cancer, 172
turmeric, 126, 154
TV watching, 27, 31, 41

Twists, 204
type 2 diabetes. *See* diabetes

ulcerative colitis, 118
ultra-processed foods, 114–15, 122
unsaturated fats, 91, 107, 110, 112, 123, 223
upright rows, 199
uric acid, 21
urinary incontinence, 181, 232, 234
urinary tract infections (UTIs), 18, 119
"use it or lose it," 185, 186–87
uterine fibroids, 233–34

vaccines (vaccinations), 293
    COVID-19, 6, 130, 131–32, 270
    flu, 6, 263, 270
    shingles, 288
vaginal bleeding, 229
vaginal dryness, 229, 252, 279
vaginal symptoms, 229
vaginitis, 229
valerian root, 53
vascular dementia, 32, 39
vegan powders, 249
vegetables. *See also specific vegetables*
    for brain health, 34, 35
    for cancer, 161, 178, 179–80
    in DASH diet, 32, 102, 103, 104,
        106, 111, 118, 177, 179
    eating the rainbow, 127
    eating when dining out, 106
    fiber in, 68–69
    frozen vs. fresh myth, 123
    green leafy, 34, 35, 104, 120, 127,
        217, 230, 296
    for heart health, 110
vegetarian/vegan diet. *See* plant-based
        diet
Victoza, 264, 265–66
vinyasa yoga, 212
visceral fat, 178, 216, 243, 246–47, 249
viscous fiber, 68, 69
vision. *See* eyes and vision
visualization, 143
vitamin A, 107, 221
vitamin B6, 118
vitamin B12, 116, 118, 287

vitamin D, 118, 260–61
VO2 max, 180
volatile organic compounds (VOCs),
        162–63
volunteering, 8, 9, 14, 17, 31, 46–47, 99
    resources, 47
vulnerability, 44, 49–50, 51, 98–99, 131,
        146
vulvodynia, 231

waist size, 178, 216, 243, 246, 247
waist-to-hip ratio, 216, 249
walking, 95–96, 186, 205–7
    for brain health, 34
    with friends, 3, 14–15
    for men, 243, 262
    pace, 15, 205, 209
    physician-led, 25–26
    step counters, 187, 206, 291
walking clubs, 33, 207
walking poles, 16, 205, 207
Walk with a Doc, 25–26
wall slides, 27
wall squats, 59, 77–78, 198
walnuts, 7, 68, 90, 105, 110
warm-ups, 196–97, 215
water, drinking. *See* hydration
water bottles, 97, 196, 208, 263
water workouts, 185, 201–4
"weak ties," 33
wearable tech, 187, 193, 263, 271–72
weekend warriors, 189–90
weight
    reviewing, 290
    wellness myths about, 241
weighted backpacks, 206
weight gain. *See also* obesity
    men and, 245–47
    middle-age, 18
weight loss
    apple cider vinegar and, 126
    for arthritis, 21
    for autoimmune diseases, 136
    for heartburn, 149
    for hot flashes, 219
    intuitive eating for, 121–23
    medications, 112–13, 263, 264–68
    for men, 244–45, 246

    for metabolic syndrome, 88
    for prostate cancer, 161, 178–79
weight training. *See* strength training
wellness myths, 241–42
wellness technology. *See* health
        technology
wellness visits, 291
whey protein powder, 249
white-coat hypertension, 294–95
white noise, 152, 276
women (women's health), 217–42. *See
        also* breast cancer; menopause;
        pregnancy
    5 healthy habits, 217
    alcohol and, 217, 234, 235–36
    back pain and, 233, 234, 237–38
    diet for, 217, 223–25, 230, 242
    exercise for, 230, 232–33, 238, 241
    falls and falling, 232–33
    heart disease and pregnancy
        complications, 227–28
    long COVID and, 132
    pain gap, 231
    sex life and, 252–54
    vaginal symptoms, 229
    wellness myths and, 241–42
wooziness. *See* dizziness
worthlessness, 42

yoga, 185, 211–12
    benefits of, 45, 54, 136, 153, 211–12
    for blood pressure, 64
    DANCERS and dementia, 38
    for heart health, 136
    for mood, 45, 54
    for pain management, 142, 143, 153
    for posture, 27
    for sleep, 147
    for stress, 147, 152
    for stress and PTSD, 147
    styles of, 212
yoga classes, 4, 212

zilebesiran, 67, 284
zinc oxide, 168
zoledronic acid (Reclast), 261
zolpidem (Ambien), 312
zuranolone (Zurzuvae), 226